CLINICAL BEHAVIORAL MEDICINE

Some Concepts and Procedures

CLINICAL BEHAVIORAL MEDICINE
Some Concepts and Procedures

Ian E. Wickramasekera, Ph.D.

Professor of Psychiatry and Behavioral Sciences
Director, Behavioral Medicine Clinic and
Stress Disorders Research Laboratory
Eastern Virginia Medical School
Norfolk, Virginia

PLENUM PRESS • NEW YORK AND LONDON

Library of Congress Cataloging in Publication Data

Wickramasekera, Ian E.
   Clinical behavioral medicine: some concepts and procedures / Ian E.
Wickramasekera.
      p.   cm.
   Includes bibliographies and index.
   ISBN 0-306-42734-6
   1. Clinical health psychology. 2. Behavior therapy. 3. Biofeedback training. 4.
Hypnotism. I. Title. [DNLM: 1. Behavior Therapy. 2. Biofeedback (Psychology) 3.
Hypnosis. WM 425 W637c]
R726.7.W53   1988
616.89'14—dc19   88-1055
                                                                       CIP

© 1988 Plenum Press, New York
A Division of Plenum Publishing Corporation
233 Spring Street, New York, N.Y. 10013

Printed in the United States of America

"Two things fill the mind with ever new and increasing wonder and awe— the starry heavens above me and the moral law within me."

—Immanuel Kant
Critique of Pure Reason, 1781

PREFACE

This book is an effort to integrate some clinical observations, theoretical concepts, and promising clinical procedures that relate psychological variables to physiological variables. My primary emphasis is on what psychological and behavioral concepts and procedures are most likely to enable us to influence physiological functions. The book covers questions that have fascinated me and with which I have struggled in daily clinical practice. What types of people are most at risk for physical disorders or dysfunctions? Why do some people present psychosocial conflicts somatically and others behaviorally? What is the placebo effect and how does it work? How do you arrange the conditions to alter maladaptive belief systems that contribute to psychopathology and pathophysiology? Do beliefs have biological consequences?

When I was in private clinical practice, and even today in my medical school clinical practice situation, I set aside one day each week to puzzle over the theoretical questions that my clinical experience generates. Often isolating these underlying theoretical questions provides guidance into the most relevant empirical literature. I have found that this weekly ritual, which I started in private practice many years ago, appears to increase my clinical efficacy or at least makes clinical work more exciting. I find the unexamined clinical practice hard to endure. Kurt Lewin once said, "There is nothing so practical as a good theory." A good theory tells you what to notice, where to look for it, when to look for it, and how to look for it. Nothing can be more useful to the practicing clinician. The practicing clinician, even more than the research scientist, is concerned daily with the control and prediction of the behavior of individual people in their natural environments. The corrective feedback from patients can sustain humility. Predicting and controlling clinical symptoms is a very challenging task, even in the circumscribed area of clinical psychophysiology.

This is not a cookbook on clinical health psychology. This book deals directly with some salient issues in the field of clinical health psychology and risks explicit experimental predictions from new concepts and procedures relevant to some big clinical questions. Without risking empirical disconfirmation or confirmation, there can be no advancement in theories or procedures. For example, what factors place people at risk for chronic stress-related somatic symptoms and what are the implications for primary prevention? What is the most effective procedure to lead the somatizing patient out of the somatic closet and into psychotherapy? What is the placebo effect and how can conditions be arranged to potentiate placebo effects? This book does not deal with some important issues framed as compliance, Type A behavior, and smoking cessation, and so on, because I do not think that anything profound or potent can be said about these topics as they are framed today. In fact, I do not think that anything important can be said about those topics outside the context of individual differences and specific procedures that engage those individual differences. For example, our lack of clinical efficacy in modifying those problems has much, but not all, to do with using the wrong key to open those doors. If your car does not start when I insert my car key into your ignition, I will not be so foolish as to accuse your car of "resistance." I will simply recognize that I failed to secure or copy your key. Human nature is usually responsive to a judicious combination of structural and functional approaches to disrobing her. This book, like Jerome Frank's *Persuasion and Healing*, is littered with promising theories and clinical procedures that need independent replication, empirical testing, and refinement and revision. This book is for all curious practicing clinicians, the academic researcher who is not willing to spend his life in the methodologically sophisticated investigation of trivia, and the graduate student who wants to know some of the salient questions in the field of clinical health psychology. There may be several important issues in clinical health psychology that I have ignored because I do not have anything particularly profound or potent to say about them.

This book contains several experimentally testable minitheories. Good theories are useful to a clinician in a medical setting because they help him to quickly and confidently intervene to relieve pain and suffering. When interventions derived from theories fail, clinical wisdom and humility can begin. A good theory directs clinical observation to those sources of variance that account for the largest chunks of variability in clinical symptoms. As my clinical experience grows I have found Lewin's comment on the practical value of theory to be profoundly true. Each patient I see is a unique configuration of myriad psychological, social, and biological factors (independent variables), and each patient is immobilized to varying degrees in his capacity to work and play; by psychological, behavioral, or psychophysiological symptoms (dependent variables). My clinical efficacy is a function of how rapidly, accurately, and powerfully I can help each patient control and predict his clinical symptoms. A good theory tells me what of the myriad available types of information to collect and how to use it to ensure maximum control and prediction of symptoms. A good theory not only tells me what to observe, but where to observe it, when to observe it, and how to observe it. When confronted with a complex and multifaceted clinical field, nothing is so practical as the ability to quickly recognize patterns and to understand the relationship between them. Delays in the clinician's pattern recognition time costs the patient money, pain, and suffering. To the clinician with limited time and energy, good theory is even more important than to the researcher.

This book deals with observations, theories, and procedures that are pertinent to *effective* practice in select areas of health psychology and behavioral medicine. The areas are selected for having procedures of known efficacy. Tautological as it might appear, the ability to *reliably* deliver effective clinical outcomes ("cures") is the *essential* and *sufficient* condition to generate powerful placebo effects (see Chapter 5). Some of the concepts and procedures in this book are new and represent fresh and complex ways of approaching common but difficult clinical phenomena.

I propose in Chapter 1 a theory of what factors predispose people to develop chronic stress disorders. The theory proposes a small number of underlying mechanisms that can account for a wide variety of presenting clinical complaints and to which etiology-specific therapies can be directed.

Chapter 2 is about how and why the profile of illness presented to physicians has changed in the last 50 years and about the implications of this change for the training of future M.D.s and professional psychologists. It points out that therapy for the new chronic disorders cannot be limited to drugs and surgery. With the development of preventive behavioral techniques and psychophysiological skills for the therapy of physical disorders and diseases (not mental symptoms) the mind–body dichotomy is no longer simply a philosophical debate. Drugs and surgery are not the only effective therapies for physical disease today. There is now a practical debate over the wisdom of refusing insurance reimbursement for, for example, a conservative and promising psychophysiological therapy for chronic pain versus ready insurance reimbursement for predominantly ineffective mutilating surgery for chronic pain. There are also now effective psychological and behavioral therapies for other physical diseases and disorders (e.g., common and classic migraine). Psychologists are now involved in areas of therapy that were once the practice of medicine. From a legal viewpoint, are clinical health psychologists today practicing as physicians? What are the common features of the three behavioral technologies (biofeedback, hypnosis, and behavior therapy) that are the most promising alternatives to drugs and surgery for certain stress-related chronic disorders?

Chapter 3 suggests that we need to stop thinking of hypnosis as something that happens to some people after a hypnotic induction, but rather as a mode of information processing into which most people can drift to varying degrees under even several naturalistic conditions (sensory restriction, high and low physiological arousal, dependency relationships, etc.) It also suggests that the hypnotic mode of information processing may have survival value for humans but that it also has implications in conjunction with other factors, for the development of psychopathology and pathophysiology.

Chapter 4 is about a subset of patients who present physical complaints without physical findings or without pathophysiology for which there is specific therapy. This challenging group of patients, called "crocks," provoke anger in many MDs. Crocks are often the recipients of iatrogenic disease because of their insistence on a medical "cure" when no treatable pathophysiology can be identified. This growing group of patients (crocks) are a major factor in escalating health care costs. These patients require a systematic approach that leads them out of the somatic closet and on to the psychotherapy couch. The outlines of an effective approach (the Trojan Horse Procedure) are broadly sketched in this chapter and elaborated in Chapters 6 and 7.

In Chapter 5, I propose a new experimentally testable Pavlovian theory of the placebo effect. In fact, at least one doctoral dissertation in Australia (Voudouris, 1986) and several animal studies in psychoneuroimmunology (Ader, 1981) have already verified some predictions from the theory. My conditioned response model of the placebo proposes several counterintuitive predictions. For example, it predicts that therapists who routinely use only active ingredients will, in fact, get stronger placebo effects than therapists who use mainly inert ingredients. The model also predicts that as science advances and therapies become increasingly specific we will get stronger placebo effects! The model identifies several conditions that will enhance placebo effects and predicts that individual differences in hypnotic ability will in the clinical situation enhance placebo responding.

Chapter 6 focuses on why patients are referred to a clinical health psychologist and on the top priorities in the initial interview. It is critical to assess the patient's subjective perception of his or her presenting complaints, to engage the patient in a therapeutic alliance and to secure the patient's commitment to work on change. It is critical to secure the above objectives in the first one or two sessions and to engage the patient in an aggressive therapeutic alliance focused on commitment to freedom from constraining clinical symptoms.

Chapter 7 describes the Trojan Horse Procedure I have developed to lead the somaticizing patient out of the somatic closet. This procedure involves psychophysiological demonstrations, a redefinition of the problem and eventually a coinvestigational model of therapy. I also present some empirical evidence for the efficacy of the Trojan Horse Procedure.

Chapter 8 makes clinically important distinctions between acute and chronic pain and proposes a new theory of the acquisition of some types of chronic pain and anxiety. It presents a case study of chronic pain with long-term follow-up.

Chapter 9 focuses on how to use the High Risk Profile clinically to provide patient feedback and to plan therapy. It also focuses on the need to identify any unconscious and overlearned beliefs and behavioral responses which may inhibit the assimilation of current life changes. This chapter includes two case studies demonstrating the therapy of high and low hypnotizable patients.

Chapter 10 examines the seven common features of several procedures (meditation, autogenic training, relaxation, systematic desensitization, EMG frontal biofeedback, etc.) developed to control psychophysiological stress reactions. It points out that empirical work on self-hypnosis marks self-hypnosis as a prototype of these psychophysiological stress-reduction procedures. The chapter concludes with a new theory of three therapeutic mechanisms (enhanced hypnotizability, entry into the "allocentric" mode of perception and cognitive control of physiological functions) associated with the practice of most psychophysiological stress-reduction procedures.

References

Ader, R. (Ed.) *Psychoneuroimmunology*. New York: Academic Press, 1981.
Voudouris, N. J. *The role of conditioning and expectancy in placebo analgesia: An experimental analogue study.* Unpublished doctoral dissertation. La Trobe University, Australia, June, 1987.

ACKNOWLEDGMENTS

There are some people who have expanded and differentiated my intellectual world, and some who have done so for my emotional life, and even a few who have indirectly contributed to the expansion and clarity of both my ability to know and to love. Their light will always shine for me like a few bright stars on a clear dark wintry night.

First, I want to thank my mother, Maude, for the faith and self-sacrifice which made it possible for me to be a student and scholar. To my father, my family, and the atmosphere of my childhood and adolescence, I owe the inspiration to recognize that while the "unexamined life is not worth living," philosophy is best appreciated with an inheritance. I want to thank Sally, Barbara, Decia, Nancylew, Vanessa, and Susan for the emotional learning they provided at various times during the 10 years this book was in preparation or in limbo. My relationships with them provoked some of my most fundamental inquiries into priorities, faith keeping, bonding, and destiny. Poetry and philosophy originate in "emotion recollected in tranquility."

Next, I want to acknowledge my gratitude to Professors O. H. Mowrer and C. H. Patterson for the intellectual challenge and emotional support they provided when I was a graduate student. Dr. Mowrer validated some of my early thoughts, when I was still an intern, on the relevance of learning theory to the analysis of psychopathology and hope. He also reviewed my first publication on a learning theory approach to analysis and therapy of a paranoid schizophrenic. Dr. Patterson nourished my lifelong preoccupation with "nonspecific factors" in clinical practice and the critical clinical sense of the big picture. During my introspective adolescence, two men, Mr. T. Kurivila and Mr. D. Bartholomeusz, led me into the world of literature and philosophy. I still continue to draw on the investments they encouraged me to make when I was an adolescent.

More recently the thoughts and support of several distinguished colleagues have influenced my intellectual and professional life. These people include Sidney Bijou, Neal Miller, Martin Orne, Elmer and Alice Green, Thomas Budzynski, Charles and Elizabeth Stroebel, Ted Barber, Erika Fromm, and Stanley Krippner. The Greens and the Strobels have provided inspiring personal relationships which they may not have recognized "rallied the red squadron of my dreams, when my spent-out heart had beaten its own retreat." Tom Budzynski has been an inspiring role model of an engineer turned clinician, who was brilliant but not afraid to be vulnerable. Professors Neal Miller, Jack Hilgard, and Martin Orne demonstrated through their work that scientific discipline could be productively invested in clinically important questions. Important questions in creative hands can generate new methodology. They were not intimidated by the big questions. Their example has shown me that a good clinician is both a hypothesis generator and a hypothesis tester.

Finally, I owe much to my boyhood heroes because in understanding anybody's work it is important to know who their boyhood heroes were. In some sense, as I grow older, I am already returning to those playgrounds of the mind where my boyhood heroes wait. My heroes were Bertrand Russell, Arnold Toynbee, T. S. Eliot, and Thomas Aquinas. Because I was not particularly athletic as a boy, I spent much time in libraries climbing on the shoulders of my heroes. This helped me to see further than most of my peers which further alienated me from them. This radical sense of alienation and anguish about which Muriac and Sartre have written does not motivate mountaineering as much as it did when I was a boy, nor does it disturb me as deeply. In conclusion, I want to thank my mindful colleague, Ron Giannetti, and my research assistants, Ellen Atkins and Marsha Turner, who kept me working on the revisions of the manuscript. Marsha particularly helped me wrap up this book.

CONTENTS

Appendixes   *255*

Selected Bibliography   *297*

Index   *301*

1

WHAT KINDS OF PEOPLE ARE AT HIGH RISK TO DEVELOP CHRONIC STRESS-RELATED SYMPTOMS?

Sometimes it is more important to know what kind of patient has a disease than what kind of disease the patient has.
—Sir William Osler

Every affection of the mind that is attended with either pain or pleasure, hope, fear is the cause of an agitation whose influence extends to the heart.
—Sir William Harvey
Exercitatio Anatomica de Motu Cordis et Sanguinis in Animalibus, 1628

Sir William Osler had to rely on intuition to identify subject features that could potentiate or attenuate either the symptoms or the etiology, or both, of a disease. The first goal of the present chapter is to specify a promising set of empirically identifiable individual differences and also a set of situational events that increase the risk of developing stress-related physical symptoms. The second goal is to present evidence from my clinical practice and the research literature to support this model of the patient at high risk to develop chronic stress-related illness. The third goal of this chapter is tentatively to suggest some procedures to quantify these subject dimensions and these situational conditions. The present model (Wickramasekera, 1979, 1980b,d, 1983) is based on clinical observations in an increasingly specialized clinical practice, theoretical spec-

An earlier version of this chapter was first presented at the Biofeedback Society of America, 1979, San Diego, and the International Stress and Tension-Control Society, England, 1983.

ulations, and empirical data from several disparate lines of controlled research.

Today the discrimination of psychophysiological or functional somatic disorders from physically based disorders is accomplished almost entirely by the exclusion of physical explanations of the patient's somatic complaints. This procedure unrealistically assumes that physical and psychological processes that result in somatic symptoms must be mutually exclusive. That is, if a physical process is found that explains the symptoms, then psychological factors must not be involved. If a physical process is not found, then psychological factors must be involved, even if no specific psychopathological process that can independently account for the symptoms is identified and to which therapy can be directed. This logic presumes a complete mind–body dichotomy and does not correspond to empirical facts.

This process of diagnosis by exclusion is practiced by default because there has been little systematic effort (Sternbach, 1966) devoted to the identification of specific, experimentally testable, and positive psychological/psychophysiological findings that can account for physical symptoms independently of physical findings. General theories of predisposition to disease have been proposed, but they have been difficult to test in predictive and mechanism-oriented experimental studies. Examples of these theories include the work of Alexander (1950) on the choice of disease, Engel (1968) on the generalized sense of actual, potential, or imaginary loss, Wolff (1953) on the failure to adapt, and Mason (1971, 1972) on the emotional response to the perception of threat. Recently, more operationally defined and experimentally testable risk factors like Type A behavior (Friedman & Rosenman, 1974) and life change (Holmes & Rahe, 1967) have been proposed. The identification of such high-risk variables have profound implications for diagnostic practice as well as for therapy and for primary prevention. For example, the presence of positive psychological findings in a patient can help the clinician inhibit his or her tendency to submit the patient to extensive physical investigations that could increase the probability of identifying and then treating a false positive physical etiology and producing an iatrogenic condition. An example of this would be unnecessary back surgery for benign and self-limiting back pain (Barton, Haight, Marsland, & Temple, 1976; Fordyce, 1980). The coexistence of positive psychological and physical findings might suggest that complaints having a physical etiology are being exacerbated by psychological factors. Effective intervention would require attention to both aspects of the condition.

Basing the diagnosis of psychophysiological disorders mainly on the exclusion of physical findings is a less than rational procedure because it is possible that the appropriate physical investigation was not done (Hall, Popkin, Devaul, Faillace, & Stickney, 1978). In fact, this approach implies that patients with physical complaints who lack positive and independent psychophysiological findings should receive the most complete and careful physical investigations.

Some physical complaints (e.g., headaches, backaches, etc.) can be accounted for by either positive physical findings like a brain tumor, a herniated disc, or alternatively by positive psychophysiological findings like functionally based high levels of muscle tension (Flor, Turk, & Birbaumer, 1985) and neuroticism (Eysenck, 1960). It is hypothesized that the five high-risk factors alone, in the absence of physical findings, can independently account for stress-related physical symptoms. Patients who present physical complaints can be divided into four cells (see Figure 1) based on the demonstrated presence or absence of identifiable physical findings (based on physical examination and laboratory tests) or identifiable psychophysiological findings (based on psychological and psychophysiological tests).

The purpose of the present chapter is to propose a set of definable, discrete, and measurable positive psychophysiological risk factors that constitute positive psychophysiological findings sufficient alone to account for physical complaints, or to account for the psychological amplification of positive physical findings. The empirical validity of these risk factors is critically evaluated as each risk factor is presented and discussed. (See Figure 1).

Cell 1 is an instance of positive physical findings and positive psychophysiological findings. This patient presents headaches and on investigation is found to have a brain tumor and to be anxious and depressed. The anxiety and depression could be amplifying (Melzack, 1973) the sensory pain component that results from the brain tumor. The acute psychological symptoms (e.g., anxiety, depression) often clear up

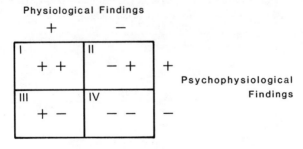

Figure 1. A model of the relationship between physical and psychophysiological data.

after removal of the tumor and the headache pain disappears. Physicians generally find patients in Group 1 easy to manage if the acute psychological reactions disappear after removal of the tumor and physical healing. But in certain people (identified by the high-risk model) the anxiety, the depression, and the pain may persist even after the brain tumor is removed.

An instance of Cell 2 is the patient who presents chronic low back pain in the absence of a herniated disc or other appropriate physical findings, but who is depressed, anxious, and sleeps poorly at night. These patients' therapeutic response frustrates the best diagnostic, surgical, and chemical efforts of physicians. These patients end up irritating and alienating many physicians (primary care and specialists) because of their dissatisfied and demanding manner and eventually become doctor shoppers. Physicians find patients in Cell 2 the most difficult to manage.

A patient in Cell 3 can present acute low back pain secondary to a herniated disc without enough time for psychological amplification of the back pain. Surgical repair is followed by rapid resolution of the physical complaint. Physicians manage patients in Group 3 very rapidly and effectively. These are the patients they are specifically trained to treat in their medical education.

A patient in Cell 4 may present headache pain in the absence of positive physical or psychophysiological findings. These negative findings (Hall et al., 1978) may result from insensitive or inappropriate physical and psychophysiological tests and examinations.

Five factors are hypothesized to increase the risk of stress-related physical symptoms. The first three risk factors are subject variables primarily related to the predisposition to illness. The last two are situational variables primarily related to the precipitation of the illness. The three predisposing factors are (a) either high- or low-hypnotic ability; (b) autonomic lability (neuroticism) and more specifically autonomic response specificity; and (c) the habitual cognitive tendency to catastrophize. The precipitating factors are (d) psychosocial stressors in the form of major life changes and/or minor hassles over a short period of time in the presence of (e) deficits in adaptive support systems or coping skills needed to manage the stressors.

Hypnotic Ability

The first risk factor is both extremes (e.g., high or low) of hypnotic ability (Wickramasekera, 1979, 1983). Hypnotic ability is a normally distributed, stable individual difference variable (Barber, 1969; Hilgard,

1965) that appears to be partly genetically based (Morgan, 1973; Morgan, Hilgard, & Davert, 1970). Hypnosis can be defined as a psychophysiological condition in which attention is focused to the point where there is a relative reduction of peripheral awareness and critical-analytic mentation, leading to major distortions in perception, mood, and memory sufficent to produce significant behavioral and biological changes. Hypnotic ability is measured with procedures of known reliability and validity, such as the Stanford and Harvard Scales (Barber, 1969; Hilgard, 1965). Current research suggests that hypnotic ability is best considered a mode of information processing (uncritical-holistic-visual-emotional) that can occur in a variety of situations (e.g., hypnotic induction, sensory restriction, transference, etc.) but particularly under conditions of high or low physiological arousal (Wickramasekera, 1971, 1972, 1973, 1976b, 1977a, 1980a). It is most important to stop thinking of hypnosis as an event that occurs only during a hypnotic induction, in the same way that we do not think of intelligence as an event that occurs only during an intelligence test. About 10% of the population are able very readily and profoundly to access the hypnotic mode of information processing and an equal percentage are almost never able to do so, except under a set of special conditions that include high (fight or flight response) or low (hypnogogic or hypnopompic) physiological arousal (Wickramasekera, 1977a).

There are three features of the high ability to use this mode of information processing and three features of the inability to use this mode of information processing that place people at high risk for developing somatic symptoms. Wickramasekera (1983) found that 85% of a sample of 103 patients with primary psychophysiological diagnosis were either very high or very low on hypnotic ability as rated by the Stanford, Harvard, or Spiegel Scales. In a general way it appears that people of high-hypnotic ability can attend too much, and sometimes in a negative way (catastrophizing cognitions), consequently amplifying even minimal unpleasant sensations in their bodies. Whereas people of low-hypnotic ability attend too little to the emotional-verbal correlates of physiological responses. (See Table 1.)

High-Hypnotic Ability

The first feature of the high-hypnotic ability that contributes to risk is the ability to hallucinate voluntarily. Unlike the high hypnotizable, the psychotic does not have voluntary control of his hallucinatory process. Factor analytic studies of hypnotic behavior indicate that this capacity for generating rich images and fantasies is a major factor in hyp-

Table 1. Characteristics of High and Low Hypnotizables

High-hypnotic ability
  1. Ability to voluntarily hallucinate in the absence of mental disorder.
  2. Hypersensitivity to psychological and physiological changes.
  3. Ability to alter memory functions and states of consciousness.

Low-hypnotic ability
  1. Hyposensitivity to psychological and physiological changes.
  2. Denial of psychological causation.
  3. Delay in seeking medical investigation.

---

nosis, accounting for close to 50% of the variance on standardized tests of hypnosis (Hilgard, 1982). Wilson and Barber's (1982) report comparing female high-hypnotizable subjects to a control group of moderate and low responders, provides numerous examples of these abilities. High-hypnotizable persons spend a great deal of time, up to 50% of waking time, in fantasy activity. The images produced in these fantasies are frequently reported to be indistinguishable from real events. Images could reach hallucinatory intensity in all sensory modalities. Recall of past events could achieve these same qualities. Actual, external, nonfantasized events could be experienced intensely. For example, high hypnotizable persons could "see," "hear," "feel," and "smell" what was being talked about during simple social conversations.

The relevance of these fantasies for stress-related disorder is that they have corresponding physiological consequences. Beliefs, irrespective of their objective validity, are more likely to have biological consequences for the superior hypnotic subject (Wickramasekera, 1979). Eighty-six percent of Wilson and Barber's subjects reported frequent experiences throughout their lifetimes of having illnesses or physical symptoms directly related to their thoughts, fantasies, or memories. Only 8% of the contrast group reported this. For example, 60% of them reported false pregnancies, including breast changes, abdominal enlargement, morning sickness, and fetal movements in response to the belief that they were pregnant. Only 16% of the comparison group reported false pregnancy. It is hypothesized that the rich and convincing perceptual and cognitive experiences of the highly hypnotizable subject, together with the physiological consequences of these experiences, can provide a foundation for the development of more chronic symptomatology.

A second feature of high-hypnotic ability that can contribute to risk is hypersensitivity to psychological and physiological changes. The following loosely related but converging empirical findings relate to the hypersensitivity hypothesis. Hypersensitivity is demonstrated by features of the high-hypnotizable person's learning process. A first learning mechanism of symptom induction in high-hypnotic-ability subjects is a *superior sensory memory* and a superior ability to transfer information from sensory to short-term memory (Ingram, Saccuzzo, McNeil, & McDonald, 1979; Saccuzzo, Safnan, Anderson, & McNeill, 1982). This ability could be used to rapidly learn and retain respondent and operant pain and anxiety. It is likely that high-hypnotizable subjects learn, remember, and incubate (Eysenck, 1968; Wickramasekera, 1970b) too well the experience of acute pain, permitting it too easily to become a chronic pain disorder. Studies of simple operant verbal conditioning (King & McDonald, 1976; Webb, 1962; Weiss, Ullman, & Krasner, 1960; Wickramasekera, 1970a), respondent conditioning (Das 1958a,b), and complex social-psychological influence procedures like short-term psychotherapy (Larsen, 1966; Nace, Warwick, Kelley, & Evans, 1982), demonstrate that the high-hypnotic-ability subject learns and conditions more rapidly than the low-hypnotic-ability subject. It is likely that they too easily learn and retain in memory pain and fear experiences.

A second learning mechanism of symptom induction is that the high-hypnotic-ability person may be *hypersensitive to sensory stimuli* and a superior discriminator of visceral sensations (Hantas, Katkin, & Reed, 1984). Clinically, it is likely that without analgesic suggestions, people of high hypnotic ability are less tolerant of pain than are people of low-hypnotic ability (Barabasz, 1982; Shor, 1964; Stam, McGrath, Brooke, & Cosier, 1986). It is known that people of high-hypnotic ability have an unusual capacity for attention to and absorption in subjective events (Tellegen & Atkinson, 1974; Wilson & Barber, 1982) like pain and fear, and perhaps this ability can be used to amplify their response to even minimal sensory and visceral stimuli. A recent study (Harsher-Towe, 1983) of normal volunteer undergraduate and medical students serendipitously found that frontal EMG levels of high-hypnotic ability subjects were significantly higher ($p < .001$) than those of low-hypnotic ability subjects during final exam week. This suggests that high-hypnotic-ability subjects may show an amplified physiological reactivity to even transient stressors. Because hypnotic ability is also positively correlated with standardized tests of creativity (Bowers & Bowers, 1979), it is possible that this creative ability is at times used to elaborate maladaptive meanings, thereby amplifying minimal sensations. It is also now well established that people of high-hypnotic ability are very much more likely to develop clinical phobias than people of low- or moderate-hypnotic ability (Foenander, Burrows, Gerschman, & Horne, 1980; Frankel & Orne, 1976; Gerschman, Burrows, Reade, & Foenander, 1979; Kelly, 1984; Perry, John, & Hollander, 1982). It has been found that an unexpectedly large number (48% to 58%) of clinical phobics (N=20 to 40) are highly hypnotizable. It is also known that in a subset of high-hypnotizable subjects, the severity of childhood punishment (including abuse) is correlated positively with high-hypnotic ability (Hilgard, 1979; Nash, Lynn, & Givers, 1984). The hypnotic ability may be developed to cope with the punishment. It is likely that the hypersensitivity to sensory stimuli of the highly hypnotizable subject provides the basis for the development of pain, anxiety, dissociative (multiple personality), and phobic disorders.

It is known that people in the hypnotic condition or people high in hypnotic ability are also more likely to report and believe that they are hypersensitive to extrasensory stimuli (Honorton & Krippner, 1969; Van De Castle, 1969). Patients who are high on hypnotic ability were very likely to report psychic experiences (Wickramasekera, 1979). Wilson and Barber (1982) reported that a sample of normal highly hypnotizable subjects (92%, N=27) were far more likely to report psychic experiences compared to low hypnotizable controls (16%, N = 25). They report experiences of precognition, telepathy, out-of-the-body experiences, or nonpsychotic hallucinatory experiences (Wilson & Barber, 1982). At least some of these people can be defined as prone to cognitive flooding or psychological pollution because they can voluntarily and temporarily reset their perceptual filters outside the constraints of rational-logical-critical analytic brain functions. This vulnerability to psychological pollution may be the basis of certain very rare psychophysiological phenomena, such as stigmata and possession. These psychic experiences, regardless of their objective validity, have the most profound subjective significance to many of these people with stress-related physical illness. It is very important clinically to give such patients permission to talk about these experiences, which they have learned to conceal lest they be regarded as insane. In each case I have found these patients to have resistant "medical" problems with multiple exploratory surgical histories. When given permission to talk about and to find meaning (reframe) or to assimilate (McReynolds, 1960) these experiences, and to integrate them into everyday life, remarkable and durable symptomatic recovery has always been observed. Today the mechanisms of this healing are obscure but they may eventually have naturalistic explanations.

A third and final feature of high-hypnotic ability is the ability voluntarily to alter their stream of consciousness (Evans, 1977) and memory functions (Kihlstrom, 1985). It is becoming clear that the highly hypnotizable subject has superior voluntary control of altered states of consciousness (Evans, 1977). This ability to alter the stream of consciousness may be a protective reflex developed to deal with biological hypersensitivity. Many subjects of high-hypnotic ability can voluntarily and easily initiate sleep during the day or night in multiple locations (e.g., sleep lab, work, classroom, on a plane or bus) and can wake up at a preselected time without an alarm. They can also learn during sleep (e.g., REM) without waking up, and demonstrate retention of simple information several days, weeks, or 6 months later (Evans 1977). Such learning is called state dependent because it can be demonstrated only by returning the subjects to the EEG sleep state in which the learning occurred in the first place. Maladaptive and/or aversive physiological responses like muscular bracing (Whatmore & Kohli, 1974) can be learned in states of hyperarousal (sexual trauma, automobile or industrial accident) or states of hypoarousal like nightmares or the sleep states that are not accessible to verbal analysis in states of moderate arousal (e.g., everyday consciousness). Clinically, it appears that sexual trauma or near-fatal industrial accidents (e.g., railroad, mining) can induce dissociative states (Hilgard, 1977) in which overlearned and incubated (Eysenck, 1968; Wickramasekera, 1970b) abnormal muscular responses (Whatmore & Kohli, 1974) can be acquired. Phenomena like incidental learning and pseudo or constructed memories (Dywan & Bowers, 1983; Laurence & Perry, 1983) acquired in unrecognized hypnotic states induced by high physiological arousal (stress of automobile or industrial accident), are particularly likely in subjects of high-hypnotic ability who present chronic pain or other somatic symptoms. It is also now known that superior hypnotic subjects, as opposed to poor hypnotic subjects, can alter the content of their night REM dreams by simply instructing themselves to do so prior to sleep (Belicki & Bowers, 1982; Tart, 1964, 1966; Stoyva, 1965). Perhaps waking negative-aversive expectations can alter the content of REM dreams and establish maladaptive patterns of muscular and vascular response in sleep. Often patients will wake up from sleep with a sudden onset of chronic pain or severe muscular or vascular headache. Hilgard (1977) has cogently documented the ability of high-hypnotizable subjects to process information outside of their own awareness to an extent that the low-hypnotizable subject cannot. Hilgard (1977) has termed this phenomena *dissociation*. Hence the high-hypnotic-ability person can very rapidly learn fear and pain responses and be unaware of what was learned and where it was learned.

The phenomena of incidental learning, source amnesia, or state-dependent learning may be the basis of the strong resistance to extinction of the bulimic syndrome. Bulimia often involves the voluntary control of a normally involuntary response (reverse peristalsis). If bulimic behaviors are in fact enacted in a totally or partially dissociated state, the critical cognitive cues that initiate bulimia may be incompletely or totally unavailable in the normal waking state. A recent study ($N=54$) showed that 57% of bulimics were high on hypnotic ability and 0% were low (Pettinatti, Horne & Staats, 1982). Also, a subset of anorexics who used purging as opposed to abstention from food were also high on hypnotic ability. These findings have recently been replicated and extended (Pettinati, Horne, & Staats, 1985). Hence, it is likely that a subset of some eating disorders may be learned and enacted in a dissociated state. Because of the phenomenon of state-dependent learning, the perceptions and cognitions that trigger some forms of bulimia may be relatively insulated from interventions (e.g., conventional psychotherapy) initiated outside of their state-dependent conditions of acquisition and maintenance.

It is known that a feature of high-hypnotic ability that can contribute to development of symptoms is *amnesic ability* (Dywan & Bowers, 1983; Kihlstrom, 1985; Laurence & Perry, 1983). The previously mentioned factor analytic studies have found that the second major factor in hypnotic ability is the capacity to make the mind blank and that this factor is orthogonal to the fantasy factor. This amnesic ability may be used to avoid or delay the recognition of organically based somatic stimuli in the acute phase of a disease, resulting in the postponement of treatment until the chronic phase. Amnesic ability may also result in decoupling the verbal subjective response system (contents of verbally mediated consciousness) from the motor or physiological response systems, resulting in somatization or conversion symptoms (Bendefeldt, Miller, & Ludwig, 1976).

Low-Hypnotic Ability

There are three features of low hypnotizability that are hypothesized to increase risk. These are hyposensitivity to psychological and physiological changes, a tendency to deny psychological causation of behavior, and to delay seeking medical investigation. Much less is known about these individuals, so these remarks should be considered as more speculative. Basically the low-hypnotic-ability subject is vulnerable to stress disorders because he or she is relatively insensitive to or deficient in attention to relationships between psychological (verbal-emotional) states and physiological (proprioceptive or interoceptive visceral) states. The low-hypnotizable subject's psychological insensitivity to changes in mood and feelings may be a liability from the viewpoint of preventive health care, because studies have suggested that changes in mood and feelings can precede the onset of even established infection (Canter, 1972; Hall *et al.*, 1978). People of low-hypnotic ability are nearly always limited to a skeptical, critical, and analytic mode of information processing; hence, they tend to negate (deny) or attenuate minimal sensory cues from their bodies. They are unwilling or unable to use verbal fantasy and imagination. It also appears that they prefer to think in concrete and discrete terms. Biofeedback instruments are helpful to low-hypnotizable subjects because they put their "insides" on the "outside" in observable, concrete, amplified, quantitative forms, such as meters that track the physiological correlates of psychological changes in ways that are harder to deny and dispute.

The low-hypnotic-ability person's hypothesized hyposensitivity to psychological and physiological changes overlaps with the concept of alexithymia. *Alexithymia* is defined as lacking "words for moods" (Sifneos, 1972) and it was first identified in individuals with psychosomatic disorders. It is also strongly related to low hypnotizability. One study (Frankel, Apfel-Savitz, Nemiah, & Sifneos, 1977), ($N=32$) found that 73% of subjects demonstrating low hypnotizability were rated as alexithymic and only 27% were rated as nonalexithymic. Only 8% of subjects of superior hypnotic ability were rated alexithymic and 92% of them were rated nonalexithymic. The average hypnotizability score on the Harvard Scale was a very low 2.7 for alexithymics. For nonalexithymics the mean score was 6.9, which is much closer to the general

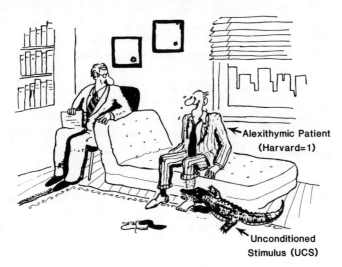

Figure 2. "This is incredible, doctor. I haven't been able to cry in years."

population mean of 7.4. It is likely that most people labeled as alexithymic are actually people who are low in hypnotic ability. For the
present, I prefer to identify alexithymia with hypnotic ability measures.
Hypnotic ability is well defined and reliably measured, whereas alexithymia is poorly defined and no reliable measure of it has been developed (Lesser, 1981; Lesser & Lesser, 1983).

Alexithymics' thinking is relatively unresponsive to psychological
events, and, I predict, to symbolic or conditioned stimuli (CS), but their
concepts will be very responsive to unconditioned stimuli (UCS) that are
concrete and objective. They either lack or fail to use a rich vocabulary to
label and discriminate among feelings and moods. They tend to attribute
psychological changes to external physical (UCS) changes (the "weather," "something I ate") and to express psychological states (e.g., depression) in somatic language (e.g., pain). When low-hypnotizable subjects
are exposed to a traumatic event (e.g., auto or industrial acident) that
causes physiological arousal, they are very likely verbally to inhibit or
deny their feelings (fear, terror, rage, anxiety, depression) associated
with the trauma. There is now some fresh evidence (Pennebaker, 1985)
that verbal and behavioral inhibition of trauma is associated with higher
levels of physiological arousal (Jones, 1960; Weinberger, Schwartz, &
Davidson, 1979), somatic complaints (Pennebaker, 1985), and even
physical diseases (Blackburn, 1965) like cancer (Kissen, 1966) and hypertension (Davies, 1970). Hence very often for the low-hypnotizable subject, somatic complaints are the final common pathway for unverbalized
psychosocial conflicts. I hypothesize that external stimuli (UCS) through
receptors may directly and reflexively change ANS functions and motor
responses in low-hypnotic ability persons, bypassing consciousness
(CNS) and the opportunity for the symbolic mediation (CS) and potential attenuation through procedures like reframing of these visceral or
motor changes. These people will present their psychological conflicts in
somatic forms and present them in medical and not psychiatric settings.

The hyposensitivity of the low-hypnotizable subject is associated
with poor anticipatory conditioning and relative weakness in voluntary
access to altered states of consciousness. Low-hypnotizable subjects
condition more poorly in both the operant (King & MacDonald, 1976;
Webb, 1962) and respondent (Das, 1958a,b) modes and probably are
slow in forming conditioned anticipatory responses. It is not the sight
(CS) or sound (CS, rustling of leaves) of the tiger that is dangerous to the
deer, but the tiger's teeth (UCS) and claws (UCS). The low-hypnotizable
subject has to wait till he or she feels the canines (UCS) in his or her
jugular before responding (see Figure 2, p. 11). The ability easily to form

conditioned anticipatory defensive responses (CR) to neutral stimuli (CS, rustling leaves) is self-preservative and biologically adaptive up to a point (this point is exceeded by the high hypnotizables). The low-hyp-notizable subjects' slow respondent conditioning may be an ANS corre-late of the inability readily to alter their states of consciousness. The immune system has recently been shown to be responsive to psycholog-ical events (Ader, 1981) and in fact subject to respondent conditioning. The respondent conditionability of the immune system (Ader, 1981) is probably an adaptive function that is relatively sluggish in low-hypnot-ic-ability people because of their slow conditioning. If the mechanism of the placebo response is respondent conditioning (Wickramesekera, 1977b, 1980c) and *immunopotentiation*, then low-hypnotic-ability people, because of their poor conditionability, will be poor placebo responders. The experience of aversive emotions and stress can inhibit the immune system, facilitating disease, or can potentiate the immune system, pro-tecting us from disease (Levy, Herberman, Macnish, Schlien, & Lip-pman, 1985; Sklar & Anisman, 1981). Within limits, the ability to form conditioned anticipatory responses and the ability easily to enter altered states of consciousness may be useful in the conditioning of the immune system.

A deficit in hypnotic ability may also inhibit the neurogenic reset-ting of dysfunctional (hypothalmic-pituitary-adrenal) feedback systems when the stress abates (e.g., after an auto or industrial trauma). The ability to enter altered states of consciousness, like hypnosis, may facili-tate the use of central (CNS) mechanisms like suggestion to reset dys-functional peripheral (ANS) feedback systems. For example, neurogenic regulation of blood pressure (Kezdi, 1967), perhaps through the reset-ting of baroreceptors, restores the body after stress to a state of home-ostasis (Cannon, 1932).

Hence, in summary, people of low-hypnotic ability may be more vulnerable to psychosocially induced stress disorders because they are less aware of psychological distress and deny the role of psychological causes of physical dysfunction. These patients are apt to deny recogniz-ing the psychological distress that may come before established infection (Canter, 1972; Canter, Imboden, & Cluff, 1966; Canter, Cluff, & Im-boden, 1972; Imboden, Canter, & Cluff, 1959, 1961) or tissue damage (UCR) and they delay seeking medical help. Physicians tend to attribute their somatic complaints to undetected organic pathology and tend to overinvestigate these patients in ways that add iatrogenic complications to the original somatic complaint. The poor conditionability of the low-hypnotic-ability subject may reduce the rate of immunopotentiation and placebo responding. Finally, low-hypnotic ability inhibits entry into altered states of consciousness useful in cognitively resetting dysfunctional peripheral feedback systems (e.g., baroreceptors).

Presently, I measure the hypnotic ability construct in three modes. Behaviorally, hypnotic performance is measured by the Harvard Scale (Shor & Orne, 1962), which is an established screening instrument of known high reliability and validity. It is measured verbally-subjectively with a self-report scale called the Absorption Scale (Tellegen & Atkinson, 1974) and the physiological potential for hypnotic behavior is measured with the conjugate lateral eye movement test (Bakan, 1969; Gur & Gur, 1974).

Habitual Catastrophizing (Panicking) Cognitions

Several large-scale prospective longitudinal studies (Hinkle, 1961; Stewart, 1962; Valliant, 1978) have shown that pessimism, self-doubt, passivity, and dependency are modest predictors of subsequent complaints of psychosomatic illness. A paper-and-pencil test of optimism as a causal factor or enduring disposition is associated with lower physical symptom checklist scores (Scheier & Carver, 1985). But there have been methodological problems in the assessment of these constructs. Ellis (1962) elucidated the role of habitual catastrophizing cognitions in the acquisition and maintenance of psychopathology. Catastrophizing is an orientation toward the future characterized by anticipating the most aversive outcomes. Catastrophizing can also be defined as becoming intensely and frequently absorbed in a negative psychological or sensory event and talking to one's self about it in ways that potentiate its aversive properties. For example, panic ("Oh my God I am dying") during a myocardial infarction can potentiate the event through inducing vasoconstriction that increases cardiac load (McKinney, Hofschive, Buell, & Eliot, 1984). It is likely that the cognitive tendency to catastrophize is at least partly based on either a generalized or situation-specific pessimistic and/or nihilistic belief system. It is likely that catastrophizing also plays a major role in attending to symptoms, altering sensory thresholds, and escalating the levels of sympathetic arousal in stress-related disorders. When catastrophizers encounter a negative experience, they typically and reflexively think thoughts like "I can't stand this" or "this is killing me," "this should not be happening to me, this is not fair." These thoughts amplify their misery and may increase sympathetic activation.

Catastrophizing has at least two response components. First, keeping the attentional focus on the sensory or visceral events that are antecedents or consequences of symptoms and, second, remembering or anticipating a wide range of negative physical and psychosocial consequences and antecedents of the aversive or symptomatic event. It is very likely that many of the internal and/or external cues that trigger the negative cognitive appraisal (catastrophizing) are outside of awareness (Dixon, 1981; Mathews & MacLeod, 1986). This preattentive bias operating outside of awareness may require special modification techniques, like dichotic listening or subliminal stimulation (Dixon, 1981; Forster & Govier, 1978) There are a number of studies relating catastrophizing to somatic complaints. At present, the assessment of catastrophizing is limited to interjudge agreement and *ad hoc* self-report scales. Chaves and Brown (1978) found that dental patients could be divided into catastrophizers and copers during an injection or extraction. Catastrophizing ideation was reliably associated with higher levels of distress and pain in the dental situation. Brown (1979) replicated the previously cited clinical finding with experimentally produced pain. Brown and Chaves (1980) found that the bulk of chronic pain patients (low back and headache) are catastrophizers. Catastrophizers have significantly higher pain ratings than copers. Eighty-six percent of catastrophizers were prescribed antianxiety or antidepressant medication, whereas only 12% of copers were on this type of medication. The clinical literature of phobias suggests that a psychophysiological predisposition to experience spontaneous panic attacks is the central and primary factor in the formation of phobias (Barlow & Mavissakalian, 1981). Conditioned anticipatory anxiety and avoidance behavior are respectively secondary and tertiary clinical phenomena. Subjectively spiralling panic and "depersonalization phenomena" (Barlow & Mavissakalian, 1981) are core components of phobic disorder and they appear to be directly reduced by antidepressant (e.g., tricyclic) medication. High levels of sympathetic activation may temporarily increase a person's hypnotic ability (Wickramasekera, 1977a) and tendency to depersonalization. The clinical observation that chronic pain (Sternbach, Janowsky, Huey, & Segal, 1976), panic or fear disorders, and depression are all partly responsive to tricyclic medication suggests that catastrophizing cognitions that subjectively reduce pain tolerance, spiral anxiety, and generate self-statements of hopelessness, may have common biological bases involving serotonin and norepinephrine metabolism. Spanos, Radtke-Bodonik, Ferguson, and Jones (1979) also found that catastrophizers had higher pain ratings than copers. Copers can be defined as people who use pleasant or positive cognitive distractions to attenuate their response to unpleasant sensory events. Spanos, Brown, Jones, and Horner (1981) found that catas-

trophizing (exaggerating) self-statements increased pain reports in experimental pain situations. Presently I measure catastrophizing with the
Zocco (1984) Scale. This scale was developed to measure catastrophizing
in phobic patients. It is not a totally adequate measure of catastrophizing
in patients presenting physical symptoms. I also use a clinical rating of
low, moderate, and high catastrophizing.

Sympathetic Reactivity/Negative Affectivity (Neuroticism)

High neuroticism (N) is a self-report dimension of personality that
is marked by a tendency to recognize and recall predominantly past
aversive memories. High N (neuroticism) scores indicate a tendency to
more negative affect (NA) across time and across situations independent
of objective stress. Neuroticism or NA is estimated on the basis of verbal
reports of distress. In clinical samples there is nearly always a large
incongruence between verbal report measures of distress and direct
physiological measures (e.g., EMG, heart rate, etc.) of distress. In fact
the goal of psychophysiological therapy is to reduce this incongruence
or dissociation. Neuroticism or NA is supposed to be based on autonomic lability (Eysenck, 1960; Wenger, 1948, 1966) or, more specifically, the
degree of reactivity of subsystems of the sympathetic division of the
ANS. Like hypnotizability, neuroticism seems to have a genetic basis
(Shields, 1962) and is known to decline with age. I predict that people
high or low on hypnotizability are more likely to show incongruence
between verbal report and direct physiological measures of distress. The
literature linking high self-report N scores to the limbic system is still
ambiguous because of methodological and other problems (Eysenck,
1983). Initially elevated baselines and measures of "delay" in returning
to baseline after stressful stimulation appear to be the most promising
physiological correlates of high N scores (Eysenck, 1983). Several retrospective studies reviewed by Jenkins (1971) and Steptoe (1981) reveal an
association between coronary artery disease and neuroticism. Two large-
scale (12,000 men) prospective studies (Medalie et al., 1976; Ostfeld,
Lebovits, Shekelle, & Paul, 1964) found a strong relationship between
neuroticism and the later development of angina pectoris but not myocardial infarction. Neuroticism appears to be related to the number of
physical complaints reported (Costa & McCrae, 1985) and the tendency
to report negative or aversive feelings (negative affectivity) across numerous places and times (Watson & Clark, 1984). Negative affectivity
should be recorded as an amplification of physical concerns rather than
as a sign of organic disease. Cross cultural and other factor analytic

studies establish negative affectivity (NA) as a stable dimension of mood that is universal and fundamental (Watson & Tellegen, 1985). I use the neuroticism scale from the Eysenck Personality Inventory (Eysenck & Eysenck, 1968) to take a brief paper-and-pencil assessment of negative affectivity.

Clinically, the most promising aspect of sympathetic reactivity is autonomic response specificity (ARS). *ARS* (Lacey, 1967; Sternbach, 1966) refers to the frequent observation of a stable profile of sympathetic response regardless of variations in the character of the stressor (e.g., mental arithmetic or cold pressor). This phenomena may have clinical implications (Sternbach, 1966). For example, people who show maximum reactivity in the cardiovascular system may be at high risk for angina pectoris, myocardial infarction, or stroke (Krantz & Manuck, 1984). Whereas those who show the strongest response on an EMG measure may be at greater risk of tension headache or low back pain (Flor *et al.*, 1985; Philips, 1977). The physiological system that is most strongly reactive (latency, elevated baseline), or delayed in returning to baseline can be termed the person's window of maximum vulnerability or the organ system in which he will develop clinical symptoms when under stress. (See Figures 3a, 3b, p. 18)

The analysis of autonomic response specificity appears to provide a promising approach to the prediction of somatic symptoms or windows of vulnerability. For example, a subset of people may respond most rapidly and strongly with their musculoskeletal system. Such people may be at high risk for developing musculo-skeletal disorders if exposed to chronic stress. Another subset may respond most strongly with their gastrointestinal system and may be at higher risk for peptic ulcer or colitis in response to chronic stress.

The Psychophysiological Stress Profile (Wickramasekera, 1976a,b) based on the ARS concept is a standardized testing procedure developed to measure directly the magnitude and duration of a patient's physiological response to a standardized psychosocial stressor. As on-line computer collects, reduces, and prints data (high–low, numbers of data points, mean and standard deviation) on heart rate, blood pressure, frontalis EMG, skin conductance, respiration, and peripheral skin temperature under three conditions. The first condition is a 15-minute habituation period, the second for patients with somatic presentations is a 3 minute period of stress (mental arithmetic problems), and finally, a 15-minute recovery or instructed return-to-baseline period. The patient is asked to give a subjective (on a visual analogue scale) rating of his or her level of muscle tension, on a subjective unit of disturbance scale (SUDS) ranging from 0 to 50 SUDS prior to actual physiological (inte-

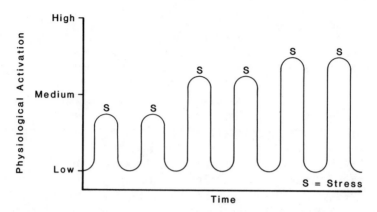

Figure 3a. Hypothetical normal pattern: no delay in return to baseline.

grated EMG) monitoring. In patients with chronic stress-related disorders (headaches, back pain, etc.) there is nearly always a marked discrepancy between the verbal report measure (much lower) and the frontalis physiological measure (0–50 microvolts EMG) on the strip chart recorder. The verbal report measure nearly always underestimates the actual frontalis EMG measure of muscle tension. This observation is used to suggest to the patient that he has psychologically habituated to a physiologically abnormal state.

Presently, I measure autonomic lability/neuroticism in two channels. A verbal report measure with the Eysenck Personality Inventory (Eysenck & Eysenck, 1968) and the psychophysiological stress profile (Wickramasekera, 1976a).

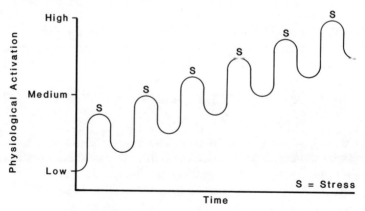

Figure 3b. Hypothetical abnormal pattern: acute stress becomes chronic pattern of bracing caused by delay in return to baseline. Elevating baseline pattern above.

Major Life Changes and/or Daily Hassles

Major Life Change

Major life changes like a new job, a divorce, the birth of a new child, and so forth, can be potent sources of psychosocial stress and precursors of somatic illness (Holmes & Rahe, 1967) because they challenge the person's capacity to adjust to change. In general, retrospective and prospective studies have shown a modest correlation (approximately .30) between increasing life change and the onset of mental or physical illness (DePue & Monroe, 1986; Rabkin & Struening, 1976). In modern industrialized society major psychosocial stressors are probably the primary class of stressors that activate the fight or flight response (Cannon, 1932) and/or the general adaptation syndrome (Selye, 1956). As Mason (1971) suggested, physical (e.g., hunger) and psychological stressors may operate through a common psychological mechanism: the perception of threat to the well-being of the animal. In fact, his research shows that in the absence of the perception of threat, biological changes (hypothalamic-pituitary-adrenal axis) may not occur in spite of physical stressors (Mason, 1971). Because the perception of threat is a learned response it can occur chronically and intermittently in response to such conditioned stimuli (CS) as cognition and images in the total absence of any UCR (tissue damage).

Psychosocial stressors, such as a problem child, an unhappy marriage, the death of a spouse, an unpleasant job, an aging parent who resides with you, etc., have certain unique and different features from physical stressors. First, psychosocial stressors commonly elicit both avoidance and approach tendencies whether sequentially or simultaneously. For example, a divorce after many years of marriage can be both a relief and a regret. Second, the sources of psychosocial stress are often nebulous and difficult to recognize, and even harder to define, unlike the threat from a saber-toothed tiger. Third, psychosocial stressors tend to be intermittent, chronic, and resistant to rapid or final resolution by primitive defenses like either fight or flight. For example, the problems posed by an adolescent or an aging parent who lives with you cannot be resolved by either physical attack or flight and they tend to hang around. In summary then, (a) ambivalence, (b) ambiguity, and (c) chronicity are three special features of psychosocial stressors that interact with the special features of people at high risk, potentiating the probability of somatic disorders and disease.

A massing of major life event changes appears to be associated with a higher probability of illness onset. A method of assessing the impact of situational stress on health is the measurement of major life changes (Dohrenwend & Dohrenwend, 1978; Holmes & Rahe, 1967). The major weakness of this method is the empirical finding that the relationship between life event change scores and health outcomes is too weak for individual prediction (DeLongis, Coyne, Dakof, Folkman, & Lazarus, 1982). Major life changes are infrequent events and are confounded with other variables (Rabkin & Struening, 1976). It appears that the features of life change that are most crucial for illness onset are (a) undesirability, (b) magnitude of change, (c) time clustering, and (d) uncontrollability (Thoits, 1983).

Daily Hassles

I have supplemented the major life change procedure with the Hassles Scale (Kanner, Coyne, Shaefer, & Lazarus, 1981). The Hassles Scale assesses the ongoing daily stresses and strains of everyday life, also called microstressors or chronic role strains. For example, getting caught in rush hour traffic, running out of gas, noise, work overload, and unexpected company. The research of Kanner *et al.* (1981) and De Longis *et al.* (1982) has demonstrated that massing of daily hassles is strongly related to somatic health outcomes and that this effect remained even after the effects of major life events was statistically removed (De Longis *et al.*, 1982; Lazarus, De Longis, Folkman, & Given, 1985; Zarski, 1984). Patients who have in the last 6 months experienced important life changes (e.g., divorce, death of a wife) may be exposed to a wave of minor hassles (paying bills, dressing children, cooking, laundry, etc.) because of one or more role changes (e.g., from husband to husband *and* housekeeper). These patients may develop complaints of back pain, headaches, stomach distress, or chest pain, and these complaints should first be evaluated in this situational context. Identification of major or microstressors is crucial of course for the therapeutic management of the individual.

Social Support Systems and Coping Skills

Social Support

Social support (Caplan, 1974) is the comfort, material help, and information one gets through formal or informal enduring contact with individuals or groups. Social support can be instrumental (material aid like money or food) or expressive (e.g., acceptance, empathy). Numerous studies reviewed by Cohen and Wills (1985) indicate that people with spouses, friends, and family members who provide psychological and material resources are in better health than those with less supportive social contacts. The best evidence for the potency of social support comes from studies of recovery, rehabilitation, and adaptation to illness (Wallston, Alagna, DeVellis, & DeVellis, 1983). There is a clear link between social support and mortality (Berkman & Syme, 1979; Blazer, 1982; House, Robbins, & Metzner, 1982). The most effective social support is likely to come from people who have similar backgrounds and values, who provide empathic understanding, and are calmly facing or have faced similar stressors (Thoits, 1986). It is important to realize that the evidence, to date, for the relationship between support systems and health is correlational and not experimental. The impact of a massing of major life event changes or minor hassles or both, will depend not only on the degree of the perception of psychological threat (Mason, 1971) provoked by life changes and hassles, but also by access to and the effective use by the patient of support systems and coping skills (Cassel, 1976; Medalie & Goldbount, 1976; Nuckolls, Cassel, & Kaplan, 1972). Support systems are essentially psychological resources (wife, siblings, psychotherapist, church, friends) on which the patient can lean and with whom he can abreact to cushion the impact of stressors. Social support probably operates through helping the person to (a) remove or alter the threat, (b) change the meaning of the threat, or (c) change his emotional reactions to the threat. Social support can be classified into the (a) number of support persons (mother, wife, brother, etc.); (b) availability of support persons (personal visits, long distance calls, etc.); and (c) satisfaction with support persons. The perceived availability and satisfaction with social support can buffer the impact of stressors (Cohen & Willis, 1985).

Coping Skills

There are probably at least three kinds of coping, namely (a) problem-focused, (b) emotion-focused, and (c) perception-focused coping. Problem-focused coping is taking direct action on the environment or self to remove or alter the threat. Emotion-focused coping consists of actions or thoughts to control the undesirable feelings provoked by the threat. Perception-focused coping consists of cognitive attempts to reduce or alter the importance of the threat.

The major elicitor of the fight or flight response today is psychological stress or chronic problematic psychosocial relationships; hence, coping skills and/or social competence can be a major factor in reducing excessive and sustained sympathetic reactivity. Social competence can be defined as a composite of social skills that reduce chronic psychophysiological arousal by resolving social and intrapersonal conflicts. Social competence (Argyle, 1981; Wine & Smye, 1981) is more than the absence of mental or physical illness. The components of social competence may include overt behavior, cognitive processes, and structures (Meichenbaum, Butler, & Gruson, 1981) that either resolve or palliate problems. Coping methods include information seeking, inhibition of action, and cognitive coping skills that alter attentional focus on the perception of problems (Wrubel, Benner, & Lazarus, 1981). Rosenbaum (1980) defined coping skills as learned resourcefulness or a compendium of skills by which an individual controls the interfering effects that certain internal events (emotion, pain, or undesired thoughts) have on the smooth execution of desired behavior. Rosenbaum (1980) defined the four component skills of learned resourcefulness as (a) the use of cognition and self instructions to cope with emotional and physiological responses; (b) the application of problem-solving strategies (such as planning, problem definition, evaluating alternatives, and anticipation of consequences; (c) the ability to delay immediate gratification; and (d) a general belief in one's ability to self-regulate internal events (i.e., self-efficacy).

The concepts of coping competence and coping skills originates in the animal learning and psychoanalytic ego psychology literature. Lazarus and Folkman (1984) discussed the complexity and clinical value of these concepts. Coping skills (religion, projection, information seeking, intellectualization, humor, repression, sublimation, escape through fantasy or reading, work, jogging, recreation, relaxation, meditation, etc.) can also be used to distract the patient, change (reframe) the aversive meaning of events, and lower the level of physiological arousal during the acute and chronic phases of the stressor's impact. Patients who lack coping skills or social support systems are at much higher risk of ego fragmentation and clinical symptoms.

Currently, we assess support systems with the Social Support Questionnaire (Sarason, Levine, Basham, & Sarason, 1983), and coping skills with a standardized clinical interview and the Ways of Coping (revised) Scale of Lazarus and Folkman (1984).

Discussion

This multidimensional model is composed of quantifiable components that separately may be weak predictors of clinical outcome, but when considered together are potent predictors that recognize the complexity of interactions between mind and body in real clinical situations (see Figure 4). The model accounts for the observation that some people with clear physical findings who get specific medical remediation can

Factors That Will Attenuate
Relationship Between Stress And Symptoms

    1. High Social Support
    2. High Satisfaction With Social Support
    3. High Coping Skills

Density Of
1) Major Life Changes --------> Mental or Physical Symptoms
    or
2) Minor Hassles (Micro-stressors)

Factors That Will Potentiate
Relationship Between Stress And Symptoms

    1. High or Low Hypnotic Ability
    2. High Catastrophizing
    3. High Neuroticism

Figure 4. Factors that moderate the relationship between stress and symptoms.

continue to have symptoms. The model provides broad targets (underlying mechanisms, not symptoms) for psychophysiological therapy in general (e.g., increase or decrease hypnotic ability, decrease catastrophizing, increase coping skills and support systems) and particularly for the patient who has not responded to the specific but exclusively medical intervention. The model is experimentally testable with pre–post measures of the five high-risk variables.

Clinical observation suggests that the impact of multiple major life changes or multiple minor hassles will depend not only on personality traits (high- or low-hypnotic ability, autonomic response specificity/neuroticism, and habitual catastrophizing ideation), but also on the patient's access to, and effective use of, social support systems and personal coping skills. For example, Nuckolls *et al.* (1972) found that 90% of women with high life change scores but low social support scores had one or more complications in pregnancy, whereas only 33% of women with equally high life change scores but with high social support scores had any complication in pregnancy. The patient at greatest risk is the one who is positive for all the predisposing features, who is deficient in support systems and coping skills, and who has experienced a massing of multiple major life changes and/or hassles. The person at lowest risk is the patient who has none of these personality features and who has effective use of multiple support systems and coping skills. In the absence of positive physical findings, but in the presence of two or more of the previously cited psychophysiological findings, one may consider a diagnosis of psychophysiological disorder. Even when there are positive physical findings, the identification of two or more of the risk factors can be regarded as likely to potentiate an illness due to a pathogen or to tissue damage. Clinical observations over the last 15 years have directed our attention to and confirmed the importance of the high-risk factors. We have continued to focus on these five constructs over the years and attempted clinically to assess or quantify them with procedures of increasing validity and reliability. Hypnotic ability is adequately measured today, but ANS lability, catastrophizing, major life change/minor hassles, coping skills, and social support systems are either poorly conceptualized or inadequately assessed by available scales today. These five risk factors have been clinically important in that they have clarified difficult diagnoses, enhanced the prediction of clinical outcome, and, most importantly, have provided broad targets for heuristic diagnostic investigation and clinical intervention. These five risk factors, after further refinement and validation, may some day be the focus of primary prevention efforts starting in childhood or adolescence. For example, we may need to reduce hypnotic ability in some people and increase (Wickramasekera, 1977a) it in others (e.g., alexithymics). We may need to reduce catastrophizing verbalizations in some patients (Ellis, 1962) while concurrently increasing the probability of coping verbalizations in them.

Some Predictions from the Model

1. Many people who present with chronic physical symptoms without physical findings or with only marginal physical findings will be found to be either low (Harvard Hypnotic Scale 0–4) or high (Harvard Hypnotic Scale 8–12) on hypnotic ability.

2. Those who are high on hypnotic ability will make physical and psychological symptom presentations in either medical or psychiatric settings, but those who are low on hypnotic ability will make mainly physical presentations and almost exclusively in medical settings (e.g., medical centers).

3. People high on hypnotic ability and neuroticism (ANS lability) will respond most strongly and recover most slowly from stressful stimulation and they will be found to have lower sensory thresholds for aversive stimulation.

4. People low on hypnotic ability will respond slowly (if at all) but consistently to stress-management therapies (e.g., biofeedback, relaxation therapy, systematic desensitization) as opposed to high hypnotizables, who will respond rapidly, and if high on neuroticism, inconsistently to psychophysiological therapy (Wickramasekera, 1976a).

5. A simple somatic checklist will show that people (nonpatients) high or low on hypnotic ability over age 35 will have a higher incidence of somatic complaints than people of moderate-hypnotic ability. The number of somatic complaints reported by low-hypnotic-ability people may need a K correction factor for denial.

6. People low on hypnotic ability *and* neuroticism because they are relatively insensitive to the psychological precursors (change in mood and feelings) of physical disease or dysfunction, will be at greater risk for developing physical disease (cancer, myocardial infarction, etc.) and they will delay longer seeking medical investigation than people high on both hypnotic ability and neuroticism.

7. People low on hypnotic ability who respond positively to psychophysiological therapy will show a tendency to increase in hypnotic ability and people high on hypnotic ability will show a tendency to reduce in hypnotic ability. People low in hypnotic ability will, through biofeedback or relaxation therapy, learn to identify and verbally discriminate physical sensations and their emotional correlates. The changes in internal attention and verbal sensitivity will tend to increase hypnotic ability (Wickramasekera, 1977a). The high-hypnotic-ability person will learn to process their internal world (sensations, emotions) through a more rational left hemisphere brain program (critical, analytical-sequential) that organizes it objectively and quantitatively. The quantitative, critical analytic mode of processing personal information may reduce or lead to a more discriminating use of hypnotic ability.

8. People high on hypnotic ability *and* neuroticism, particularly if they are also elevated on catastrophizing, are likely to be heavy users of medical and/or psychiatric services.

9. When people are sorted into low- and high-hypnotic ability groups and are required to attend (with appropriate controls for attention and hearing) to the same sensory stimulus (UCS) of known magnitude, the high-hypnotic-ability person will show a higher event-related brain potentials (ERPs) than the low-hypnotic-ability person.

10. High neuroticism scores or ANS lability will tend to inhibit the reliability of scores on tests of hypnotic ability both inside and outside the clinic.

11. People high or low on hypnotic ability are more likely to show incongruence between verbal report and direct physiological measures of distress or anxiety.

References

Ader, R. (Ed.) *Psychoneuroimmunology*. New York: Academic Press, 1981.

Alexander, F. *Psychosomatic medicine*. New York: Norton, 1950.

Argyle, M. The contribution of social interaction research to social skills training. In J. D. Wine & M. D. Syme (Eds.), *Social competence*. New York: Guilford Press, 1981.

Bakan, P. Hypnotizability, laterality of eye movements and functional brain asymmetry. *Perceptual and Motor Skills*, 1969, *28*, 927–932.

Barabasz, A. Restricted environmental stimulation and the enhancement of hypnotizability: Pain, EEG alpha, skin conductance and temperature responses. *International Journal of Clinical and Experimental Hypnosis*, 1983, *31*, 235–238.

Barber, T. X. *Hypnosis: A scientific approach*. New York: Van Nostrand Reinhold, 1969.

Barlow, D. H., & Mavissakalian, M. Directions in the assessment and treatment of phobia: The next decade. In D. H. Barlow & M. Mavissakalian (Eds.), *Phobia: Psychological and pharmacological treatment*. New York: Guilford Press, 1981.

Barton, J., Haight, R., Marsland, D., & Temple, T. Low back pain in the primary care setting. *Journal of Family Practice*, 1976, *3*, 363–366.

Belicki, K., & Bowers, P. The role of demand characteristics and hypnotic ability in dream change following a presleep instruction. *Journal of Abnormal Psychology*, 1982, *91*(6), 426–432.

Bendefeldt, F., Miller, T., & Ludwig, A. Cognitive performance in conversion hysteria. *Archives of General Psychiatry* 1976, *33*, 1250–1254.

Berkman, L. F., & Syme, S. L. Social networks, host resistance, and mortality: A nine-year follow-up study of Alameda County residents. *American Journal of Epidemiology*, 1979, *109*, 186–204.

Blackburn, R. Emotionality, repression-sensitization, and maladjustment. *British Journal of Psychiatry*, 1965, *111*, 399–400.

Blazer, D. G. Social support and mortality in an elderly community population. *American Journal of Epidemiology*, 1982, *115*, 684–694.

Bowers, P. E., & Bowers, K. S. Hypnosis and creativity. In E. Fromm & R. E. Shor (Eds.), *Hypnosis: Development in research and new perspectives* (2nd ed.), New York: Aldine, 1979.

Brown, J. M. *Cognitive activity, pain perception and hypnotic susceptibility*. Presented at the Annual Meeting of the American Psychological Association, September 1979, New York.

Brown, J. M., & Chaves, J. F. *Cognitive activity, perception, and hypnotic susceptibility in chronic pain patients*. Paper presented at Annual Meeting of the American Psychological Association, Montreal, Quebec, September 1980.

Cannon, W. B. *The wisdom of the body*. New York: Appleton-Century Crofts, 1932.

Canter, A. Changes in mood during incubation of acute febrile disease and the effects of pre-exposure psychologic states. *Psychosomatic Medicine*, 1972, *34*, 424–430.

Canter, A., Imboden, J. B., & Cluff, L. E. The frequency of physical illness as a function of prior psychological vulnerability and contemporary stress. *Psychosomatic Medicine*, 1966, *28*, 344–350.

Canter, A., Cluff, L. E., & Imboden, J. B. Hypersensitive reactions to immunization innoculations and antecedent psychological vulnerability. *Journal of Psychosomatic Research*, 1972, *16*, 99–101.

Caplan, G. *Support systems and community mental health*. New York: Behavioral Publications, 1974.

Cassel, J. C. The contribution of the social environment to host resistance. *American Journal of Epidemiology*, 1976, *104*, 107–123.

Chaves, J. F., & Brown, J. M. *Self-generated strategies for the control of pain and stress.* Presented at the Annual Meeting of the American Psychological Association, Toronto, Canada, August, 1978.

Cohen, S., & Wills, T. A. Stress, social support, and the buffering hypothesis. *Psychological Bulletin*, 1985, *98*, 310–357.

Costa, P. T., Jr., & McCrae, R. R. Hypochondriasis, neuroticism, and aging: When are somatic complaints unfounded? *American Psychologist*, 1985, *40*, 19–28.

Das, J. P. The Pavlovian theory of hypnosis: An evaluation. *Journal of Mental Sciences*, 1958a, *104*, 82–90.

Das, J. P. Conditioning and hypnosis. *Journal of Experimental Psychology*, 1958b, *56*, 110–113.

Davies, M. Blood pressure and personality. *Journal of Psychosomatic Research*, 1970, *14*, 89–104.

DeLongis, A., Coyne, J. C., Dakof, G., Folkman, S., & Lazarus, R. S. Relationship of daily hassles, uplifts and major life events to health status. *Health Psychology*, 1982, *1*(2), 119–136.

Depue, R. A., & Monroe, S. M. Conceptualization and measurement of human disorder in life stress research: The problem of chronic disturbance. *Psychological Bulletin*, 1986, *99*, 36–51.

Dixon, N. F. *Preconscious processing*, Chichester, England: Wiley, 1981.

Dohrenwend, B. S., & Dohrenwend, B. P. Some issues in research on stressful life events. *Journal of Nervous and Mental Disease*, 1978, *166*, 7–15.

Dywan, J., & Bowers, K. The use of hypnosis to enhance recall. *Science*, 1983, *22*, 184–185.

Ellis, A. *Reason and emotion in psychotherapy*. New York: Lyle Stuart, 1962.

Engel, G. L. A life setting conducive to illness: The giving up–given up complex. *Bulletin of the Meninger Clinic*, 1968, *32*, 355–365.

Evans, F. J. Hypnosis and sleep: The control of altered states of consciousness. *Annals of the New York Academy of Sciences*, 1977, *296*, 162–174.

Eysenck, H. J. *The structure of human personality* (2nd ed.). London: Methuen, 1960.

Eysenck, H. J. A theory of the incubation of anxiety/fear responses. *Behavior Research and Therapy*, 1968, *6*, 309–321.

Eysenck, H. J., & Eysenck, S. B. G. *Eysenck Personality Inventory, Form A*, San Diego, CA: Educational and Industrial Testing Service, 1968.

Eysenck, H. J. Psychophysiology and personality. In A Galse & J. A. Edward (Eds.), *Physiological correlates of human behavior*. London: Academic Press, 1983.

Flor, H., Turk, D. C., & Birbaumer, N. Assessment of stress-related psychophysiological reactions in chronic back pain patients. *Journal of Consulting and Clinical Psychology*, 1985, *53*, 354–364.

Foenander, G., Burrows, G. D., Gerschman, J., & Horne, D. J. Phobic behavior and hypnotic susceptibility. *Australian Journal of Clinical and Experimental Hypnosis*, 1980, *8*, 41–46.

Fordyce, A behavioral perspective on chronic pain. In J. J. Bonica & K. K. Y. Ng (Eds.), *Pain, discomfort and humanitarian care*. New York: Elsevier/North-Holland, 1980.

Forster, P. M. & Govier, E. Discrimination without awareness? *Quarterly Journal of Experimental Psychology*, 1978, *30*, 282–295.

Frankel, F. H., & Orne, M. T. Hypnotizability and phobic behavior. *Archives of General Psychiatry*, 1976, *33*, 1259–1261.

Frankel, F. H., Apfel-Savitz, R., Nemiah, J. C., & Sifneos, P. E. The relationship between hypnotizability and alexithymia. *Psychotherapy and Psychosomatics*, 1977, *8*, 172–178.

Friedman, M., & Rosenman, R. H. *Type A behavior and your heart*. New York: Knopf, 1974.

Gerschman, J., Burrows, G. D., Reade, P., & Foenander, G. Hypnotizability and the treatment of dental phobic behavior. In G. D. Burrows, D. R. Collison & L. Dennerstein (Eds.), *Hypnosis*. New York: Elsevier, 1979.

Gur, R. C., & Gur, R. E. Handedness, sex, and eyedness as moderating variables in the relationship between hypnotic susceptibility and functional brain asymmetry. *Journal of Abnormal Psychology*, 1974, *83*, 635–643.

Hall, R. C. W., Popkin, M. K., Devaul, R. A., Faillace, L. A., & Stickney, S. K. Physical illness presenting as psychiatric disease. *Archives of General Psychiatry*, 1978, *35*, 1315–1320.

Hantas, M. N., Katin, E. S., & Reed, S. D. Cerebral lateralization and heart beat discrimination. *Psychophysiology* 1984, 3(21), 274–278.

Harsher-Towe, D. *Control of EMG activity in subjects demonstrating high and low levels of hypnotizability*. Unpublished doctoral dissertation, Virginia Consortium for Professional Psychology, 1983.

Hilgard, E. R. *Hypnotic susceptibility*. New York: Harcourt, Brace & World, 1965.

Hilgard, E. R. *Divided consciousness: Multiple controls in human thought and action*. New York: Wiley Interscience, 1977.

Hilgard, J. R. *Personality and hypnosis: A study of imaginative involvement*. Chicago: University of Chicago Press, 1979.

Hilgard, E. R. Hypnotic susceptibility: Implications for measurement. *International Journal of Experimental and Clinical Hypnosis*, 1982, *30*, 394–403.

Hinkle, L. E. Ecological observations on the relation of physical illness, mental illness and the social environment. *Psychosomatic Medicine*, 1961, *23*, 289–296.

Holmes, T. H. *Schedule of recent events*. University of Washington Press, 1981.

Holmes, T. H., & Rahe, R. H. The social readjustment rating scale. *Journal of Psychosomatic Research*, 1967, *11*, 213–218.

Honorton, C., & Krippner, S. Hypnosis and ESP performance: A review of the experimental literature. *Journal of the American Society for Psychical Research*, 1969, *63*, 214–252.

Horder, T. J. cited in M. S. Straus (Ed.), *Familiar medical quotations*. Boston: Little, Brown & Company, 1968.

House, J. S., Robbins, C., & Metzner, H. L. The association of social relationships and activities with mortality: Prospective evidence from the Tecumseh Community Health Study. *American Journal of Epidemiology*, 1982, *116*, 123–140.

Imboden, J. B., Canter, A., & Cluff, L. E. Brucellosis. *Archives of Internal Medicine*, 1959, *103*, 406–414.

Imboden, J. B., Canter, A., & Cluff, L. E. Convalescence from influenza. *Archives of Internal Medicine*, 1961, *198*, 393–399.

Ingram, R. E., Saccuzzo, D. P., McNeil, B. W., & McDonald, R. Speed of information processing in high and low susceptible subjects: A preliminary study. *International Journal of Clinical and Experimental Hypnosis*, 1979, 27(1), 42–47.

Jenkins, C. D. Psychologic and social precursors of coronary disease. *New England Journal of Medicine*, 1971, *284*, 244–255.

Jones, H. E. The longitudinal method in the study of personality. In I. Iscoe & H. W. Stevenson (Eds.), *Personality development in children*. Chicago: University of Chicago Press, 1960.

Kanner, A. D., Coyne, J. C., Schaefer, C., & Lazarus, R. S. Comparison of two modes of stress measurement: Daily hassles and uplifts versus major life events. *Journal of Behavioral Medicine*, 1981, *4*, 1–39.

Kelly, S. F. Measured hypnotic response and phobic behavior. *International Journal of Clinical and Experimental Hypnosis*, 1984, *32*, 1–5.

Kezdi, P. Neurogenic control of blood pressure in hypertension. *Cardiologia*, 1967, *51*, 193–203.

Kihlstrom, J. F. Hypnosis. In M. S. Rosenzweig & L. W. Porter (Eds.), *Annual review of psychology*. Palo Alto: Annual Reviews, 1985.

King, D. R., & McDonald, R. D. Hypnotic susceptibility and verbal conditioning. *International Journal of Clinical and Experimental Hypnosis*, 1976, *24*, 29–37.

Kissen, D. M. The significance of personality in lung cancer in men. *Annals of the New York Academy of Science*, 1966, *125*, 820–826.

Krantz, D. S., & Manuck, S. B. Acute psychophysiologic reactivity and risk of cardiovascular disease: A review and methodologic critique. *Psychological Bulletin*, 1984, *96*(3), 435–464.

Lacey, J. I. Somatic response patterning and stress: Some revisions of activation theory. In M. H. Appley & R. Trumball (Eds.), *Psychological stress*. New York: Appleton-Century Cofts, 1967.

Larsen, S. Strategies for reducing phobic behavior. *Dissertation Abstracts*, 1966, *26*, 6850.

Laurence, J. R., & Perry, C. Hypnotically created memory among highly hypnotizable subjects. *Science*, 1983, *222*, 523–524.

Lazarus, R. S., & Folkman, S. *Stress, appraisal and coping*. New York: Stringer, 1984.

Lazarus, R. S., DeLongis, A., Folkman, S., Given, R. Stress and adaptational outcomes: The problem of confounded measures. *American Psychologist*, 1985, *40*(7), 770–779.

Lesser, I. M. A review of the alexithymia concept. *Psychosomatic Medicine*, 1981, *43*(6), 531–543.

Lesser, I. M., & Lesser, B. Z. Alexithymia: Examining the development of a psychological concept. *American Journal of Psychiatry*, 1983, *140*, 10.

Levy, S. M., Herberman, R. B., Macnish, A. M., Schlien, B., & Lippman, M. Prognostic risk assessment in primary breast cancer by behavioral and immunological parameters. *Health Psychology*, 1985, *4*, 99–113.

Mason, J. W. A re-evaluation of the concept of "non-specificity" in stress theory. *Journal of Psychiatric Research*, 1971, *8*, 323–333.

Mason, J. W. Organization of psychoendocrine mechanisms: A review and reconsideration of research. In N. S. Greenfield & R. S. Sternbach (Eds.), *Handbook of psychophysiology*. New York: Holt, Reinhart & Winston, 1972.

Mathews, A., & Macleod, C. Discrimination of threat cues without awareness in anxiety states. *Journal of Abnormal Psychology*, 1986, *95*(2), 131–138.

McKinney, M. E., Hofschive, P. J., Buell, J. C., & Eliot, R. S. Hemodynamic and biochemical responses to stress: The necessary link between Type A behavior and cardiovascular disease. *Behavioral Medicine Update*, 1984, *6*, 16–21.

McReynolds, P. Anxiety, perception, and schizophrenia. In D. D. Jackson (Ed.), *The etiology of schizophrenia*. New York: Basic Books, 1960.

Medalie, J. H., & Goldbount, U. Angina pectoris among 10,000 men: II. Psychosocial and other risk factors as evidenced by a multivariate analysis of a five year incidence study. *American Journal of Medicine*, 1976, *60*, 910–921.

Medalie, J. H., Snyder, M., Groen, J. J., Neufeld, H. N., Goldbourt, U., & Riss, E. Angina pectoris among 10,000 men: 5 year incidence and univariate analysis. *American Journal of Medicine*, 1973, *55*, 583–594.

Meichenbaum, D., Butler, L., & Gruson, L. Toward a conceptual model of social competence. In J. D. Wine & M. D. Syme (Eds.), *Social competence*. New York: Guilford Press, 1981.

Melzack, R. *The puzzle of pain*. New York: Basic Books, 1973.

Morgan, A. H. The heritability of hypnotic susceptibility in twins. *Journal of Abnormal Psychology*, 1973, *82*, 55–66.

Morgan, A. H., Hilgard, E. R., & Davert, E. C. The heritability of hypnotic susceptibility of twins: A preliminary report. *Behavioral Genetics*, 1970, *1*, 213–224.

Nace, E. P., Warwick, A. M., Kelley, R. L., & Evans, F. J. Hypnotizability and outcome in brief psychotherapy. *Journal of Clinical Psychiatry*, 1982, *43*, 129–133.

Nash, M. R., Lynn, J. S., & Givers, D. L. Adult hypnotic susceptibility, childhood punishment and child abuse. *International Journal of Clinical and Experimental Hypnosis*, 1984, *32*, 6–11.

Nuckolls, K. B., Cassel, J., & Kaplan, B. H. Psychological assets, life crisis, and the prognosis of pregnancy. *American Journal of Epidemiology*, 1972, *95*, 431–441.

Ostfeld, A. M., Lebovits, B. Z., Shekelle, R. B., & Paul, O. A. Prospective study of the relationship between personality and coronary heart disease. *Journal of Chronic Disease*, 1964, *17*, 265–276.

Pennebaker, J. W. Traumatic experience and psychosomatic disease: Exploring the roles of behavioral inhibition, obsession, and confiding. *Canadian Psychology*, 1985, *26*, 82–95.

Perry, C., John, R., & Hollander, B. *Hypnotizability and phobic behavior.* Paper presented at the 34th Annual S.E.C.H. Convention, Indianapolis, October 1982.

Pettinati, H., Horne, R. L., & Staats, J. M. *Assessment of hypnotic capacity in patients with anorexia nervosa.* Paper presented at the 90th Annual Convention of the American Psychological Association, Washington, D.C., August 1982.

Pettinati, H., Horne, R. L., & Staats, J. M. Hypnotizability in patients with anorexia nervosa and bulimia. *Archives of General Psychiatry*, 1985, *42*, 1014–1016.

Phillips, C. A psychological analysis of tension headache. In S. Rachman (Ed.), *Contributions to medical psychology.* Oxford, United Kingdom: Pergamon Press, 1977.

Rabkin, J. G., & Struening, E. L. Life events, stress, and illness. *Science*, 1976, *194*, 1013–1020.

Rosenbaum, M. A schedule of assessing self-control behaviors: Preliminary findings. *Behavior Therapy*, 1980, *11*, 109–121.

Saccuzzo, D. P., Safnan, D., Anderson, V., & NcNeill, B. Visual information processing in high and low susceptible subjects. *International Journal of Clinical and Experimental Hypnosis*, 1982, *30*, 32–44.

Sarason, I. G., Levine, H. M., Basham, R. B., & Sarason, B. R. Assessing social support: The social support questionnaire. *Journal of Personality and Social Psychology*, 1983, *44*(1), 127–139.

Scheier, M. F., & Carver, C. S. Optimism, coping and health: Assessment and implications of generalized outcome expectancies. *Health Psychology*, 1985, *4*(3), 219–247.

Selye, H. *Stress and disease.* New York: McGraw-Hill, 1956.

Shields, J. *Monozygotic twins brought up apart and brought up together.* New York: Oxford University Press, 1962.

Shor, R. E. A note on the shock tolerance of real and simulating hypnotic subjects. *International Journal of Clinical and Experimental Hypnosis*, 1964, *12*, 258–262.

Shor, R. E., & Orne, E. C. *Harvard Group Scale of Hypnotic Susceptibility, Form A.* Palo Alto, CA: Consulting Psychologist Press, 1962.

Sklar, L. S., & Anisman, H. Stress and cancer. *Psychological Bulletin*, 1981, *89*(3), 369–406.

Sifneos, P. M. *Short-term psychotherapy and emotional crisis.* Cambridge: Harvard University Press, 1972.

Spanos, N. P., Radtke-Bodonik, L., Ferguson, J. D., & Jones, B. The effects of hypnotic susceptibility, suggestions for analgesia, and the utilization of cognitive strategies on the reduction of pain. *Journal of Abnormal Psychology*, 1979, *88*(3), 282–292.

Spanos, N. P., Brown, J. M., Jones, B., & Horner, D. Cognitive activity and suggestions for analgesia in the reduction of reported pain. *Journal of Abnormal Psychology*, 1981, *90*(6), 554–561.

Stam, H., McGrath, P., Brooke, R., & Cosier, F. Hypnotizability and the treatment of chronic facial pain. *International Journal of Clinical and Experimental Hypnosis*, 1986, *34*, 182–191.

Steptoe, A. *Psychological factors in cardiovascular disorders.* New York: Academic Press, 1981.

Sternbach, R. A. *Principles of psychophysiology.* London: Academic Press, 1966.

Sternbach, R. A., Janowsky, D. S., Huey, L. Y., & Segal, D. S. Effects of altering brain serotonin activity on human chronic pain. In J. J. Bonica & D. Albe-Fessard (Eds.), *Proceedings on the First World Congress on Pain:* Vol. 1. Advances in pain research and therapy. New York: Raven Press, 1976.

Stewart, L. H. Social and emotional adjustment during adolescence as related to the development of psychosomatic illness and adulthood. *Genetic Psychology Monographs*, 1962, 175–215.

Stoyva, J. M. Posthypnotically suggested dreams and the sleep cycle. *Archives of General Psychiatry*, 1965, *12*, 287–294.

Tart, C. A comparison of suggested dreams occuring in hypnosis and sleep. *International Journal of Clinical and Experimental Hypnosis*, 1964, *12*, 263–289.

Tart, C. Some effects of posthypnotic suggestions on the process of dreaming. *International Journal of Clinical and Experimental Hypnosis*, 1966, *14*, 30–46.

Tellegen, A., & Atkinson, G. Openness to absorbing and self-altering experiences ("absorption"), a trait related to hypnotic susceptibility. *Journal of Abnormal Psychology*, 1974, *83*, 268–277.

Thoits, P. A. Dimensions of life events that influence psychological distress: An evaluation and synthesis of the literature. In H. B. Kaplan (Ed.), *Psychosocial stress: Trends in theory and research.* New York: Academic Press, 1983.

Thoits, P. A. Social support as coping assistance. *Journal of Consulting and Clinical Psychology*, 1986, *54*, 416–423.

Valliant, G. E. Natural history of male psychological health: IV. What kind of men do not get psychosomatic illness. *Psychosomatic Medicine*, 1978, *40*, 420–431.

Van De Castle, R. L. The facilitation of ESP through hypnosis. *American Journal of Clinical Hypnosis*, 1969, *12*(1), 37–56.

Wallston, B. S., Alagna, S. W., DeVellis, B. M., & DeVellis, R. F. Social support and physical health. *Health Psychology*, 1983, *2*, 367–391.

Watson, D., & Clark, L. A. Negative affectivity: The disposition to experience aversive emotional states. *Psychological Bulletin*, 1984, *96*, 465–490.

Watson, D., & Tellegen, A. Toward a consensual structure of mood. *Psychological Bulletin*, 1985, *98*(2), 219–235.

Webb, R. A. Suggestibility and verbal conditioning. *International Journal of Clinical and Experimental Hypnosis*, 1962, *10*, 275–279.

Weinberger, D. A., Schwartz, G. E., & Davidson, R. J. Low-anxious, high-anxious, and repressive coping styles: Psychometric patterns and behavioral and physiological responses to stress. *Journal of Abnormal Psychology*, 1979, *88*, 369–380.

Weiss, R. L., Ullman, L. P., & Krasner, L. On the relationship between hypnotizability and response to verbal operant conditioning. *Psychological Reports*, 1960, 59–60.

Wenger, M. A. Studies of autonomic balance in USAF personnel. *Comparative Psycholology Monographs*, 1948, *19*, 4.

Wenger, M. A. Studies of autonomic balance: A summary. *Psychophysiology*, 1966, *2*, 173–186.

Whatmore, G. B., & Kohli, D. R. *The physiopathology and treatment of functional disorders.* New York: Grune & Stratton, 1974.

Wickramasekera, I. *The effects of hypnosis and a control procedure on verbal conditioning.* Paper presented at the meeting of the American Psychological Association, Miami, September 1970.(a)

Wickramasekera, I. Desensitization, re-sensitization and desensitization again: A preliminary study. *Journal of Behavior Therapy and Experimental Psychiatry.* 1970b, *1,* 257–262.

Wickramasekera, I. Effects of EMG feedback training on susceptibility to hypnosis: preliminary observations. *Proceedings of the 79th Annual Convention of the American Psychological Association,* 1971, *6,* 785–787. (Summary)

Wickramasekera, I. A technique for controlling a certain type of sexual exhibitionism. *Psychotherapy: Theory, Research, and Practice,* 1972, *9,* 207–210.

Wickramasekera, I. The effects of EMG feedback on hypnotic susceptibility: More preliminary data. *Journal of Abnormal Psychology,* 1973, *82,* 74–77.

Wickramasekera, I. (Ed.). *Biofeedback, behavior therapy, and hypnosis,* Chicago: Nelson-Hall, 1976.(a)

Wickramasekera, I. Aversive behavior rehearsal for sexual exhibitionism. *Behavior Therapy,* 1976b, *7,* 167–176.

Wickramasekera, I. On attempts to modify hypnotic susceptibility: some psychophysiological procedures and promising directions. *Annals of the New York Academy of Sciences,* 1977a, *296,* 143–153.

Wickramasekera, I. The placebo effect and biofeedback for headache pain. *Proceedings of the San Diego Biomedical Symposium.* New York: Academic Press, 1977b.

Wickramasekera, I. *A model of the patient at high risk for chronic stress-related disorders. Do beliefs have biological consequences?* Paper presented at Annual Convention of the Biofeedback Society of America, San Diego, California, 1979.

Wickramasekera, I. Aversive behavior rehearsal: A cognitive-behavioral procedure. In D. J. Cox & R. J. Daitzman (Eds.), *Exhibitionism: Description, assessment and treatment.* New York: Harland, 1980.(a)

Wickramesekera, I. *Principles of psychophysiology and the high risk patient.* Invited address, University of Illinois College of Medicine, Peoria, July 1980.(b)

Wickramasekera, I. A conditioned response model of the placebo effect: Predictions from the model. *Biofeedback and Self-Regulation,* 1980c, *5*(1), 5–18.

Wickramasekera, I. *Patient variables in behavioral medicine, and the psychological aspects of health care.* Invited address, Veterans Administration, North Central Regional Medical Education Center, May 1980.(d)

Wickramasekera, I. *A model of people at high risk.* Paper presented at the International Stress and Tension Control Society, Brighton, England, August 1983.

Wilson, S. C., & Barber, T. X. The fantasy-prone personality: Implications for understanding imagery, hypnosis and parapsychological phenomena. In A. A. Shiekh (Ed.), *Imagery: Current theory research and application.* New York: Wiley, 1982.

Wine, J. D., & Smye, M. D. (Eds.). *Social competence.* New York: Guilford Press, 1981.

Wolff, H. G. *Stress and disease.* Springfield: Charles C. Thomas, 1953.

Wrubel, J., Benner, P., & Lazarus, R. S. Social competence from the perspective of stress and coping. In J. D. Wine & M. D. Smye (Eds.), *Social competence.* New York: Guilford Press, 1981.

Zarski, J. J. Hassles and health: A replication. *Health Psychology,* 1984, *33,* 243–251.

Zocco, L. *The development of a self-report inventory to assess dysfunctional cognitions in phobics.* Unpublished dissertation, Virginia Consortium for Professional Psychology, 1984.

2

CLINICAL BEHAVIORAL MEDICINE AND ITS CUTTING EDGES
Biofeedback, Behavior Therapy, and Hypnosis

> *Inevitably, the doctor's work in the future will be more and more educational and less and less curative. More and more will he deal with the physiology and psychology of his patient, less and less with his pathology. He will spend his time keeping the fit fit, rather then trying to make the unfit fit.*
> —Thomas Lord Horder
> in *Familiar Medical Quotations*

> *Nowhere are the needs and opportunities for progress in the biobehavioral sciences clearer than in problems of health and behavior. Behavioral factors contribute to much of our burden of illness. Half of the mortality from the ten leading causes of death in the United States is strongly influenced by life-style.*
> —David A. Hamburg, M.D.
> President, Institute of Medicine
> National Academy of Science
> *Science*, 1982

Profound changes have been occurring in health care, particularly in terms of the types of diseases presented to physicians today, and the recognition of the inadequacies of conventional medical treatments for these disorders. Acute infectious diseases, like pneumonia and tuberculosis, no longer kill or cripple citizens of the United States so frequently as they did in 1900. Instead, chronic stress-related multifactorial conditions, like cardiovascular disease, cancer, and auto accidents, are today's major killers and cripplers. These diseases cannot be traced to a single pathogen, but behavioral and environmental factors can increase vulnerability to the disease (Califano, 1979). Eighty percent of the problems presented to physicians today are chronic diseases, such as colitis, arthritis, asthma, diabetes, and cardiovascular disease. These are diseases of choice, not chance, because life-style and behavioral factors, such as diet, smoking, and exercise, are major risk factors for the prevention of these disorders. With the chronicity of disease, behavioral factors become even more crucial to prognosis and to effective therapy (compliance with medication, depression, etc.). In 1979 the Surgeon General's Report attributed 50% of all deaths to unhealthy behaviors. The profile of illness today is marked by chronic-stress-related multifactorial diseases in which behavioral and psychological variables and issues of choice are crucial to prevention, therapy, and prognosis. It is worth noting that even for a new infectious disease, AIDS, behavior is a major risk factor and in fact a specific type of behavior, sexual behavior. (See Figure 5.)

The joint impact of the previously cited changes may lead to a revolution in health care. This revolution, which can be labeled behav-

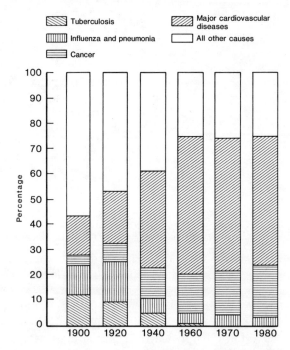

Figure 5. Deaths for selected causes as a percentage of all deaths: United States, selected years, 1900–1980. Source: National Center for Health Statistics, Division of Vital Statistics.

ioral medicine, is based on the growing recognition that behavioral and cognitive factors may be crucial to the etiology, prevention, and therapy of physical diseases like lung cancer and heart disease. Cigarette smoking, diet, exercise, Type A behavior, and obesity are risk factors for lung cancer and heart disease. The behavioral medicine revolution is also based on the recognition that there are now promising behavioral treatments for physical disorders such as muscular and vascular headaches (Budzynski, Stoyva, & Ader, 1970; Sargent, Green, & Walters, 1973; Wickramasekera, 1972), primary Raynauds disease (Surwit, 1973), and primary hypertension (Patel, 1977). The behavioral medicine revolution may approach the importance of the antibiotic revolution that occurred approximately 50 years ago because it signals the demise of the mind–body dichotomy in practical matters like therapy and preventative health care. Behaviors, and, as I will later show, beliefs that select and mobilize behavior can have biological consequences (Wickramasekera, 1979a). If psychological techniques can reliably and effectively alter some biological functions, should health psychologists then be defined as *physicians* (Wickramasekera, 1984b)? Does the legal definition of physician require revision now that therapies other than drugs and surgery can heal physical dysfunctions?

There have been several efforts to define behavioral medicine (Matarazzo, 1979; Pomerleau & Brady, 1979; Schwartz & Weiss, 1977), and it seems that these definitions have been either too narrow or too broad. In an elementary sense, *behavioral medicine* can be defined as the interfacing of behavioral and biomedical sciences in the areas of research, diagnosis, prevention, and therapy of physical diseases and dysfunctions. This integration started much earlier in the research domain, and is now extending into the clinical arena, primarily because of recent advances in three psychological technologies of stress management: biofeedback, behavior therapy, and hypnosis. These behavioral and psychological technologies have two important features. First, they enable a substitution of skills for pills, and second, they make the patient an active participant in identifying, treating, and preventing the patient's own disease process. In the biomedical model the patient is a passive recipient of services and interventions. In contrast, replicated experimental research in hypnosis, for example, has shown during the last 30 years that hypnotic behavior depends primarily on the subject's ability or talent and only to a small extent on the hypnotist's skill (Fromm & Shor, 1979; Hilgard, 1965). Proficiency in biofeedback and behavior therapy skills seem to depend on the degree of patient participation with homework practice. Biofeedback, behavior therapy, and hypnosis (Wickramasekera, 1976) follow an educational model, teaching the patient to identify stressors and to practice skills that can be used to cope with stress.

> I believe the idea of a "right" to health should be replaced by that of a moral obligation to preserve one's own health. The individual then has the "right" to expect help with information, accessible services of good quality, and minimum financial barriers. Meanwhile the people have been led to believe that national health insurance, more doctors, and greater use of high-cost, hospital-based technologies will improve health. Unfortunately, none of them will. (Knowles, 1977)

As the quotations from the eminent medical philosophers Horder and Knowles indicate, the educational model is still relevant to health care. The word *doctor* originally meant teacher, and the best patient is an actively learning and participating student, not a passive decorticate animal preparation in a bed. The business of health care today is too heavy and complex a burden to be borne by medical doctors alone. As Franz J. Ingelfinger, M.D., editor emeritus of the *New England Journal of Medicine* stated, preventive health measures are much more influenced by occupations that can shape social attitudes rather than by individual doctors (Ingelfinger, 1978). Patients, health psychologists, environmen-

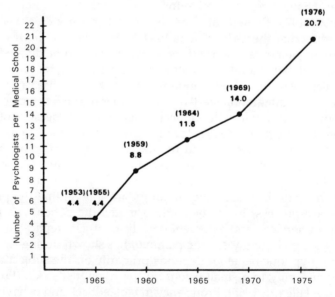

Figure 6. Average number of psychologists in American medical schools from 1953 to 1976. (Numbers in parentheses are the years for which the averages apply.) *Note:* These trends outstrip the growth rates of other factors, such as the numbers of medical schools and medical students (Lubin, Nathan, & Matarazzo, 1978).

talists, and medical doctors will all have to work together as a team to resolve the new health care problems. Behavioral medicine promises to improve the efficacy and quality of contemporary health care for chronic diseases, while significantly reducing its currently escalating cost by giving patients major responsibility for their own health care. In the clinical arena, behavioral medicine started with an uneasy flirtation between psychology and medicine, which is now growing into a marriage forced by therapeutic, economic, and political factors. This uneasy marriage has several important implications for scientific and professional psychology to which I will return later. One simple fact of employment data that demonstrates the recognition of the importance of behavioral and psychological factors in health care education, research, and therapy is illustrated by the following graph on the employment of psychologists in medical schools. (See Figure 6.)

The Origins of Behavioral Medicine

The behavioral medicine revolution stems from several specific and salient changes that have occurred in the profile of health care in the last 75 years. First, most death and disability in the United States today are not caused by acute infectious diseases (e.g., plague, smallpox, polio, etc.); the introduction of sterile procedures into surgery, the public health treatment of water and sewage, immunization measures, and the introduction of antibiotics have nearly eradicated these diseases. Today's death and disabilities are caused by chronic-stress-related conditions, such as heart attacks, strokes, cancer, pulmonary diseases, diabetes, automobile accidents, and alcoholism (Gori & Richter, 1978). Stress refers to an abnormal neuroendocrine state associated with alterations in tissue functions that occur when people perceive threats to their physical or mental well-being (Mason, 1972). The choices people make about how to cope with threats to their well-being have consequences for physical health (e.g., smoking, alcoholism, Type A behavior, etc.). There is growing evidence that a patient's cognitive, emotional, and behavioral life-style responses can potentiate, maintain, or attenuate these chronic physical disorders (Engel, 1977; Glass, 1977; Jemmott & Locke, 1984; Weiner, 1977). The previous acute infectious diseases were mainly diseases of chance, because choice and volition were trivial factors in the prevention, diagnosis, and therapy of these diseases. Mechanisms relating behavior to physical disease today include (a) stress (Selye, 1976); (b) maladaptive methods of coping with stress (e.g., smoking, drug and alcohol abuse); (c) bad health habits (diet, lack of exercise);

and, (d) psychological reactions to illness, such as denial of symptoms, noncompliance, etc. (Lazarus & Folkman, 1984). For example, estimates of behavioral noncompliance with long-term medical regimens range from 25% to 80% for chronic disease (Haynes, Taylor, & Sackett, 1979). In fact, for chronic diseases the mean rate of noncompliance is over 50% (Epstein & Cluss, 1982; Sackett & Haynes, 1976). Efficacious medications are ineffective unless they are used. The best combination of standard risk factors accounts for only 50% of the incidence of coronary heart disease (Glass, 1977). Several of the standard risk factors for coronary disease are behaviors, or have large behavioral components (smoking, diet, alcohol consumption, physical inactivity, etc.). The medical philosopher, John H. Knowles (1977) recognized that, as never before, the prevention of disease and death involves forsaking bad habits that many people enjoy: "overeating, too much drinking, taking pills, staying up at night, engaging in promiscuous sex, driving too fast, and smoking cigarettes." There is serious doubt today that a strictly unifactorial biomedical model (Engel, 1977; Lipowski, 1977) of diseases that ignores cognitive, emotional, and behavioral factors can adequately explain, predict, prevent, and lead to the control of the chronic-stress-related disorders that cripple and kill Americans today. Behavioral medicine proposes a multifactorial model of diseases for chronic-stress-related diseases of choice.

Second, chronic anxiety (Tallman, Paul, Skolnick, & Gallager, 1980), chronic pain (Fordyce, 1976; Ng & Bonica, 1980), insominia, and depression are probably the largest components in the profile of illness presented to physicians today. More recently, Inderal, Tagamet, and Valium are among the seven most frequently prescribed drugs in the United States ("Top 200 Drugs," 1985). Pills alone cannot be the long-term solution to these chronic psychophysiological symptoms because of problems created by drug tolerance, physical and psychological dependency on drugs, and the negative physical and psychological side effects of long-term use of drugs (hyperalgesia, interference with normal physiological functions). It is becoming clear that psychophysiological skills (e.g., relaxation, coping, etc.) may have to replace pills as therapy for many of the chronic-stress-related diseases. Psychological stress (Lazarus, 1966; Mason, 1972) triggered by the perception of threat appears to be a large component in the etiology and maintenance of most chronic anxiety, pain, and insomnia complaints. There is growing evidence of a correlational and now an experimental nature (Ader, 1981) that cognitive expectancy and behavioral factors, such as depression and anxiety, can influence the immune system and physical disease susceptibility through neuroendocrine mechanisms (Ader, 1981; Jemmott &

Locke, 1984; Rasmussen, 1969; Rogers, Dubey, & Reich, 1979; Solomon, Amkraut, & Kasper, 1974) and that these effects may also be true for the geriatric population (Kielot-Glaser *et al.*, 1985). The over 100-year-old dogma that the immune system is insulated from the brain (mind) is untenable today. This is a threat to the doctrine of mind–body dichotomy on which the biomedical model has rested. Beliefs and behaviors may have biological consequences (Wickramasekera, 1979a) for degrees of vulnerability even to acute infectious diseases (Canter, Imboden, & Cluff, 1966; Canter, Cluff, & Imboden, 1972).

Third, conventional unifactorial biomedical treatment models used by physicians to treat the previously cited conditions are of limited efficacy, and, in fact, create new behavioral and biological problems. The biomedical model ignores psychological stress, regards it as trivial and epiphenomenal, and depends exclusively on chemical and surgical solutions to complex, multifactorial human problems. It is clear that for many modern diseases and for some patients, psychological factors are neither trivial nor unreliable. The assessment and treatment of psychological stress (Lazarus, 1966; Lazarus & Folkman, 1984; Woolfolk & Lehrer, 1984) requires sophistication in psychology and behavioral science. Behavioral science training is the least popular, weakest, and smallest portion of a contemporary physician's education (Institute of Medicine–National Academy of Sciences, 1979a; Orleans, George, Houpt, & Brodie, 1985). Consequently, physicians rely primarily on drugs and surgery to treat the symptoms of psychological stress, such as anxiety, insomnia, and chronic pain (Orleans *et al.*, 1985). Approximately 50% of the patients seated in a general practitioner's office present physical complaints without "physical findings" (Fink & Shapiro, 1966; Hilkevitch, 1965). Eighty percent of the visits to emergency rooms are not strictly medical emergencies (Gibson, Bugbee, & Anderson, 1970). These statistics are supported by the findings that at least 8,000 tons of benzodiazepines (Valium, Librium, and Dalmane, etc.) were prescribed by physicians and consumed by patients in the United States in 1977 (Tallman *et al.*, 1980). Minor tranquilizers and sleep medications (Smith, 1979) are among the most frequently prescribed medications in the United States, and if the current rate of prescription writing for these drugs continues, by the year 2000 most of the nation will be on antianxiety agents (Blackwell, 1975).

According to HEW, "50 million Americans have trouble sleeping in a given year" (Institute of Medicine–National Academy of Sciences, 1979b), and 10 million people in the United States consult a physician about the problem. According to an Institute of Medicine–National Academy of Sciences (1979b) study, 25 million prescriptions are written annually in the United States for sleep medication. The psychophysiological functions of sleep are exquisitely sensitive to psychological and environmental stress. Approximately 2 million people use these pills nightly for more than 2 months at a time. Clinical trials cited in the study show that the efficacy of most of the pills falls off after 4 weeks (Hauri, 1982). Prolonged use is even more likely among the elderly, particularly those in nursing homes, where prescriptions are made for reasons of behavioral control. The hazards of long-term use of sleep medication are just beginning to be recognized (Institute of Medicine–National Academy of Sciences, 1979b). Sleeping pills as a remedy for chronic-stress-related insomnia is even worse than the disease. Kales & Kales (1984) described three types of insomnia that are related to the withdrawal of hypnotic drugs: drug withdrawal insomnia, early morning insomnia, and rebound insomnia. Sleeping pills, one of the most prescribed medications in the world, are more dangerous and less useful than either physicians or patients realize, according to a recent report by the Institute of Medicine–National Academy of Sciences (Smith, 1979).

In 1978 alone, physicians prescribed Darvon 31 million times, making it the third most frequently prescribed drug in 1978 (Smith, 1979). Darvon was found in several double-blind studies not to be significantly more effective than the safer nonprescription medication, aspirin (Moertel, Ahman, Taylor, & Schwartau, 1972). However, patients may, on a placebo (psychological) basis alone, respond better to an analgesic like Darvon that is medically prescribed. Our growing reliance on strictly chemical solutions (Cummings, 1979) to common and chronic human problems is problematic.

A recent study cited by Benson (1979) from the *Journal of the American Medical Association* states that 6,000 to 12,000 deaths each year are related to prescription drugs. Pills can be a solution to short-term psychosocial stress but they only exacerbate chronic psychosocial stress-related physical symptoms. Chemicals alone cannot be long-term solutions to the complex chronic psychosocial problems presented by the bulk of patients with depression, anxiety, chronic pain, GI tract distress, essential hypertension, and sleep disturbances.

Fourth, alcohol, tobacco, food, and drug abuse (legal and illegal) are other mind- and mood-altering techniques patients themselves use to cope with psychological stress and behavioral inadequacies. But these short-sighted, nonprescription remedies for psychological stress increase the rate of disease and medical utilization, and cost employers major losses in terms of absenteeism and lost production (Jones & Vischi, 1979). It is estimated that one-fifth of the cost of medical care is due to tobacco and alcohol abuse (Ball, 1978). The combined economic cost of drug abuse and alcoholism is estimated at $50 billion (Barchas, Akil, Elliott, Holman, & Watson, 1978).

Fifth, there has been a rapid increase in medical costs without a comparable improvement in health status, and it is likely we have reached the top of the cost-benefit curve with expensive biomedical technology (DeLeon & VandenBos, 1983). Frazier and Hiatt (1978) of Harvard Medical School say,

> Fineberg has described the proliferating laboratory tests that in 1977 accounted for in excess of $11 billion of our health resource expenditures. He pointed out that there is evidence that much laboratory usage, which is increasing at a rate of 14 percent annually, has little or no beneficial effect on patient care. (p. 875)

Although definite evidence is not yet in, several studies cited by Tancredi and Barondess (1978) point out that some of this increased utilization of tests is in response to the fear of malpractice lawsuits, and that these tests expose patients to significant "risks of harm from unnecessary procedures." Ingelfinger (1978), and Benson (1979) have also recently elaborated on the abuses of medical diagnostic test procedures. In spite of these massive expenditures and increasingly sophisticated medical instrumentation, there is little evidence that the United States public is any more healthy today (Knowles, 1977). Although patients demand and many physicians continue to provide expensive and strictly medical solutions to complex human problems, the cost of health care continues to rise in the United States. In 1950 health care was only 4.6% of the gross national product, and in 1983 it had escalated to 10.8% of the gross national product or $355.4 billion (Cohen, 1985). Hospital costs account for 40% of the health care bill and these costs have recently been inflating at an annual average of 17.3% (Culliton, 1978; Hamburg & Brown, 1978).

Psychophysiological Stress Management Skills for Pain, Anxiety, and Sleep Disorders

Pills cannot be a long-term solution to chronic pain, anxiety, and sleep disorders because of problems with tolerance, negative physical and psychological side effects, and dependency. Stress management techniques developed with biofeedback, behavior therapy and hypnosis technologies constitute the best available cost-effective (Blanchard, Jaccard, Andrsik, Guarnieri, & Jurish, 1985) alternatives to pills today (Wickramasekera, 1976; Woolfolk & Lehrer, 1984). Psychologists and psychiatrists have developed some behavioral techniques that are in fact currently the most promising therapies for some physical presentations. Recent developments in the fields of biofeedback (Birk, 1973; Green & Green, 1977; Wickramasekera, 1976), behavior therapy (Wolpe, 1982), and hypnosis (Barber, 1969; Fromm & Shor, 1979) have provided psychologists with credible, safe, and promising alternative therapies to the standard medical treatments (drugs and surgery) for several chronic and unresponsive psychophysiological problems, such as chronic pain (Fordyce, 1976), functional vascular and muscular headache (Blanchard & Andrsik, 1982; Budzynski et al., 1970; Cox, Freundlich, & Meyer, 1975; Wickramasekera, 1972), insomnia (Borkovec, 1982), primary Raynaud's syndrome (Surwit, 1982), essential hypertension, (Patel, 1977; Shapiro & Goldstein, 1982) and coronary prone behavior (Suinn, 1982). These stress-reduction therapies include EMG, biofeedback, systematic desensitization, autogenic therapy, meditation, and progressive muscular relaxation (Wickramasekera, 1977; Woolfolk & Lehrer, 1984). Numerous independent replications (Blanchard, 1982) with clinical samples have demonstrated that these technologies stemming from biofeedback, behavior therapy, and hypnosis can produce not merely statistically significant but also clinically significant treatment effects with some patients under some conditions with certain problems. The specific mechanisms through which these treatment effects are generated is unknown (Fuller, 1978; Roberts, 1985; Stroebel & Glueck, 1973; Wickramasekera, 1977a). It is my view that most of the variance will eventually be accounted for by recognizing that these technologies have contributed to specifying the nonspecific aspects of the placebo effect (Wickramasekera, 1977a, 1978, 1980, 1985). In other words, we are learning in clinical behavioral medicine how to arrange the psychological, behavioral, and situational conditions to produce more powerful, reliable, and durable psychophysiological effects. The implications of this statement will be elaborated on in Chapter 5, which deals with the placebo effect. These psychological and behavioral procedures have no serious side effects, seem cost-effective, are either curative or palliative, and can be adjunctive or primary interventions. Behavioral procedures have also been proposed to reduce obesity, smoking, and noncompliance with medication, but efficacy and reliability demonstrated in these areas have not yet reached satisfactory levels for routine clinical application.

Biofeedback, behavior therapy, and hypnosis (Wickramasekera, 1976) are empirically and procedurally oriented technologies; they tend to be symptomatic and short term in treatment focus. These four features make them acceptable to, and consistent with, the values of the pragmatically oriented physicians who dominate the health care system and with whom health psychologists have to work. Psychologists seem to be developing effective, durable, safe, and cheap skill alternatives to pills such as minor tranquilizers, sleep, and pain medications. If these alternative psychophysiological skill therapies, which stem from biofeedback, behavior therapy, and hypnosis, become reimbursable by health insurance companies, the groundwork will be laid for profound long-term changes in the practice and role of primary care physicians. Currently, patients who present chronic-stress-related physical symptoms constitute a large component of patients who visit primary care physicians (Cummings, 1977; Houpt *et al.*, 1980) and are treated with drugs and surgery. Health care psychologists can today treat or palliate many of these physical conditions with effective behavioral and psychological techniques (Blanchard, 1982). If psychologists can treat physical disorders with psychological techniques, are these health psychologists practices calling for a legal redefinition and expansion of the word *physician* (Wickramasekera, 1984)? This substitution of skills for pills is the first practical demonstration of the growing erosion of the mind–body dichotomy in health care and it has the most profound economic, political, and legal implications for psychology and medicine. How will these alternative skill therapies offered by clinical health psychologists impact the income and the demand for the services of primary care physicians (Wickramasekera, 1979b)? Will clinical health care psychologists and primary care physicians work next to each other in the same office complex, or will they work independently across town? These are all practical questions that will shortly have salient implications for the education, training, and practice of clinical health psychologists and physicians in the twenty-first century. There has been a tremendous increase in the use of psychologists in medical settings and schools (Lubin, Nathan, & Matarazzo, 1978; Matarazzo, 1980), demonstrating that organized medicine recognizes that psychologists have concepts and skills useful to physicians. How cost-effective is it to have expensive, highly trained specialists in medicine and surgery teaching patients with complex psychosocial problems equally complex psychosocial and psychophysiological skills? Does it not make more sense for medical doctors to limit their practice to diagnosing and treating acute, life-threatening diseases for which they are exceptionally well trained? Many problems have arisen because medical doctors have been pressured into treating complex chronic-stress-related disorders as if they were acute medical emergencies. A statement by Ingelfinger is pertinent to this point.

> Nobody would argue that treatment of a disease is preferable to its prevention. Comprehensive prevention, however, entails skills and efforts that are beyond the capabilities of many a good doctor. Preventive health measures are much more influenced by occupations that can shape social attitudes

rather than by individual doctors who categorically instruct, "Smoke and drink less." The doctor should not be expected to play a major role in changing whatever lifestyles may be seriously detrimental. He has enough to do if he takes care of the crisis illnesses that do occur, and if he keeps up to date with the various scientific facts known about their nature and management. Hence, I would not consider the failure of the doctor to practice holistic medicine as substantive evidence of inferior medical practice. (1978, p. 944)

Psychologists, like physicians, also have to recognize the present limitations of their education. Unfortunately, there are no indications that physicians are increasingly involved in the education of psychologists. Physician involvement in the education of clinical health care psychologists may improve the quality of training and reduce our vulnerability to future malpractice lawsuits (Wickramasekera, 1979b; 1984).

Common Features of Biofeedback, Behavior Therapy, and Hypnosis

Because it is likely that in the near future the most clinically important contributions to behavioral medicine will come from the technologies of biofeedback, behavior therapy, and hypnosis, it will be useful to look at the common features of these three domains. Wickramasekera (1976) previously identified and elaborated on several common features of these technologies that today provide the routine clinical tools in behavioral medicine.

Roots in the Experimental Laboratory. The clinical procedures in biofeedback, behavior therapy, and hypnosis can be related to an already large and growing body of experimentally established information. The experimental tradition in hypnosis, for example, ranges from Pavlov (1927) and Hull (1933) to Hilgard (1965) and Barber (1969), with a degree of emphasis on methodological rigor that may surprise most experimental psychologists and other scientists. All three technologies have roots in the experimental psychology laboratory, and have been pioneered by, or stem from, the concepts and procedures of experimental psychologists like Pavlov (conditioning and hypnosis), Skinner (behavior therapy), Mowrer (behavior therapy), Hilgard (hypnosis, conditioning), Barber (hypnosis), and N. E. Miller (behavior therapy and biofeedback). The experimental method tends to generate replicable knowledge. Knowledge based on the repeated confirmation of expectancies under specifiable conditions generates faith and confidence in the clinical investigator and patient.

Potentiating the Placebo Effect. Because the experimental method that marks scientific knowledge tends to generate replicable observations that repeatedly confirm expectancies under conditions confidently specifiable in advance, it is one of the most potent methods of creating belief and faith in the clinical investigator and patient. Faith and feelings of competence inhibit skeptical internal dialogue that can distract both the therapist and the patient from the optimal mobilization of their energy, creativity, and therapeutic skills. This faith and confidence can be the basis of powerful placebo effects (Wickramasekera, 1977a). In fact it is very likely that the general public has more faith in science today than in the God of traditional religions because it believes that science reliably delivers the goods. The fruits of scientific knowledge touch our lives daily and in reliably positive forms that range from electric light switches to our automobiles. In fact, each time we step into an elevator in our office building we are implicitly making an act of faith in science.

Biofeedback, behavior therapy, and hypnosis use the methods and technological hardware of science. All three technologies have potentiated the placebo effect or at least contributed to the investigation and specification of previously unspecified components of the placebo effect in healing (Stroebel & Glueck, 1973; Wickramasekera, 1976, 1977a, 1985). For example, the concept *demand characteristics* (Orne, 1962) came into the literature from hypnosis. The recognition of the importance of equating treatments for credibility (Borkovec & Nau, 1972; Kirsch & Henry, 1977) and the recognition that self-monitoring is a reactive process, came into the psychological literature through behavior therapy. The behavior therapy rituals of self-monitoring, counting, and graphing subjective events (fear, pain, anxiety, pleasure, images, etc.) are clearly empirically useful (Mahoney & Arnkoff, 1979) in generating a subjective sense of control. But graphing and quantifying rituals are also neutral conditioned stimuli (CS) associated with the faith and confidence that science and objectivity generate (Wickramasekera, 1977a, 1980). Biofeedback, which uses powerful faith generating biomedical instruments (Wickramasekera, 1977a, 1978, 1980) has itself been labeled an "ultimate placebo" (Stroebel & Glueck, 1973) because it appears to trigger the patient's inherent self-regulatory ability (Green & Green, 1977).

Independent Variables. All three technologies specify their independent variables (treatment components) in ways that enable independent replication and evaluation of their alleged clinical efficacy. This is particularly true of the explicit component-analysis approach that Barber (1969) has taken to hypnosis, the component-analysis work on systematic desensitization (Lang, 1969), and the analytical approach to biofeedback (Taub, 1977). This component-analysis approach has led, for example, to the multiple channel (verbal-subjective, physiological, and motor) analysis of anxiety, fear, relaxation, acute pain, and other salient clinical phenomena. In fact, Hilgard's hidden observer technique (1977) is an approach to carving the verbal-subjective channel into independent components that may have some nonoverlapping parameters. The technique may illuminate some paradoxical clinical phenomena, such as dissociative states. All of this provides a differentiated and less simplistic approach to the investigation and observation of complex clinical phenomena and enables independent clinical investigators to take a treatment component approach to testing the efficacy of therapeutic packages.

Quantitative Dependent Variables. All three technologies specify their dependent variables (target symptoms, e.g., fear, pain, or warts) in circumscribed ways that permit objective and quantitative evaluation. This is in contrast to other psychotherapies that focus on target symptoms that are nebulous dependent variables, such as self-esteem, growth, or making the unconscious conscious. This circumscribed and objective approach encourages hypothesis testing, experimental manipulation of therapy components, and corrective empirical feedback that confirms or disconfirms treatment hypotheses. Because the target symptoms or dependent variables are observable and quantifiable (e.g., number of feet from phobic object or number of hours of "up" time for chronic pain patients), it is much harder to practice self-deception and convince oneself that the therapy is effective if the target symptoms do not reduce in frequency or intensity (Wickramasekera, 1981).

Psychophysiological Focus. All three technologies have had a psychophysiological focus. Hypnosis, for example, was one of the earliest psychological techniques used systematically to treat organic disorders (e.g. allergies, etc.) with careful scientific controls (Black, 1963a,b; Mason, 1952, 1955), and its psychophysiological correlates were studied quite early (Sarbin & Slagle, 1972). The psychophysiological emphasis in behavior therapy was pioneered by Wolpe (1958) and Paul (1966), and was explicit in the early laboratory study of phobias (Lang, 1969). Biofeedback, with its emphasis on the remission of physical symptoms, is, of course, the most explicitly psychophysiological of these three behavioral technologies.

Self-Regulation. All three technologies have contributed to expanding the boundaries of the self-regulation of clinically salient cognitive, physiological, and motor behaviors. In biofeedback the patient is an active participant in learning complex psychophysiological skills to alter, for example, his or her EMG or skin temperature in therapy. In those clinically effective behavior therapy techniques, such as systematic desensitization, the patient learns complex cognitive and motor skills (e.g., graduated approach, muscular relaxation) that make them active participants in their own therapy. Recent efforts even moderately to increase baseline hypnotic ability have used an explicit skill training methodology (Diamond, 1977) or have made us aware of psychophysiological skills and methods (sensory deprivation, EMG, or theta biofeedback) that we can use even temporarily to increase hypnotic ability (Wickramasekera, 1977). These technologies place primary responsibility on the patient for changing his or her verbal and behavioral responses in ways that increase the probability of positive clinical outcomes. But for some patients, in the early stages of hypnotherapy, it is necessary to preserve the illusion of external or hypnotist control. The recent experimental investigations (Fromm et al., 1981; Johnson, 1979) of self-hypnosis are quite promising and may illuminate individual differences in clinical efficacy rates when other self-control procedures (meditation, relaxation training, etc.) not labeled self-hypnosis are used. The investigation of stable (Hilgard, 1965) and partly genetically based individual differences in hypnotizability (Morgan, 1973; Morgan, Hilgard, & Davert, 1970) is starting to permit a rational matching of patient types to types of treatments (Qualls & Sheenan, 1979; Wickramasekera, 1979a, 1983, 1984a) and information about voluntary control of altered states of consciousness (Evans, 1977).

Wider Application. These three technologies apply to more types of patients than conventional psychotherapy or psychoanalysis. The treatment focus is short term and symptomatic. The first goal of these three technologies is to return the patient to his nonsymptomatic or at least premorbid functional status. Hypnosis, for example, is often the treatment of choice of the poor, the illiterate, and those patients who are functionally immobilized by their clinical symptoms (e.g., anxiety, pain) and who cannot afford long-term personality reconstruction or "psychoarcheology."

Procedural Handle on Cognition. All three technologies either explicitly or implicitly manipulate cognition by arranging (a) physical environments, (b) informational input, or (c) psychophysiological procedures. For example, the study by Orne and Scheibe (1976) on the contribution of nondeprivation factors to the production of sensory deprivation effects illustrates how the design of physical environments and informational scripts can be covertly utilized to alter cognitions. Information about the alleged laws of learning and conditioning rationales for the efficacy of systematic desensitization are used in behavior therapy. The quest for quantifiable physiological correlates of imagery (Lang, 1979), and the systematic induction of low physiological arousal states to improve cognitive control of physiology demonstrate a psychophysiological approach to enhance the control of cognition (Wickramasekera, 1977). Others in hypnosis and behavior therapy have used sensory restriction (Suedfeld, 1980; Wickramsekera, 1969, 1970) procedures to alter cognitions and to enhance therapeutic messages. Impressive biomedical and electronic instruments (Wickramasekera, 1977) are used credibly to structure expectancies in biofeedback and fixation objects in hypnosis. This systematic manipulation of information, environmental designs, and procedural variables can potentiate the manipulation of cognitive responses, fantasies, and belief systems in patients (Wickramsekera, 1970, 1977a,b). In summary then, these three technologies seek to put a procedural handle on cognition or, at least, to index its quantifiable correlates, and are more subtle and indirect techniques of altering beliefs than procedures as transparent as psychotherapy.

Biofeedback, behavior therapy, and hypnosis, because of their technological emphasis, circumscribed and quantifiable goals, and origins in the experimental laboratory, provide the primitive but promising cutting edge of useful tools for clinical behavioral medicine. These technologies provide the roots of a systematic approach to the behavioral investigation, assessment, and management of chronic-stress-related physical disorders that are replacing acute infectious diseases as the major cause of death and disability today.

References

Ader, R. Behavioral influences on immune responses. In S. Weiss, A. Herd, & B. Fox (Eds.), *Perspectives on behavioral medicine*. New York: Academic Press, 1981.

Aronoff, G. M. [Editorial]. *The Clinical Journal of Pain*, 1985, *1*, 1–3.

Ball, R. M. National health insurance: Comments on selected issues. *Science*, 1978, *200*, 864–870.

Barber, T. X. *Hypnosis: A scientific approach*. New York: Van Nostrand Reinhold, 1969.

Barchas, J. D., Akil, H., Elliott, G. R., Holman, R. B., & Watson, S. Behavioral neurochemistry: Neuroregulators and behavioral states. *Science*, 1978, *200*, 964–973.

Benson, H. *The mind–body effect*. New York: Simon & Schuster, 1979.

Birk, L. (Ed.). *Biofeedback: Behavioral medicine*. New York: Grune & Stratton, 1973.

Black, S. Inhibition of immediate-type hypersensitivity response by direct suggestion under hypnosis. *British Medical Journal*, 1963, *1*, 925–929. (a)

Black, S. Shift in dose-response curve of Prausnitz-Kustner reaction by direct suggestion under hypnosis. *British Medical Journal*, 1963, *1*, 990–992. (b)

Blackwell, B. Minor tranquilizers: Use, misuse or overuse? *Psychosomatics*, 1975, *16*, 28–31.

Blanchard, E. B. Behavioral medicine: Past, present and future. *Journal of Consulting and Clinical Psychology*, 1982, *50*, 795–803.

Blanchard, E. B., & Andrsik, F. Psychological assessment and treatment of headache: Recent developments and emerging issues. *Journal of Consulting and Clinical Psychology*, 1982, *50*, 859–879.

Blanchard, E. B., Jaccard, J., Andrsik, F., Guarnieri, P., & Jurish, S. Reduction in headache patients medical expenses associated with biofeedback and relaxation treatments. *Biofeedback and Self-Regulation*, 1985, *10*, 63–68.

Borkovec, T. D. Insomnia. *Journal of Consulting and Clinical Psychology*, 1982, *50*, 880–895.

Borkovec, T. D., & Nau, S. D. Credibility of analogue therapy rationales. *Journal of Behavior Therapy and Experimental Psychiatry*, 1972, *3*, 257–260.

Budzynski, T., Stoyva, J., & Ader, C. Feedback-induced relaxation: Application to tension headache. *Journal of Behavior Therapy and Experimental Psychiatry*, 1970, *1*, 205–211.

Califano, J. A. *Healthy people: The Surgeon General's report on health promotion and disease prevention.* Washington D.C: U.S. Government Printing Office, 1979.

Canter, A., Imboden, J. B., & Cluff, L. E. The frequency of physical illness as a function of prior psychological vulnerability and contemporary stress. *Psychosomatic Medicine*, 1966, *28*, 344–350.

Canter, A., Cluff, L. E., & Imboden, J. B. Hypersensitive reactions to immunization innoculations and antecedent psychological vulnerability. *Journal of Psychosomatic Research*, 1972, *16*, 99–101.

Cohen, W. S. Health promotion in the workplace: A prescription for good health. *American Psychologist*, 1985, *40*, 213–216.

Cox, D. J., Freundlich, A., & Meyer, R. G. Differential effectiveness of relaxation techniques and placebo with tension headaches. *Journal of Consulting and Clinical Psychology*, 1975, *43*, 892–898.

Culliton, B. J. Health care economics: The high cost of getting well. *Science*, 1978, *196*, 129–136.

Cummings, N. A. The anatomy of psychotherapy under national health insurance. *American Psychologists*, 1977, *32*, 711–718.

Cummings, N. A. Turning bread into stones: Our modern antimiracle. *American Psychologist*, 1979, *34*,(12), 1119–1129.

DeLeon, P. H., & VandenBos, G. R. The new federal health care frontiers: Cost containment and "Wellness". *Psychotherapy in Private Practice*, 1983, *1*(2), 17–32.

Diamond, M. J. Hypnotizability is modifiable: An alternative approach. *International Journal of Clinical and Experimental Hypnosis*, 1977, *25*, 147–166.

Engel, G. L. The need for a new medical model: A challenge for biomedicine. *Science*, 1977, *196*, 129–136.

Epstein, L. H., & Cluss, P. A. A behavioral medicine perspective on adherence to long-term medical regimens. *Journal of Consulting and Clinical Psychology*, 1982, *50*, 950–971.

Evans, F. J. Subjective characteristics of sleep efficiency. *Journal of Abnormal Psychology*, 1977, *86*, 561–564.

Fink, R., & Shapiro, S. Patterns of medical care related to mental illness. *Journal of Health and Human Behavior*, 1966, *7*, 98–105.

Fordyce, W. E. *Behavioral methods for chronic pain and illness.* St. Louis: C. V. Mosby, 1976.

Frazier, H. S., & Hiatt, H. H. Evaluation of medical practices. *Science*, 1978, *200*, 875–878.

Fromm, E., & Shor, R. E. (Eds.). *Hypnosis: Developments in research and new perspectives* (2nd ed.). New York: Aldine, 1979.

Fromm, E., Brown, D. P., Hurt, S. W., Overlander, J. Z., Boxer, A. M., & Pfeifer, G. The phenomena and characteristics of self-hypnosis. *International Journal of Clinical and Experimental Hypnosis,* 1981, *29*, 189–246.

Fuller, G. D. Current status of biofeedback in clinical practice. *American Psychologist*, 1978, *33*, 1, 39–48.

Gibson, C., Bugbee, C., & Anderson, O. W. *Emergency medical services in the Chicago area.* Chicago: Center for Health Administration Studies, University of Chicago, 1970.

Glass, D. C. *Behavior patterns, stress, and coronary disease*. Hillsdale: Erlbaum, 1977.

Gori, G. B., & Richter, B. J. Macroeconomics of disease prevention in the United States. *Science*, 1978, *200*(9), 1124–1130.

Green, E., & Green, A. *Beyond biofeedback*. New York: Dell, 1977.

Hamburg, D. A. Frontiers of research in neurobiology [Editorial]. *Science*, 1983, *222*, 969.

Hamburg, D. A., & Brown, S. S. The science base and social context of health maintenance: An overview. *Science*, 1978, *200*, 847–849.

Hauri, P. *The sleep disorders*. Kalamazoo: Upjohn, 1982.

Haynes, R. B., Taylor, D. W., & Sackett, D. L. *Compliance in health care*. Baltimore: Johns Hopkins University Press, 1979.

Hilgard, E. R. *Hypnotic susceptibility*. New York: Harcourt, Brace & World, 1965.

Hilgard, E. R. *Divided consciousness*. New York: Wiley, 1977.

Hilgard, E. R., & Bentler, P. M. Predicting hypnotizability from the Maudsley Personality Inventory. *British Journal of Psychology*, 1963, *54*, 63–69.

Hilkevitch, A. Psychiatric disturbances in outpatients of a general medical outpatient clinic. *International Journal of Neuropsychiatry*, 1965, *1*, 371–375.

Horder, T. J. Cited in M. S. Straus (Ed.), *Familiar medical quotations*. Boston: Little, Brown & Company, 1968.

Houpt, J. L., Orleans, C. S., George, L. K., Keith, H., Brodie, H. K. The role of psychiatric and behavioral factors in the practice of medicine. *American Journal of Psychiatry*, 1980, *137*, 37–47.

Hull, C. L. *Hypnosis and suggestibility: An experimental approach*. New York: Appleton Century, 1933.

Inglefinger, F. J. Medicine: Meritorius and meretricious. *Science*, 1978, *200*, 942–946.

Institute of Medicine. *DHEW's research planning principles: A review*. Washington, D.C.: National Academy of Sciences, 1979. (a)

Institute of Medicine. *Report of a study: Sleeping pills, insomnia, and medical practice*. Washington, D.C.: National Academy of Sciences, 1979. (b)

Jemmott, J. B., & Locke, S. E. Psychosocial factors, immunologic mediation, and human susceptibility to infectious diseases: How much do we know? *Psychological Bulletin*, 1984, *95*, 52–77.

Johnson, L. S. Self hypnosis: Behavioral and phenomenological comparisons with heterohypnosis. *International Journal of Clinical and Experimental Hypnosis*, 1979, *27*, 246–249.

Jones, K., & Vischi, J. *Impact of alcohol, drug abuse, and mental health treatment on medical care utilization—A review of the literature* (Unpublished report). Alcohol, Drug Abuse, and Mental Health Administration, Rockville, MD, 1979.

Kales, A. & Kales, J. D. *Evaluation and treatment of insomnia*. New York: Oxford University Press, 1984.

Kielolt-Glaser, J. K., Glaser, R., Williger, D., Stout, J., Messick, G., Sheppard, S., Bonnell, G., & Donnerberg, R. Psychosocial enhancement of immunocompetence in a geriatric population. *Health Psychology*, 1985, *4*(1), 25–41.

Kirsch, I., & Henry, D. Extinction versus credibility in the desensitization of speech anxiety. *Journal of Consulting and Clinical Psychology*, 1977, *45*, 1052–1059.

Knowles, J. H. The responsibility of the individual. In J. H. Knowles (Ed.), *Doing better and feeling worse: Health in the United States*. New York: Norton, 1977.

Lang, P. J. The mechanics of desensitization and the laboratory study of human fear. In C. Franks (Ed.), *Behavior therapy: Appraisal and status*. New York: McGraw-Hill, 1969.

Lang, P. J. A bio-informational theory of emotional imagery. *Psychophysiology*, 1979, *6*, 495–512.

Lazarus, R. S. *Psychological stress and the coping process*. New York: McGraw-Hill, 1966.

Lazarus, R. S., & Folkman, S. *Stress, appraisal and coping*. New York: Springer, 1984.

Lipowski, Z. J. Psychosomatic medicine in the seventies: An overview. *American Journal of Psychiatry*, 1977, *134*, 233–244.

Lubin, B., Nathan, R. G., & Matarazzo, J. D. Psychologists in medical education: 1976. *American Psychologist*, 1978, *33*(4), 339–343.

Mahoney, M. J., & Arnkoff, O. B. Self-management. In O. F. Pomerleau & J. P. Brady (Eds.), *Behavioral medicine: Theory and practice*. Baltimore: Williams and Wilkins, 1979.

Mason, A. A. A case of congenital Ichthyosiform Erythrodermia of Brocq treated by hypnosis. *British Medical Journal*, 1952, August 23, 422–423.

Mason, A. A. Ichthyosis and hypnosis. *British Medical Journal*, 1955, *2*, July 2, 57–58.

Mason, J. W. Organization of psychoendocrine mechanisms: A review and reconsideration of research. In N. S. Greenfield & R. S. Sternbach (Eds.), *Handbook of psychophysiology*. New York: Holt, Reinhart & Winston, 1972.

Matarazzo, J. D. Health psychology: APA's newest division. *The Health Psychologist*, 1979, *1*, 1–3.

Matarazzo, J. D. Behavioral health and behavioral medicine: Frontiers for a new health psychology. *American Psychologist*, 1980, *35*, 807–817.

Moertel, C. G., Ahman, D. L., Taylor, W. F., & Schwartau, N. A comparative evaluation of marketed analgesic drugs. *Journal of the American Medical Association*, 1972, *286*, 813–815.

Morgan, A. H. The heritability of hypnotic susceptibility in twins. *Journal of Abnormal Psychology*, 1973, *82*, 55–66.

Morgan, A. H., Hilgard, E. R., & Davert, E. C. The heritability of hypnotic susceptibility of twins: A preliminary report. *Behavioral Genetics*, 1970, *1*, 213–224.

Ng, L. K. Y., & Bonica, J. J. (Eds.). *Pain, discomfort and humanitarian care*. New York: Elsevier/North Holland, 1980.

Orleans, C. T., George, L. K., Houpt, J. L., & Brodie, H. K. How primary care physicians treat psychiatric disorders: A national survey of family practioners. *American Journal of Psychiatry*, 1985, *142*(1), 52–57.

Orne, M. T. On the social psychology of the psychological experiment: With particular reference to demand characteristics and their implications. *American Psychologist*, 1962, *17*, 776–783.

Orne, M. T., & Scheibe, K. E. The contribution of nondeprivation factors in the production of sensory deprivation effects: The psychology of the "panic button." In I. Wickramasekera (Ed.), *Biofeedback, behavior therapy, and hypnosis*. Chicago: Nelson-Hall, 1976.

Patel, C. H. Biofeedback-aided relaxation in the management of hypertension. *Biofeedback and Self-Regulation*, 1977, *2*, 1–41.

Paul, G. L. *Insight versus desensitization in psychotherapy*. Stanford: Stanford University Press, 1966.

Pavlov, I. P. *Conditioned reflexes* (Translated by G. V. Annep). London: Oxford University Press, 1927.

Pomerleau, O. F., & Brady, J. P. Introduction: The scope and promise of behavioral medicine. In O. F. Pomerleau & J. P. Brady (Eds.), *Behavioral medicine: Theory and practice*. Baltimore: Williams & Wilkins, 1979.

Qualls, P. J., & Sheenan, P. W. Capacity for absorption and relaxation during EMG biofeedback and no feedback conditions. *Journal of Abnormal Psychology*, 1979, *88*(6), 652–663.

Rasmussen, A. J., Jr. Emotions and immunity. *Annals of the New York Academy of Sciences*, 1969, *164*, 458–461.

Roberts, A. H. Biofeedback: Research, training and clinical roles. *American Psychologist*, 1985, *40*, 938–941.

Rogers, M. P., Dubey, D., & Reich, P. The influence of the psyche and the brain on immunity and disease susceptibility: A critical review. *Psychosomatic Medicine*, 1979, *41*, 147–164.

Sackett, D. L., & Haynes, R. B. *Compliance with therapeutic regimens*. Baltimore: Johns Hopkins University Press, 1976.

Sarbin, T. R., & Slagle, R. W. Hypnosis and psychophysiological outcomes. In E. Fromm & R. E. Shor (Eds.), *Hypnosis: Research developments and perspectives*. Chicago: Aldine-Atherton, 1972.

Sargent, J., Green, E., & Walters, E. Preliminary report on the use of autogenic feedback techniques in treatment of migraine and tension headaches. *Psychosomatic Medicine*, 1973, *35*, 129–135.

Schwartz, G., & Weiss, S. What is behavioral medicine? *Psychosomatic Medicine*, 1977, *36*, 377–381.

Selye, H. *The stress of life* (2nd ed.). New York: McGraw-Hill, 1976.

Shapiro, D., & Goldstein, I. B. Biobehavioral perspectives on hypertension. *Journal of Consulting and Clinical Psychology*, 1982, *50*, 841–858.

Smith, R. J. Study finds sleeping pills overprescribed. *Science*, 1979, *204*, 287–288.

Solomon, G. F., Amkraut, A. A., & Kasper, P. Immunity, emotions and stress, with special references to the mechanisms of stress effects on the immune system. In H. Musaph (Ed.), *Mechanism in symptom formation*. Basel, Switzerland: S. Karger, 1974.

Stroebel, C. F., & Glueck, B. C. Biofeedback treatment in medicine and psychiatry: An ultimate placebo? *Seminars in Psychiatry*, 1973, *5*, 379–393.

Suedfeld, P. *Restricted environmental stimulation: Research and clinical applications*. New York: Wiley, 1980.

Suinn, R. M. Intervention with Type A behaviors. *Journal of Consulting and Clinical Psychology*, 1980, *50*(6), 933–949.

Surwit, R. S. *Raynaud's disease*. In L. Birk (Ed.), *Biofeedback: Behavioral medicine*. New York: Grune & Stratton, 1973.

Surwit, R. S. Behavioral treatment of Raynaud's syndrome in peripheral vascular disease. *Journal of Consulting and Clinical Psychology*, 1982, *50*(6), 922–932.

Tallman, J. F., Paul, S. M., Skolnick, P., & Gallager, D. W. Receptors for an age of anxiety: Pharmacology of the benzodiazepines. *Science*, 1980, *207*, 274–281.

Tancredi, L. R., & Barondess, J. A. The problem of defensive medicine. *Science*, 1978, *200*, 883–886.

Taub, E. Self-regulation of human tissue temperature. In G. E. Schwartz & J. Betty (Eds.), *Biofeedback theory and research*. New York: Academic Press, 1977.

Top 200 drugs of 1984: 2.1% increase in refills pushes 1984 RXs 1.7% ahead of 1983. *Pharmacy Times*, April, 1985, pp. 25–33.

Weiner, H. *Psychobiology and human disease*. New York: Elsevier, 1977.

Wickramasekera, I. Effects of sensory restriction on susceptibility to hypnosis. *International Journal of Clinical and Experimental Hypnosis*, 1969, *17*, 217–224.

Wickramasekera, I. Effects of sensory deprivation on susceptibility to hypnosis: A hypothesis and more preliminary data. *Journal of Abnormal Psychology*, 1970, 76(1), 69–75.

Wickramasekera, I. Electromyographic feedback training and tension headache: Preliminary observations. *The American Journal of Clinical Hypnosis*, 1972, 15(2), 83–85.

Wickramasekera, I. (Ed.). *Biofeedback, behavior therapy and hypnosis*. Chicago: Nelson-Hall, 1976.

Wickramasekera, I. The placebo effect and biofeedback for headache pain. *Proceedings of the San Diego Biomedical Symposium*, 1977, 2, 227–230. (a)

Wickramasekera, I. On attempts to modify hypnotic susceptibility: Some psychophysiological procedures and promising directions. *Annals of the New York Academy of Sciences*, 1977, 296, 143–153. (b)

Wickramasekera, I. (with M. T. Orne & C. Stroebel). *A conditioned response model of the placebo*. Paper presented to Biofeedback Society of America, Symposium on Nonspecific Effects in Biofeedback. Albuquerque, New Mexico, March 1978.

Wickramasekera, I. *Do beliefs have biological consequences?* Paper presented to the Biofeedback Society of America, San Diego, California, 1979. (a)

Wickramasekera, I. Implications of behavioral health for psychology. *Illinois Psychologist*, 1979, 18, 11–14. (b)

Wickramasekera, I. A conditioned response model of the placebo effect: Predictions from the model. *Biofeedback and Self Regulation*, 1980, 5, 5–18.

Wickramasekera, I. Clinical research in a behavioral medicine private practice. *Behavioral Assessment*, 1981, 3, 265–271.

Wickramasekera, I. *A model of people at high risk*. Paper presented at the International Stress and Tension Control Society, Brighton, England, August 1983.

Wickramasekera, I. A model of people at high risk to develop chronic stress-related symptoms. In F. J. McGuigan, W. Sime, & J. Macdonald Wallace (Eds.), *Stress and tension control 2*. New York: Plenum Press, 1984. (a)

Wickramasekera, I. Are health psychologists physicians? *Contemporary Psychology*, 1984, 29(10), 821. (b)

Wickramasekera, I. A conditioned response model of the placebo effect: Predictions and postdictions from the model. In L. White, B. Tursky, & G. Schwartz (Eds.), *Placebo: Clinical phenomena and new insight*. New York: Guilford Press, 1985.

Wolpe, J. *Psychotherapy by reciprocal inhibition*. Stanford: Stanford University Press, 1958.

Wolpe, J. *The practice of behavior therapy* (3rd ed.). New York: Pergamon Press, 1982.

Woolfolk, R. J., & Lehrer, P. M., (Eds.). *Principles and practice of stress management*. New York: Guilford Press, 1984.

3

HYPNOSIS
Scientific Status and Clinical Relevance

Hypnosis is a form of information processing in which voluntarily initiated suspension of peripheral awareness and critical analytic mentation can readily lead in some people to major changes in perception, memory, and mood that have important behavioral and physiological consequences. There are individual differences in how easily these voluntarily initiated changes in perception, mood, and memory can subjectively begin to seem involuntary or quasi-automatic. It appears that conditions of (a) sensory restriction and (b) very high, or (c) very low physiological arousal predispose all people toward the hypnotic mode of information processing (Wickramasekera, 1977b).

Hypnotic phenomena have been reported in all cultures across the world, across all periods of recorded history, and in various culturally conditioned forms. Manifestations of hypnotic behavior have typically occurred in either a religious or a healing (medical) context. It is important to recognize that hypnosis did not originate with the physician Anton Mesmer (1734–1815) in France 250 years ago; however, Mesmer deserves recognition as the first person known to propose a naturalistic rather than a magical or demonic explanation of hypnotic phenomena. Borrowing from contemporary physics, Mesmer formulated a theory of hypnotic behavior based on magnetism (animal) radiating from his own person.

The last 50 years of experimental hypnotic research has clearly and repeatedly established that the bulk of hypnotic response resides in the subject's natural hypnotic ability, and not in any projection from the operator or from the operator's hypnotic skill (Hilgard, 1982). In fact, a series of clever experiments done over 200 years ago, designed by a distinguished committee (Ben Franklin, Lavoisier, Guillotin, etc.) of the French Academy of Sciences appointed to investigate Mesmer, found no evidence of animal magnetism in his procedures, but did not deny the empirical reality of his cures. Hence, Mesmer was wrong with respect to the mechanism of hypnosis and the sources of hypnotic response. The committee alternatively proposed that the mechanism of his cures was "mere imagination."

We know today that the committee was partly right with respect to the alternative mechanism of imagination it proposed to account for his clinical results, but it was seriously wrong with respect to the apparent implication that the potency of imaginative and cognitive effects are trivial. I refer to this as the error of the French Academy of Sciences. It is an error that is even today commonly made by many physicians, bio-medical researchers, and other reductionistic thinkers who are committed to mind–body dualism. In fact, in certain subjects (high hypnotizables) and under certain conditions, beliefs can have potent, specific, and reliable biological consequences ranging from allergic reactions, warts, or congenital skin diseases to changes in mammary glands, burns, and the inhibition of bleeding (Barber, 1984). These effects in these subjects can be more specific and rapid than the effects of drugs. For example, one study (Maslach, Marshall, & Zimbardo, 1972) demonstrated that it is possible to suggest increases in peripheral skin temperature in one hand and to reduce it concurrently in the other hand. It would be hard to find a drug that can have such specific and arbitrarily selected effects on the body.

The English physician Braid (1795–1860) coined the term *hypnotism* or "nervous sleep," thereby proposing another naturalistic explanation of hypnosis, and he went on to demonstrate its clinical value in medical practice. This second hypothesized mechanism of hypnotic behavior has also been proved false by controlled EEG studies of hypnosis in the last 50 years. Hypnosis is definitely not sleep Stages 4, 3, or 2 (Evans, 1977).

The third naturalistic but pathological explanation of the mechanism of hypnotic behavior was proposed by the eminent French neurologist Charcot (1835–1893) of Paris. According to Charcot, hypnosis was associated with a psychopathological phenomena (hysteria) and was based on an abnormal CNS function. Bernheim, professor of medicine at Nancy, challenged Charcot's theory and proposed that hypnosis was due to normal behavioral phenomena initiated by suggestion. Based on the last 50 years of experimental research, we know today that Charcot was wrong and Bernheim was more nearly correct. People free of major psychopathology are generally better hypnotic subjects (Graham & Evans, 1977; Hilgard, 1965; Horne, Evans, & Orne, 1982; Spiegel, Detrick, & Frischolz, 1982). Serious mental disorders appear to disrupt the attentional process, which is one of the crucial preconditions for hypnotic behavior. In fact, normal (without serious psychiatric history) volunteer subjects and medical patients with circumscribed physical problems are in general probably the best adult hypnotic subjects.

The modern systematic study of hypnosis in the experimental laboratory can be dated to the psychologist Clark Hull, whose research at Yale led to a classic text, *Hypnosis and Suggestibility*, in 1933. Many physicians and psychologists are unaware of the fact that in 1955 the British Medical Association, recognizing that a large enough body of clinical observations and experimentally verified information existed about hypnosis, recommended its cautious teaching in medical schools and its use in clinical practice. In 1958, the American Medical Association went on record-making a similar recommendation. In 1960, the American Psychological Association officially recognized the American Board of Psychological Hypnosis and its authority to examine and certify diplomates in either experimental or clinical hypnosis. There are now similar national boards in medical and dental hypnosis.

Current Theories of Hypnosis

Because of prior empirical research, all scientific investigators of hypnosis are now essentially in agreement at an observational level (Spanos & Barber, 1974). For example, investigators of hypnotic ability, regardless of their theoretical orientation, report that approximately 70% of people with superior hypnotic ability can significantly reduce pain (by at least 50%) (Hilgard & Hilgard, 1975). However, at the level of explanation or mechanism there is still salient disagreement. At the explanatory level some theorists see the essence of hypnosis as motivation, or goal-oriented striving (Barber, 1969) that involves no discontinuous special state, whereas others (Hilgard, 1965; Orne, 1977), who are state theorists, see the essence of hypnosis as an altered state of consciousness (discontinuous from the waking everyday state) produced by a trait (hypnotic ability) and a procedure or induction. They consider motivation to be necessary but not a sufficient condition for the experience of profound hypnotic (e.g., amnesia, hallucinations, etc.) phenomena.

Experimental research has made it very clear in the last 25 years that hypnotic experience and behavior are primarily dependent on individual ability or talent and only secondarily on hypnotic procedure (Hilgard, 1982). In fact, most of the early controversy between state and non-state theorists was caused by the failure to control for hypnotic ability in the early studies. If subjects are not selected for hypnotic ability, no differences emerge between a hypnotic procedure and a task-motivated procedure (Barber, 1969; Hilgard, 1965). The mere performance of a hypnotic induction ritual will not guarantee hypnotic behavior. To demonstrate the potency of hypnosis we need first to identify people with hypnotic ability. Hypnotic ability, like intellectual ability, exists independently of intelligence tests and hypnotic tests, but these tests enable us accurately to identify people with these abilities. Through the identification of these people and the analytic study of their abilities, we may come to understand the mechanism on which hypnotic phenomena are based, and eventually we may be able to teach these mechanisms to others who are deficient in hypnotic talent.

Parameters of Hypnosis

Several scales of high reliability (.80 to .90) and validity have been developed to measure hypnotic ability. (See Figure 7.) These scales include the Stanford, Harvard, and Barber Scales. The scales have shown measured hypnotic ability to be very reliable across different experimenters and very stable over periods as long as 10 years (Hilgard, 1965; Hilgard & Hilgard, 1975). The predictive validity of these scales is partly documented by the numerous studies showing a high correlation between clinical and experimental outcomes with responses mediated by the autonomic nervous system and measured hypnotic ability (Bowers & Kelley, 1979; Hilgard, 1982; Perry, Gelfand, & Marcovitch, 1979), but the evidence is weaker for a relationship between hypnotic ability and operant behaviors like cigarette smoking. For example, 61% of superior hypnotic subjects and only 3% of inferior hypnotic subjects can significantly reduce experimental pain (Hilgard & Hilgard, 1975). These scales

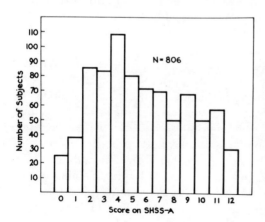

Figure 7. Hypnotic responsiveness scores of 806 college students. The scores were earned on individual tests with the Stanford Hypnotic Susceptibility Scale, Form A; the least responsive scored 0, the most responsive 12. Most scores lie between these extremes. Unpublished data, Stanford Laboratory. From *Hypnosis in the Relief of Pain* by E. R. Hilgard & J. R. Hilgard, 1975.

reveal hypnotic ability to be approximately normally distributed; approximately 10% of the population has superior hypnotic ability and an equal percentage is refractory to hypnosis (Barber, 1969; Hilgard, 1965). Hypnotic ability is also moderately and positively related to IQ, peaks in preadolescence (ages 10 to 12 years) and declines slowly with age (Morgan & Hilgard, 1973). (See Figures 8, 9.)

From studies of monozygotic twins it appears that hypnotic ability has a genetic component (Morgan, 1973; Morgan, Hilgard, & Darert, 1970) approximately equal to that of IQ. There appears to be no significant sex differences in hypnotic ability (Hilgard, 1965) but at least one large-scale ($N=653$) study (Morgan & Hilgard, 1973) indicated that only for young (age 21 to 32) females who were mothers was there a temporary recovery of adolescent level hypnotic ability during their childbearing age. If this finding is replicated it would be interesting to speculate that young mothers who do not show this temporary recovery of hypnotic ability may be at higher risk for developing stress-related psychophysiological problems either in themselves and/or in their infants. This speculation is based on the assumption that the empathic and other components (ability to regress and be playful with child or "regression in the service of the ego") of hypnotic ability facilitates "bonding" and the implementation of good child rearing practices. Mothers who feel ineffective and frustrated in their parenting skills are probably at greater risk for developing mental or physical disorders in themselves or in their children.

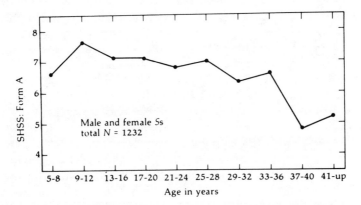

Figure 8. Mean hypnotic susceptibility scores by age. The scores recorded are all from individual hypnotic tests. From "Age Differences in Susceptibility to Hypnosis" by A. H. Morgan & E. R. Hilgard, *International Journal of Clinical and Experimental Hypnosis*, 1973, 21, 78–85. Copyright by the Society for Clinical and Experimental Hypnosis, April 1973. Reprinted by permission.

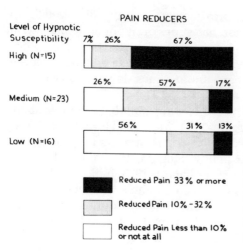

Figure 9. Reduction of pain through hypnotically suggested analgesia as related to susceptibility to hypnosis. The subjects were fifty-four university subjects whose prior experience of hypnosis was limited to a standard test of hypnotic responsiveness following a standardized induction procedure. From *Hypnosis in the Relief of Pain,* by E. R. Hilgard and J. R. Hilgard, 1975.

Behavioral response to suggestion outside of hypnosis correlates with measured hypnotizability approximately .60 (Hilgard & Tart, 1966). This correlation implies that given (a) a cooperative subject with (b) good hypnotic ability, any verbal instruction or suggestions are likely to have a significant impact regardless of whether the instructions are called propaganda, psychotherapy, or public education. This implies that some of the benefits of suggestion are available to those with hypnotic ability even without a formal prior hypnotic induction, if their therapist or physician recognizes the subject's ability and mobilizes it positively to secure compliance with psychotherapy homework or medication usage. The benefits of suggestion constitute a good reason routinely to measure the hypnotic ability of all patients even if hypnosis *per se* is not formally used in therapy.

Suggestions used in hypnosis differ from simple verbal instructions in several important ways (Bowers, 1982; Wickramasekera, 1976): (a) Responses to instructions are not dependent on a subjects hypnotic ability. For example, "Pick up your pants, Jack!", is a verbal instruction that does not presuppose hypnotic ability. Positive response to hypnotic suggestions is dependent on subject characteristics (superior hypnotic ability). For example, the simple suggestion "You will be unable to feel pain" will be effective only if given to a person with hypnotic ability. (b) A suggestion is experienced as nonvolitional (classic suggestion effect) or occurring without the subject's conscious participation. For example, "You will be unable to take your hands apart" is experienced by people with hypnotic ability as an involuntary inability to separate their hands. Instructions require only voluntary social compliance, for example in complying with the request, "Pass me the salt." (c) Suggestions are particularly effective with autonomically mediated responses (Bowers, 1982), and less effective with skeletally mediated or operant behavior. For example, suggestion is less likely to be effective with weight loss or smoking than with nausea or vomiting. Because the good hypnotic subject, when positively motivated, is cognitively flexible and profoundly empathic, he or she is more likely to be agreeable and to even be seen as compliant. In fact, a preliminary study of the relationship between hypnotic ability and annual alumni giving (money) showed a modest relationship between making financial contributions and hypnotic ability (Graham & Greene, 1981). But several studies have shown that people of superior hypnotic ability are not particularly motivated by exhortation and, in fact, on motor tasks they do not try as hard as people of low-hypnotic ability (London & Fuhrer, 1961).

Characteristics of High Hypnotizables

Hypnotic ability is not significantly correlated with any known personality variable (Barber, 1964; Hilgard, 1965). Very recently the careful study of exceptionally responsive hypnotic subjects (Hilgard, 1977; Wilson & Barber, 1982) is leading not only to further convergence at the observational level but also at the explanatory level. For example, Wilson and Barber (1982), based on a study of very superior hypnotic subjects, recently claimed that the essence of hypnosis is fantasy involvement of hallucinatory intensity. But Hilgard, a state theorist, has pointed out that at best measures of fantasy yield only a correlation of about .50 with measured hypnotizability (Hilgard, 1982; Monterio, McDonald, & Hilgard, 1980). If fantasy is the ability to furnish the mind with rich and varied images, then another major factor in hypnosis is the ability to make the mind empty or blank. This second factor, which is orthogonal to the fantasy factor, correlates with posthypnotic amnesia (Evans, 1965; Hammer, Evans, & Bartlett, 1963) and seems related to the superior hypnotic subject's ability voluntarily to control states of consciousness.

The superior hypnotic subject can voluntarily control the switches of consciousness like waking, sleeping, remembering, forgetting, and dreaming. Most superior hypnotic subjects can reliably and voluntarily fall asleep during the day or night (Evans, 1977) in a variety of situations (e.g., in EEG sleep laboratory, at lectures and plays, on a train, plane, or bus). It is likely that many chronic insomniacs are in fact poor hypnotic subjects or good ones who have inadvertently suggested themselves into chronic insomnia. The superior hypnotic subject can also demonstrate learning of simple environmental stimuli (e.g., motor response to simple verbal suggestion to touch nose) presented exclusively during EEG defined sleep (e.g., stage REM or Stage 1 alpha free sleep) and continue to show this state-specific learning for several weeks or for as much as 6 months later. In the waking state there is no evidence of state-specific learning (Evans, 1977). Superior hypnotic subjects can also often wake up at a specific preselected time before their alarm goes off. Superior hypnotic subjects can also voluntarily alter the content of their REM dreams (Stoyva, 1965). This ability voluntarily and reliably to control several important functions (sleep, waking, dreaming, etc.) or states of consciousness may have survival value. It may also permit some degree of environmental monitoring and even monitoring of stress within sleep. It may be the basis of individual differences in the ability to acquire coping skills like psychophysiological stress reduction techniques (e.g., meditation, progressive muscle relaxation). Flexibility in changing psychological states that permits a fresh look at an old problem may be a useful survival skill and an indicator of good mental health. For example, Rivers (1976) reported that superior hypnotic subjects learn meditation more rapidly than poor hypnotic subjects and they also appear to learn "lucid dreaming" very rapidly (Dane, 1984) Lucid dreams are now empirically verifiable events in which the dreamer controls the content of the ongoing REM dream (LaBerge, 1983). It may be useful routinely to screen patients for hypnotic ability even if hypnosis is never used formally in therapy, because hypnotic ability appears to be correlated with voluntary control and access to several important psychological functions like sleep onset, waking, and dreaming.

Highly hypnotizable people can reliably develop posthypnotic amnesia and on cancellation of the suggestion can accurately retrieve the lost memories (Kihlstrom, 1977). They can also readily create, mix, and merge memories (Laurence & Perry, 1983; Orne, 1986), but they can also have exceptional recall for distant events (Evans, 1983). Hence, the use of hypnosis in courtroom testimony to enhance witness recall is a complex affair and requires several control conditions beyond mere skill in hypnotic induction.

The complexity of the issue of memory creation is further documented by the fact that there is now good independently replicated evidence that superior hypnotic subjects generally score higher on a variety of standardized tests of creativity (Ashton & McDonald, 1982; Bowers & Bowers, 1979). In fact a preliminary study by Dave (1979) has shown that using the hypnotic technique of induced dreams, the creative resolution of academic, vocational, and personal problems could be enhanced over a control procedure. Unfortunately, unlike the previous authors, Dave (1979) did not control for hypnotic ability in his study.

There are three additional features of the experience of superior hynotic subjects that have clinical implications. The first is the well-established fact that subjects in hypnosis underestimate the passage of time by about 40% of clock time (St. Jean & MacLeod, 1983). The second is the fact that subjects who score high on hypnotic ability tests generally experience the suggestions as happening to them outside their voluntary control or occurring without any personal effort on their part (Bowers, 1982). The third is that subjects of superior hypnotic ability appear to process information more quickly and efficiently than subjects of low hypnotic ability (Ingram, Saccuzzo, McNeil, & McDonald, 1979; Saccuzzo, Safnan, Anderson, & McNeill, 1982). These three features can make therapeutic learning seem simple and effortless.

It has also been found that superior hypnotic subjects respond more rapidly to various types of short-term psychotherapy (Larsen, 1966; Nace, Warwick, Kelley, & Evans, 1982), meditation techniques (Benson, Greenwood, & Klemchuck, 1975; Rivers, 1976), respondent conditioning (Das, 1958a,b), operant conditioning, and operant verbal conditioning (Weiss, Ullman, & Krasner, 1960; Webb, 1962; King & McDonald, 1976; Wickramasekera, 1970b) (see Figure 10). Good hypnotic subjects also show a superior hypnotherapeutic response to allergic skin reactions (Black, 1969), asthma (Collison, 1975), and migraine headaches (Cedercreutz, 1978). The previously cited cluster of findings jointly suggests that the superior hypnotic subjects learn, become physiologically

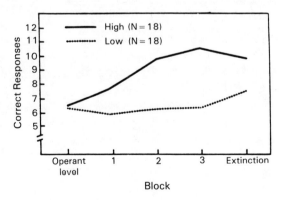

Figure 10. Verbal conditioning as a function of hypnotic susceptibility. From "Hypnotic Susceptibility and Verbal Conditioning," by D. R. King & R. D. McDonald, *International Journal of Clinical and Experimental Hypnosis,* 1976, 24.

aroused, and condition more rapidly than poor hypnotic subjects, particularly with respect to autonomically mediated functions.

Psychopathology, Pathophysiology, Healing, and Hypnotic Ability

Ironically the previously cited findings can have positive and negative consequences for the individual who has superior hypnotic ability. For superior hypnotic subjects, images, fantasies, anticipations, and ruminations can be so real as to reach hallucinatory intensity (Wilson & Barber, 1982), generating strong emotions and physiological changes. Several studies (Foenander, Burrows, Gerschman, & Horne, 1980; Frankel & Orne, 1976; Gerschman, Burrows, Reade, & Foenander, 1979; Kelley, 1984; Perry, John, & Hollander, 1982) have clearly shown that superior hypnotic ability may predispose individuals to the development of phobias. (See Table 2.) Developmental studies have also shown that in a subset of high-hypnotic-ability people there is a positive correlation with the perceived severity of childhood punishment (Hilgard, 1979) and even perceived child abuse (Nash, Lynn, & Givens, 1984). (See Table 3.) The ability of highly hypnotizable subjects to block out of mind or compartmentalize high intensity emotions may place them at higher risk for developing phobic and psychophysiological reactions (Wickramasekera, 1979). In the case of displaced fears, the actual phobic object may not be the object the patient reports he is phobic of. If a person is highly hypnotizable and also autonomically labile (sympathetically hyperactive) he may be at even higher risk for developing psychophysiological symptoms (Wickramasekera 1979, 1984) involving the ANS and certain types of psychological and behavioral symptoms

Table 2. Comparison of Phobic and Nonphobic Patients' Hypnotic Susceptibility[a]

	Hypnotic susceptibility			
	Low	Medium	High	Total
Phobic	0	4	15	19
Nonphobic	20	51	35	106
Total	20	55	50	125

[a]From Measured hypnotic response and phobic behavior: A brief communication by Sean F. Kelly, *The International Journal of Clinical and Experimental Hypnosis*, 1984, 321, 1–5.

Table 3. Experiment 2: Frequency Data[a]

	Low susceptible (HGSHS:A = 0–4)	Medium susceptible (HGSHS:A = 5–7)	High susceptible (HGSHS:A = 8–12)	Total
Nonabused	76 (25.30%)	105 (35.00%)	119 (39.70%)	300
Abused	3 (18.80%)	0 (00.0%)	13 (81.20%)	16

[a]From M. R. Nash, S. J. Lynn, & D. L. Givens (1984). Adult hypnotic susceptibility and childhood punishment, and child abuse: A brief communication. *International Journal of Clinical and Experimental Hypnosis, 32*, 1, 6–11.

(e.g., phobias, fugue, amnesia, and conversion symptoms). I believe it is that subset of high hypnotizables who are prone to excessive sympathetic reactivity and lack support systems and coping skills who develop clinical symptoms (Wickramasekera, 1979, 1984).

Recently it has been reported that those anorexia patients who purge and vomit, and most bulimic patients, are likely to have above average hypnotic ability (Pettinati, Horne, & Staats, 1985). These intriguing findings on certain eating disorders need independent replication but seem to illuminate factors that contribute to the etiology of these puzzling eating disorders. (See Table 4.) Perhaps people with high hypnotic ability learn too easily to voluntarily initiate reverse peristalsis.

Clinical experience (Wickramasekera, 1979) suggests that it is this subset of highly hypnotizables, who are also high on sympathetic reactivity (Eysenck, 1960), who are likely to become symptomatic under

Table 4. Hypnotizability of Anorectic Subgroups (Abstainers and Purgers) and Bulimic Patients[a]

	Mean score (SD)					
	Anorexic			Bulimic		
	Abstain (n = 19)		Purge (n = 46)			
Scale[b]				(n = 21)	F	p
HIP	4.66	(3.2)	4.93 (3.2)	7.13 (2.4)	4.58	<.05
HGSHS:A	6.11	(2.7)	7.1 (2.7)	8.05 (2.3)	2.74	<.10
SHSS:C	5.00	(2.3)	6.13 (2.6)	7.71 (1.7)	6.97	<.01

[a]From H. M. Pettinati, R. L. Horne, & J. M. Staats. (1985). Hypnotizability in patients in the anorexia nervosa and bulimia. *Archives of General Psychiatry, 42*, 1014–1016.
[b]HIP = Hypnotic Induction Profile (Spiegel, 1972); HGSHS:A = Harvard Group Scale of Hypnotic Susceptibility: Form A (Shor & Orne, 1962); SHSS:C = Standard Hypnotic Susceptibility Scale: Form C (Weitzenhoffer & Hilgard, 1962).

chronic stress. For example, there is some preliminary evidence (Stutman & Bliss, 1985) that people of high hypnotic ability, when placed under conditions of high chronic stress, such as warfare, are more likely to develop severe Posttraumatic Stress Disorder than people of lower hypnotic ability. (See Table 5.) The profound empathy and capacity for absorption of these superior hypnotic subjects (Hilgard, 1977) increases the probability that in significant interpersonal conflict situations their emotions are very likely to be hyperintense and associated with physiological consequences. The creativity of the superior hypnotic subject (Bowers, 1979) can also lead to potent negative cognitive elaborations (catastrophizing) that can further amplify fears and induce sustained levels of sympathetic hyperarousal. The superior dissociation abilities of the good hypnotic subject (Hilgard, 1977) may inadvertently be used to inhibit the psychological component of distress from consciousness and to transduce the psychological distress into a physiological presentation or somatization. (See case study, Chapter 8, p. 177). So that the psychological distress (e.g., fear, anger, etc.) may fade from consciousness and be replaced by a diffuse psychological feeling of emptiness or numbness, but be eventually replaced at a physiological level by a peptic ulcer, irritable bowel syndrome, or primary hypertension.

There is some uneven evidence (Bowers, 1979; Hilgard, 1977) that right-handed people of high-hypnotic ability during reflective thought

Table 5. Posttraumatic Stress Disorder, Imagery, and Hypnotizability among 26 Vietnam Veterans[a]

Item	Veterans with high posttraumatic stress disorder			Veterans with low posttraumatic stress disorder			t	df	p
	N	Mean	SE	N	Mean	SE			
Posttraumatic stress disorder score[b]	14	11.8	0.64	12	0.67	0.19	14.9	21	<.001
Percent of posttraumatic stress symptoms on self-report[c]	14	19	3	8	7	1	3.1	21	<.005
Hypnotizability score[d]	14	10.9	0.22	12	7.1	0.54	6.6	25	<.001

[a]Control subjects were men and women age 20–45 years from the general population. From R. K. Stutman & E. L. Bliss. (1985). *American Journal of Psychiatry, 142*, 6.
[b]Range = 0–15
[c]Percent of 313 possible symptoms on self-report; range = 0–7; a score below 2 indicates high imaging ability
[d]Range = 0–12; a score from 9 to 12 is very high; significantly different from score of 49 control subjects (6.6 = 0.37; p < .001).

are more likely to show left conjugate lateral eye movements (L-CLEMS) in the face-to-face situation. In fact, left CLEMs may be a crude biological test of the potential for superior hypnotic performance. It is interesting to note that the majority of the patients seen at the Behavioral Medicine Clinic at the Eastern Virginia Medical School (EVMS sample) demonstrate left CLEMs on the EVMS-CLEM test.[1] It appears that our CLEM test data confirms the prediction from the high-risk model that more people with stress-related disorders are likely to have high-hypnotic ability. The good hypnotic subject may also be vulnerable to complex subliminal perception effects. A study (Sackeim, Packer, & Gur, 1977) has shown that under conditions of "unstructured" set, right-handed subjects of high hypnotic ability (defined as left conjugate lateral eye movers or CLEMS) are more likely to experience subliminal perception effects. Hence it appears likely that people of good hypnotic ability may be more vulnerable to subliminal perception effects and to "unconsciously" motivated effects. In this context it is worth noting that there is now growing empirical and logical evidence for a "psychological unconscious" (Bowers & Meichenbaum, 1984; Shevrin & Dickman, 1980). Based on clinical observation (Wickramasekera, 1976a), it is also likely that in high-hypnotic-ability subjects images in night dreams (REM) may be transduced into physiological dysfunctions that persist even after the triggering stressful psychological component has faded from consciousness and memory in the waking state. For example, it is common for patients prone to headaches and chronic pain to wake up at night or from morning sleep with an acute attack of pain. In summary, the superior hypnotic subject's capacity for profound empathy, absorption, imagery of hallucinatory intensity, and relatively unfiltered perception may make him inadvertently more vulnerable to psychological pollution from incidental learning, dreams, and even weak sensory stimuli.

Clinical experience (Wickramasekera, 1979) and a recent study (Wilson & Barber, 1982) suggests that a subset of highly hypnotizable subjects are at higher risk for reporting parapsychological incidents. It is

[1] The hypothesis underlying the conjugate lateral eye movement test (CLEM test) is that in right-handed people during reflective thought provoked by a combination of verbal and visual task questions (Appendix C) the movement of the subject's eyes to the subject's left indicated preferential activation of the contralateral (right) cerebral hemisphere. There are several studies that with some complications suggest a fairly reliable relationship between superior hypnotic ability and a predominant tendency during reflective thought to left CLEMS in right-handed people (Bowers, 1976; Hilgard, 1977). This tendency to predominantly left CLEMS during reflective thought appears to be independent of the content of the reflective thought (visual-holistic or verbal, quantitative analytic) when provoked by questions asked by an examiner in a face-to-face situation with a symmetrical physical background.

3434

important to recognize that the previous statement does not in any way imply that these verbal reports have any objective validity, but that they are simply an interesting place (a pure culture) to start the empirical (validity) investigation of the reports of these incidents. A brief paper-and-pencil test that I developed (Wickramasekera, 1985b; Wickramasekera, 1986) to predict hypnotic ability in college undergraduates demonstrates that a large number (80%) of high-hypnotic ability people endorse previously unreported psychic experiences; whereas only a few (19%) people of low-hypnotic ability report having had these experiences. (See Table 6.) Wilson and Barber (1982) studied two matched groups of high- and low-hypnotic-ability subjects who were fully functional and nonpsychotic females. Over 90% of the high-hypnotic-ability subjects reported numerous psychic experiences (telepathic, precognitive, out-of-the-body experiences, etc.) and less than 15% of the low-hypnotic-ability subjects reported these experiences. It is likely that some of these high-hypnotic subjects learn to use their hypnotic ability to cope adaptively or maladaptively (phobias, chronic pain, etc.) with physical or sexual abuse or other types of childhood trauma (life-threat-

Table 6. Types of Test Items on the WAT Scale That Predict Hypnotic Talent and Percentage of Subjects of Low- or High-Hypnotic Ability Who Respond in Critical Direction to Eight Types of Test Items

Type of test items	True responses[a]			Hypnotic ability[b]
	1984 study (N = 64)	1986 study A (N = 53)	1986 study B (N = 30)	
Parapsychological	19	32	42	Low
experience	71	80	90	High
Absorption	34	21	33	Low
	84	70	85	High
Hypersensitivity to sensory	22	29	39	Low
stimuli	65	69	90	High
Fantasy	8	18	22	Low
	50	48	68	High
Control of altered states of	25	27	30	Low
consciousness	63	57	70	High
Hallucinations	11	10	22	Low
	42	47	70	High
Empathy	62	50	50	Low
	84	77	100	High
Memory	25	14	33	Low
	34	53	20	High

[a] As a percentage
[b] Low (Harvard:0–3); High (Harvard:9–12)

ening events, accidents, etc.). It is known that an unusually large proportion of physically abused people score high on hypnotic ability tests (Hilgard, 1979; Nash et al., 1984). They appear to have learned to use the natural superior hypnotic ability that children have to block out or psychologically exit the situation of mental or physical pain and abuse, I speculate that at other times adaptive hypnotic coping may sometimes occur, through high-hypnotic subjects using their profound capacity for emotional and cognitive empathy to identify the fears and superstitions of their aggressor. This information on fears and superstitions can then be used to manipulate the fears and weaknesses of the aggressor. Alternatively and less probably, the superior hypnotic subject may, by some still unknown mechanism, then cause the aggressor to perceive physical perturbations (telekinesis) in the environment as a means of frightening away the aggressor.

Good hypnotic ability may also be related to good placebo responding. In spite of some initial negative findings (McGlashan, Evans, & Orne, 1969) there is evidence that in real clinical situations (Evans, 1967) and properly structured experimental situations (Knox & Gekoski, 1981), good hypnotic subjects will also be good placebo responders. There are also some theoretical reasons as predicted by the conditioned response model of the placebo (Wickramasekera, 1977a, 1980b) to expect a relationship between placebo responding and hypnotizability (Wickramasekera, 1980b, 1985a). There is some preliminary evidence that people with superior hypnotic ability may be more sensitive to pain (Shor, 1964) and perhaps have lower sensory or tolerance thresholds for noxious stimuli. But if their superior hypnotic ability is mobilized, their pain tolerance threshold can be raised to surgical levels (Hilgard & Hilgard, 1975) by the suggestion of a negative hallucination ("your hand is in a leather glove") or anesthesia. In fact, for some subjects with superior hypnotic ability, suggestions of hypnotic analgesia may be more effective than even morphine (Stern, Brown, Ulett, & Sletten, 1977).

If psychotherapy is a healing process that involves learning, then the ability objectively to learn quickly and efficiently, and subjectively to perceive the learning as occurring effortlessly and more quickly than actual clock time, provides ideal conditions for human learning. These advantages may be available to good hypnotic subjects with appropriate instruction in and out of the hypnotic state (Bowers, 1982; Das, 1958a,b; Ingram et al., 1979; King & Mcdonald, 1976; Saccuzzo et al., 1982; St. Jean & MacLeod, 1983; Webb, 1962; Wickramasekera, 1970b). Hence, the identification of the subject's ability can enable a teacher or therapist to make learning for the subject appear quick and easy. In fact, it is likely that the general population's fantasy quest for learning that is quick and easy may be based on reports of learning in this small (10%) and highly select (high-hypnotic-ability) subset of the population who seem to learn more efficiently than the rest of us. The intermittent observation of the abilities of superior hypnotic subjects, by priests and physicians in the course of human history, has probably kept alive the belief in mind–body interaction. The dramatic effects that psychological variables (perception, memory, beliefs, imagination, information, etc.) can have on biological dependent variables in this small select group (10% of the population) of people is hard to miss observationally in religious or medical settings (Barber, 1984).

The previously cited cluster of empirical-clinical findings and speculations suggests that the good hypnotic subject's capacity for rapid learning and conditioning, profound empathy, absorption, creative mentation, role involvement, and subliminal perception may be a mixed blessing. A mixed blessing because this capacity for voluntarily accessing relatively unfiltered perceptions that can be creatively embellished makes the good hypnotic subject more vulnerable to psychological trauma and psychological pollutions (incidental learning) that can be compartmentalized (dissociated) from consciousness. But their empathic and creative capacities, their ability voluntarily to alter and program their states of consciousness (sleeping, waking, dreaming) and even perhaps adaptively to use their unconfirmed parapsychological ability, can make the superior hypnotic subject, who has good social and physical judgment and reliable discriminatory control of these hypnotic abilities, strong contenders in the struggle for survival.

The story is told that when Alexander the Great was a child in Macedonia, a powerful and magnificent stallion was brought to the court of his father. None of the great equestrians of the court were able to ride the bucking beast. Alexander, though still a child, was a keen observer and hypothesized that the animal's instability was a function of the fear of his own shadow. Therefore, he hypothesized that if the animal's face was turned toward the sun, its shadow would fall behind him and its energy could then be mobilized in a disciplined fashion. Alexander then turned the horse's face into the sun and rode into history.

Like Alexander the Great's horse, Bucephalus, when the highly hypnotizables' imagination, sensitivity, and tremendous energy are disciplined, they can be towers of sustained strength; but if their shadow falls in front of them, their behavior can become dysfunctional, unstable, and fragmented. Therapy for them requires turning their face into the sun (transcendent goals and ideals) and keeping their shadow behind them. Their empathic, creative, and psychic talents can give them an edge over their contemporaries of lesser hypnotic ability. If our species survives these perilous times, a subset of superior hypnotic subjects who are also high in IQ and have good social judgment, and are low on ANS lability (sympathetic reactivity) may learn to domesticate these hypnotic abilities in the services of superior adaptation and survival. Perhaps 20,000 years from now the percentage of humans with superior hypnotic ability may be 40% of the population and not 10% as they are today.

Increasing Hypnotic Ability

Even today it appears that certain promising psychophysiological procedures (Wickramasekera, 1977b) may temporarily produce large increases in the probability of hypnotic behavior by inhibiting that sequential critical-analytic brain program that is mediated by language and the left hemisphere. (See Figure 11.) These promising procedures include

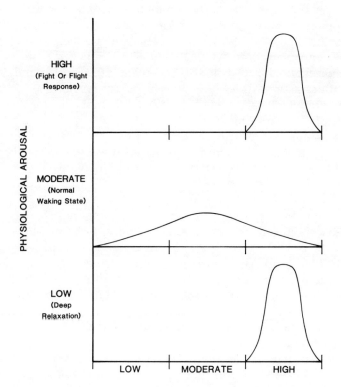

Figure 11. Hypothesized hypnotic ability in general population as a function of the level of physiological arousal.

sensory restriction (Pena, 1963; Sanders & Rehyer, 1969; Wickramase-kera, 1969, 1970a) low arousal EMG or EEG biofeedback training (Engstrom, 1976; Wickramasekera 1971, 1973, 1977b), and perhaps even high arousal induction (Gur, 1974; Wickramasekera, 1972, 1976b, 1980a). The level of physiological arousal (very low or very high) may be a critical but insufficient factor in increasing hypnotic and parapsychological suscepti-bility. Diamond (1974, 1977) has developed and presented in several well-controlled studies of "operant and informational control-based systemat-ic training" procedures that appear to produce small but more stable and generalizable increases in hypnotizability. The magnitude of these gener-alizable increases have been modest and testify to the remarkable stability of hypnotic behavior in the laboratory situation (Perry, 1977) or to the general population's relative inflexibility in switching their information processing programs under normal conditions. However, one must be cautious in assuming the cross-situational stability of personality and behavior traits (Mischel, 1968), including the hypnotic information pro-cessing style. For example, generalizing from a standardized test of hypnotic ability in a laboratory situation to a clinical situation can be hazardous. It may be much more heuristic to focus research on the mechanisms that mediate hypnotic behavior. It is very likely that the hypnosis-enhancing procedures mentioned earlier (Diamond, 1977; Wickramasekera, 1977b) will also potentiate other verbal and psycho-social influence procedures (e.g. preaching, psychoanalysis, counseling, psychotherapy, education, etc.) and even those not used for therapeutic purposes, like advertising (Wickramasekera, 1970a,c). This is particularly likely if during the course of the social-psychological influence pro-cedures the subjects experience (a) profound absorption in and (b) a sense of involuntary compliance with the verbal and nonverbal instructions of the instructor or therapist. Under such conditions we may be inclined to label the behavior of such subjects as hypnotic.

The approach outlined earlier regards hypnotic behavior as not totally discontinuous from normal social compliance, but related to hyp-nosis to the degree to which certain subject variables are activated (ab-sorption, ANS arousal, perceived involuntariness) and certain pro-cedural variables (sensory restriction, low or high arousal induction) that inhibit critical-analytic brain functions are used in the social-psychologi-cal influence procedure (Wickramasekera, 1976a). This approach to hyp-nosis is important because it restores hypnosis to the field of general psychology and encourages the investigation of its relevance to experi-mental cognitive psychology (Neisser, 1967; Nisbett & Wilson, 1977). The approach is also relevant to social psychology and the investigation of perceptual and dissociative mechanisms (Hilgard, 1977) in normal and psychopathological behavior (Kihlstrom, 1979) because it views the ability voluntarily to inhibit critical-analytic brain functions as the initial and most salient operation in hypnosis.

In conclusion, it is most important to stop thinking of hypnotic behavior as an event that only follows a hypnotic induction, in the same way one does not regard intelligent behavior as an event that only follows the administration of an intelligence test. The hypnotic mode of information processing on one hand and the rational critical-analytic mode of information processing on the other hand may be supplementary and complimentary forms of more general coping behaviors important at different stages of problem solving and with different problems.

In fact, it is likely that the hypnotic program for information processing and coping, although it is probably more primitive, has a larger channel capacity than the sequential analytic-critical brain functions program (left hemisphere) created by the development of language (Jaynes, 1977). There is some evidence that during hypnosis there is an inhibition of the left hemisphere (Gruzelier, Brow, Perry, Rhonder, & Thomas, 1984). Hypnotic ability may continue to have survival value at different stages of problem solving when judiciously blended with the objective sequential-analytic thinking characteristics of the dominant hemisphere.

Summary of Clinical Implications

What are some of the clinical implications of the experimental hypnosis research findings? First, hypnotic ability should be covertly and overtly assessed in all interpersonal healing situations regardless of whether hypnosis is formally used or not in therapy. Second, hypnosis should be presented to patients as a state of enhanced and focused concentration (like the beam of a flashlight in a dark room) in which peripheral awareness and critical-analytic mentation is temporarily suspended, in a way that permits a fresh perspective on old problems. Third, hypnotic capacity can be a positive talent or ability that has important coping and survival value for mental and physical health. But hypnotic ability can under some conditions be inadvertently used by the patient to potentiate psychosocial and other stressors. Fourth, the attainment of the hypnotic mode of information processing is the subject's achievement and only secondarily facilitated by the hypnotist. Fifth, the identification of hypnotic talent prior to therapy will facilitate a more rational matching at a baseline level of salient patient features and clinical procedures. For example, people of high-hypnotic ability can be engaged rapidly by relatively unstructured, verbally oriented therapies (gestalt, psychoanalysis, etc.) whereas people of low-hypnotic ability are more likely to be rapidly engaged by more technologically oriented and structured types of therapy (biofeedback, behavior therapy, etc.). Sixth, hypnotic ability can be an accurate predictor of the latency of symptomatic remission and a positive clinical prognosis with any interpersonal treatment modality (psychotherapy, surgery, chemotherapy, etc.), providing a good therapist–patient relationship exists. Seventh, all treatments that are learning based or have a significant learning component may profit from hypnotic-ability-enhancing procedures (Wickramasekera, 1977b).

References

Ashton, M. A. & McDonald, R. *Effect of hypnosis on verbal and non-verbal creativity*. Paper presented at American Psychological Association, Washington, DC, September, 1982.

Barber, T. X. Hypnotizability, suggestibility and personality. *Psychological Reports*, 1964, *14*, 299–320.

Barber, T. X. *Hypnosis: A scientific approach*. New York: Van Nostrand Reinhold, 1969.

Barber, T. X. Changing "unchangeable" bodily process by (hypnotic) suggestions. *Advances*, 1984, *1*, 7–40.

Benson, H., Greenwood, M. M., & Klemchuck, H. The relaxation response: Psychophysiological aspects and clinical applications. *International Journal of Psychiatric Medicine*, 1975, *6*, 87–97.

Black, S. *Mind and body*, London: William Kimber, 1969.

Bowers, K. S. *Hypnosis for the seriously curious*. New York: Norton, 1976.

Bowers, K. S., & Kelley, P. Stress, disease, psychotherapy and hypnosis. *Journal of Abnormal Psychology*, 1979, *88*, 490–505.

Bowers, K. S. & Meichenbaum, D. *Unconscious revisited*. New York: Wiley-Interscience, 1984.

Bowers, P. E. The classic suggestion effect: Relationships with scales of hypnotizability, effortless experiencing and imagery vividness. *International Journal of Clinical and Experimental Hypnosis*, 1982, *3*, 270–279.

Bowers, P. E., & Bowers, K. S. Hypnosis and creativity: A theoretical and empirical rapprochement. In E. Fromm & R. E. Shor (Eds.), *Hypnosis: developments in research and new perspectives* (2nd ed.). New York: Aldine, 1979.

Cedercreutz, C. Hypnotic treatment of 100 cases of migraines. In F. H. Frankel & H. S. Zamansky (Eds.), *Hypnosis at its bicentennial*. New York: Plenum Press, 1978.

Collison, D. A. Which asthmatic patients should be treated by hypnotherapy. *Medical Journal of Australia*, 1975, *1*, 776–781.

Dane, J. R. *A comparison of waking instructions and posthypnotic suggestion for lucid dream induction*. Unpublished doctoral dissertation, Georgia State University, Atlanta, 1984.

Das, J. P. The Pavlovian theory of hypnosis: An evaluation. *Journal of Mental Sciences*, 1958, *104*, 82–90. (a)

Das, J. P. Conditioning and hypnosis. *Journal of Experimental Psychology*, 1958, *56*, 110–113. (b)

Dave, R. Effects of hypnotically induced dreams on creative problem solving. *Journal of Abnormal Psychology*, 1979, *88*, 293–302.

Diamond, M. J. Modification of hypnotizability: A review. *Psychological Bulletin*, 1974, *81*, 180–193.

Diamond, M. J. Issues and methods for modifying responsivity to hypnosis. *Annals of the New York Academy of Sciences*, 1977, *296*, 119–128.

Engstrom, D. R. Hypnotic susceptibility, EEG-alpha and self-regulation. In G. E. Schwartz & D. Shapiro (Eds.), *Consciousness and self-regulation*. New York: Plenum Press, 1976.

Evans, F. J. *The structure of hypnosis: A factor analytic investigation*. Unpublished doctoral dissertation, University of Sydney, Sydney, Australia, 1965.

Evans, F. J. Suggestibility in the normal waking state. *Psychological Bulletin*, 1967, *2*, 114–129.

Evans, F. J. Hypnosis and sleep: The control of altered states of consciousness. *Annals of the New York Academy of Sciences*, 1977, *296*, 162–174.

Evans, F. J. Forensic uses and abuses of hypnosis. *American Psychological Association, Division 30 Newsletter*. April 1983, p. 6.

Evans, F. J., Orne, E. C., & Markowsky, P. A. *Punctuality and hypnotizability*. Paper presented at Eastern Psychological Association, Boston, Massachusetts, April 1977.

Eysenck, H. J. *The structure of human personality* (2nd ed.). London: Methuen, 1960.

Foenander, G., Burrows, G. D., Gerschman, J., & Horne, D. J. Phobic behavior and hypnotic susceptibility. *Australian Journal of Clinical and Experimental Hypnosis*, 1980, *8*, 41–46.

Frankel, F. H. & Orne, M. T. Hypnotizability and phobic behavior. *Archives of General Psychiatry*, 1976, *33*, 1259–1261.

Gerschman, J., Burrows, G. D., Reade, P., & Foenander, G. Hypnotizability and the treatment of dental phobic behavior. In G. D. Burrows, D. R. Collison, & L. Dennerstein (Eds.), *Hypnosis*. New York: Elsevier, 1979.

Graham, C., & Evans, F. J. Hypnotizability and the deployment of working attention. *Journal of Abnormal Psychology*, 1977, *86*, 631–638.

Graham, K. R., & Greene, L. D. Hypnotic susceptibility related to an independent measure of compliance—Alumni annual giving. *International Journal of Clinical and Experimental Hypnosis*, 1981, *29*, 351–354.

Gruzelier, J., Brow, T., Perry, A., Rhonder, J., & Thomas M. Hypnotic susceptibility: A lateral predisposition and altered cerebral asymmetry under hypnosis. *International Journal of Psychophysiology*, 1984, *2*, 131–139.

Gur, R. C. An attention-controlled operant procedure for enhancing hypnotic susceptibility. *Journal of Abnormal Psychology*, 1974, *83*, 644–650.

Hammer, A. G., Evans, F. J., & Bartlett, M. Factors in hypnosis and suggestion. *Journal of Abnormal and Social Psychology*, 1963, *67*, 15–23.

Hilgard, E. R. *Hypnotic susceptibility*. New York: Harcourt, Brace & World, 1965.

Hilgard, E. R. *Divided consciousness: Multiple controls in human thought and action*. New York: Wiley-Interscience, 1977.

Hilgard, E. R. Hypnotic susceptibility: Implications for measurement. *International Journal of Experimental and Clinical Hypnosis*, 1982, *30*, 394–403.

Hilgard, E. R., & Hilgard, J. R. *Hypnosis In the relief of pain*. Los Altos, CA: Kaufman, 1975.

Hilgard, E. R., & Tart, C. T. Responsiveness to suggestions following waking and imagination instructions and following induction of hypnosis. *Journal of Abnormal Psychology*, 1966, *71*, 196–208.

Hilgard, J. R. *Personality and hypnosis: A study of imaginative involvement* (rev. ed.). Chicago: University of Chicago Press, 1979.

Horne, R. L., Evans, F. J., & Orne, M. T. Random number generation, psychopathology and therapeutic change. *Archives of General Psychiatry*, 1982, *39*, 680–683.

Hull, C. *Hypnosis and suggestibility*. New York: Appleton-Century Crofts, 1933.

Ingram, R. E., Saccuzzo, D. P., McNeil, B. W., & McDonald, R. Speed of information processing in high and low susceptible subjects: A preliminary study. *International Journal of Clinical and Experimental Hypnosis*, 1979, *27*(1), 42–47.

Jaynes, J. *The origins of consciousness in the breakdown of the bicameral mind*. Boston: Houghton Mifflin, 1977.

Kelly, S. F. Measured hypnotic response and phobic behavior. *International Journal of Clinical and Experimental Hypnosis*, 1984, *32*, 1–5.

Kihlstrom, J. F. Models of posthypnotic amnesia. *Annals of the New York Academy of Sciences*, 1977, *296*, 284–301.

Kihlstrom, J. F. Hypnosis and psychopathology: Retrospect and prospect. *Journal of Abnormal Psychology*, 1979, *88*(5), 459–473.

King, D. R., & McDonald, R. D. Hypnotic susceptibility and verbal conditioning. *International Journal of Clinical and Experimental Hypnosis*, 1976, *24*, 29–37.

Knox, V. J., & Gekoski, W. L. *Analgesic effect of acupuncture in high and low hypnotizables.* Paper presented at a meeting of the Society for Clinical and Experimental Hypnosis, 1981, October.

LaBerge, S. P. *Awake in your dreams: The new world of lucid dreaming*. New York: Simon & Schuster, 1983.

Larsen, S. Strategies for reducing phobic behavior. *Dissertation Abstracts*, 1966, *26*, 6850.

Laurence, J. R., & Perry, C. Hypnotically created memory and highly hypnotizable subjects. *Science*, 1983, *222*, 523–524.

London, P., & Fuhrer, M. Hypnosis, motivation and performance. *Journal of Personality*, 1961, *29*, 321–333.

Maslach, C., Marshall, G., & Zimbardo, P. G. Hypnotic control of peripheral skin temperature: A case report. *Psychophysiology*, 1972, *9*(6), 600–605.

McGlashen, T. H., Evans, F. J., & Orne, M. T. The nature of hypnotic analgesia and placebo response to experimental pain. *Psychosomatic Medicine*, 1969, *31*, 227–246.

Mischel, W. *Personality and assessment*, New York: Wiley, 1968.

Monterio, K., McDonald, H., & Hilgard, E. R. Imagery, absorption and hypnosis: A factorial study. *Journal of Mental Imagery*, 1980, *4*, 63–81.

Morgan, A. H. The heritability of hypnotic susceptibility in twins. *Journal of Abnormal Psychology*, 1973, *82*, 55–66.

Morgan, A. H., & Hilgard, E. R. Age differences in susceptibility to hypnosis. *International Journal of Clinical and Experimental Hypnosis*, 1973, *21*, 78–85.

Morgan, A. H., Hilgard, E. R., & Darert, E. C. The heritability of hypnotic susceptibility of twins: A preliminary report. *Behavioral Genetics*, 1970, *1*, 213–224.

Nace, E. P., Warwick, A. M., Kelley, R. L., & Evans, F. J. Hypnotizability and outcome in brief psychotherapy. *Journal of Clinical Psychiatry*, 1982, *43*, 129–133.

Nash, M. R., Lynn, S. J., & Givens, D. L. Adult hypnotic susceptibility, childhood punishment, and child abuse: A brief communication. *International Journal of Clinical and Experimental Hypnosis*, 1984, *32*(1), 6–11.

Neisser, U. *Cognitive psychology*. New York: Appleton-Century Crofts, 1967.

Nisbett, R. E., & Wilson, T. D. Telling more than we know: Verbal reports on mental processes. *Psychological Review*, 1977, *84*, 231–259.

Orne, M. T. The construct of hypnosis: Implications of the definition for research and practice. *Annals of the New York Academy of Sciences*, 1977, *296*, 1–314.

Orne, M. T. (Chair). Scientific status of refreshing recollection by the use of hypnosis

(Council Report of American Medical Association). *International Journal of Clinical and Experimental Hypnosis*, 1986, *34*, 1–12.

Pena, F. *Perceptual isolation and hypnotic susceptibility*. Unpublished doctoral dissertation, Washington State University, Pullman, Washington, 1963.

Perry, C. Is hypnotizability modifiable? *International Journal of Clinical and Experimental Hypnosis*, 1977, *25*, 125–146.

Perry, C., John, R., & Hollander, B. *Hypnotizability and phobic behavior*. Paper presented at the 34th Annual S.E.C.H. Convention, Indianapolis, October, 1982.

Perry, C., Gelfand, R., & Marcovitch, P. The relevance of hypnotic susceptibility in the clinical context. *Journal of Abnormal Psychology*, 1979, *88*, 592–603.

Pettinati, H. M., Horne, R. L., & Staats, J. M. Hypnotizability in patients with anorexia nervosa and bulimia. *Archives of General Psychiatry*, 1985, *42*, 1014–1016.

Rivers, S. M. *Hypnosis and meditation*. Paper read at 84th Annual Convention of American Psychological Association, Washington, D.C., 1976.

Saccuzzo, D. P., Safnan, D., Anderson, V., & McNeill, B. Visual information processing in high and low susceptible subjects. *International Journal of Clinical and Experimental Hypnosis*, 1982, *30*, 32–44.

Sackeim, H. A., Packer, I. K., & Gur, R. C. Hemisphericity, cognitive set, and susceptibility to subliminal perception. *Journal of Abnormal Psychology*, 1977, *86*, 624–630.

Sanders, R. S., & Rehyer, J. Sensory deprivation and the enhancement of hypnotic susceptibility. *Journal of Abnormal Psychology*, 1969, *74*, 375–381.

Shevrin, H., & Dickman, S. The psychological unconscious: A necessary assumption for all psychological theory? *American Psychologist*, 1980, *35*, 421–434.

Shor, R. E. A note on the shock tolerance of real and simulating hypnotic subjects. *International Journal of Clinical and Experimental Hypnosis*, 1964, *12*, 258–262.

Shor, R. E., & Orne, E. C. *Manual: Harvard Group Scale of Hypnotic Susceptibility Form A*. Palo Alto, CA: Consulting Psychologists Press, 1962.

Spanos, N. P., & Barber, T. X. Toward a convergence in hypnosis research. *American Psychologist*, 1974, *29*, 500–511.

Spiegel, D., Detrick, D., & Frischolz, E. Hypnotizability and psychopathology. *American Journal of Psychiatry*, 1982, *139*(4), 431–437.

Spiegel, H., An eye-roll test for hypnotizability. *American Journal of Clinical Hypnosis*, 1972, *15*(1), 25–28.

Stern, J. A., Brown, M., Ulett, G. A., & Sletten, I. A comparison of hypnosis, acupuncture, morphine, valium, aspirin, and placebo in the management of experimentally induced pain. *Annals of the New York Academy of Sciences*, 1977, *296*, 175–193.

St. Jean, R., & MacLeod, C. Hypnosis, absorption and time perception. *Journal of Abnormal Psychology*, 1983, *92*, 81–86.

Stoyva, J. M. Posthypnotically suggested dreams and the sleep cycle. *Archives of General Psychiatry*, 1965, *12*, 287–294.

Webb, R. A. Suggestibility and verbal conditioning. *International Journal of Clinical and Experimental Hypnosis*, 1962, *10*, 275–279.

Weiss, R. L., Ullman, L. P., & Krasner, L. On the relationship between hypnotizability and response to verbal operant conditioning. *Psychological Reports*, 1960, 59–60.

Weitzenhoffer, A. M., & Hilgard, E. R. *Stanford Hypnotic Susceptibility Scale Form C*. Palo Alto: Consulting Psychologists Press, 1962.

Wickramasekera, I. The effects of sensory restriction on hypnotic susceptibility. *International Journal of Clinical and Experimental Hypnosis*, 1969, *17*, 217–224.

Wickramasekera, I. The effects of sensory restriction on hypnosis: A hypothesis and more preliminary data. *Journal of Abnormal Psychology*, 1970, *76*, 69–75. (a)

Wickramasekera, I. *The effects of hypnosis and a control procedure on verbal conditioning.* Paper presented at the meeting of the American Psychological Association, Miami, September 1970. (b)

Wickramasekera, I. Goals and some methods in psychotherapy: Hypnosis and isolation. *American Journal of Clinical Hypnosis,* 1970, *13*(2) 95–107. (c)

Wickramasekera, I. Reinforcement and/or transference in hypnosis and psychotherapy: A hypnothesis. *American Journal of Clinical Hypnosis.* 1970, *12*(3), 137–140. (d)

Wickramasekera, I. Effects of EMG feedback training on susceptibility to hypnosis: preliminary observations. *Proceedings of the 79th Annual Convention of the American Psychological Association,* 1971, *6*, 787–785. (Summary)

Wickramasekera, I. A technique for controlling a certain type of sexual exhibitionism. *Psychotherapy: Theory, research and practice,* 1972, *9*, 207–210.

Wickramasekera, I. The effects of EMG feedback on hypnotic susceptibility: More preliminary data. *Journal of Abnormal Psychology,* 1973, *82*, 74–77.

Wickramasekera, I. (Ed.). *Biofeedback, behavior therapy, and hypnosis.* Chicago: Nelson-Hall, 1976. (a)

Wickramasekera, I. Aversive behavior rehearsal for sexual exhibitionism. *Behavior Therapy,* 1976, *7*, 167–176. (b)

Wickramasekera, I. The placebo effect and biofeedback for headache pain. *Proceedings of the San Diego Biomedical Symposium.* New York: Academic Press, 1977. (a)

Wickramasekera, I. On attempts to modify hypnotic susceptibility: Some psychophysiological procedures and promising directions. *Annals of the New York Academy of Sciences,* 1977, *296*, 143–153. (b)

Wickramasekera, I. *A model of the patient at high risk for chronic stress-related disorders.* Paper presented at Annual Convention of the Biofeedback Society of America, San Diego, California, 1979.

Wickramasekera, I. Aversive behavior rehearsal: A cognitive behavioral procedure. In D. J. Cox & R. J. Daitzman (Eds.), *Exhibitionism: Description, assessment and treatment.* New York: Harland, 1980. (a)

Wickramasekera, I. A conditioned response model of the placebo effect: Predictions from the model. *Biofeedback and Self-Regulation,* 1980, *5*, 5–18. (b)

Wickramasekera, I. A model of people at risk to develop chronic stress related disorders. In F. J. McGuigan, W. E. Sime, J. MacDonald-Wallace (Eds.), *Stress and tension control.* New York: Plenum Press, 1984.

Wickramasekera, I. A conditioned response model of the placebo effect: Predictions and postdiction from the model. In L. White, B. Tusky, & G. Schwartz (Eds.), *Placebo: Clinical phenomena and new insights.* New York: Guilford Press, 1985. (a)

Wickramasekera, I. *Development of a self-report measure of hypnotic ability: Preliminary findings.* Paper presented at the Biofeedback Society of America, 1985, New Orleans. (b)

Wickramasekera, I. Parapsychological verbal reports, hypnotizability, and stress-related disorders. Paper invited to the *35th Annual International Conference on Parapsychology,* Washington, D. C., November, 1986.

Wilson, S. C., & Barber, T. X. The fantasy-prone personality: implications for understanding imagery, hypnosis and parapsychological phenomena. In A. A. Sheikh (Ed.), *Imagery: Current theory research and application.* New York: Wiley, 1982.

4

CROCKS, QUACKS, AND SHRINKS

*Pain syndrome patients, in their desperate search
for the elusive cure, often chase "windmills" and
convince their doctors to perform a myriad of
invasive tests and procedures. As a result of their
pain behaviors, many experience iatrogenic
complications, suffering and disability. Those
involved in their treatment must find improved
ways to detect this highly susceptible population,
establish a therapeutic alliance and short-circuit
their pain careers. . . . Do the health care
providers truly get to know the patients and their
psychosocial dilemmas which, as studies indicate,
often contribute to or cause the medical
complaints? Or is this lack of rapport an
unavoidable consequence of the increasing
depersonalization within the medical system? The
now antiquated model of the physician-healer who
visited the patient's home has been replaced by the
all too frequent scenario of the patient who takes a
tranquilizer before going to the physician's office.*
—G. M. Aronoff, M.D.,
The Clinical Journal of Pain, 1985

In 1950, health care costs accounted for 4.6% of the gross national product. In 1985, health care costs accounted for 10.8% of the gross national product (Cohen, 1985). Sophisticated biomedical technology and expensive medical tests have contributed to this cost escalation (Culliton, 1978). This massive increase in health care costs appears to have occurred without a comparable increase in health status (DeLeon & VandenBos, 1983) of United States citizens as measured by morbidity, mortality, longevity, and so on.

It appears that another major contributor to this escalating cost is the patient who presents somatic complaints without physical findings

and the patient whose somatic problems are exacerbated by psychosocial factors. "These patients are very common in general medical practices and consume a disproportionately large fraction of physician services, diagnostic procedures and therapeutic resources" (Barsky &
Klermen, 1983). Studies of primary care practice report that between
68% to 92% of patients are without serious physical disease (Brown *et
al.*, 1971; Garfield *et al.*, 1976). It has been estimated that between 30% to
80% of patients who consult a physician have functional complaints
(Lowy, 1975). Data from the National Ambulatory Medical Care Survey
(Jencks, 1985) shows a rate of recognition of mental distress for adult
patients in primary care settings of at least double the rate of diagnosis
of mental disorder in the primary care settings. For several reasons to be
presented later, primary care physicians are reluctant to make a mental
diagnosis, to use a specific mental therapy themselves, or to refer the
patient to a psychologist or psychiatrist. Previous studies of the primary
care situation have reported that 15% to 40% of these patients have
diagnosable mental disorders (Goldberg, 1980; Orleans, George, Houpt,
& Brodie, 1985). It is known that most patients with mental disorders are
seen only in the primary care sector of the medical care system (Regier,
Goldberg, & Taube, 1978). A recent national survey (Orleans *et al.*, 1985)
of 350 family practice physicians found that 75% of them blamed patient
resistance to psychiatric referral and lack of family physician time as the
major obstacles to effective management of emotional disorders presented in their practice. Insufficient physician training was also listed as a
secondary obstacle to the effective treatment of emotional disorders.
Anxiety, stress, and tension states were picked by 99% of the previously
cited physicians as among the six most commonly seen symptoms in
primary care practice. Chronic pain, gastrointestinal disorders (exclud-
ing cancer), symptoms of ill-defined conditions, and psychophysiological and pain disorders received frequency ratings of 93.4%, 82.9%,
81.1%, and 67.1% respectively. These figures clearly demonstrate how
frequently functionally based somatic or psychological symptoms are
presented to a nationwide sample of primary care physicians. Based on
a national survey of 16,576 visits to internists, family practitioners, and
general practitioners, by patients over age 15 years, Jencks (1985) concluded that physicians may fail to record a mental diagnosis for several
reasons, including the fact that physicians (a) feel unskilled in mental
diagnosis; (b) fear that the patient will be stigmatized; (c) fear that the
patient will object to the diagnosis; or (d) fear that third parties will not
reimburse for services. It is becoming increasingly clear that efforts to
treat these patients with strictly biomedical methods (drugs, surgery,

etc.) or with expensive and sophisticated tests and procedures is a costly exercise in futility.

The failures of drugs, surgery, and sophisticated medical technology to remedy current chronic-stress-related somatic illness (e.g. cardiovascular and musculoskeletal disorders, etc.) results partly from the fact that the bulk of the stressors that impinge on most of these patients seldom involves direct and clear-cut tissue damage. The triggers for these chronic disorders are psychosocial stressors that may include an unhappy marriage or the stress of a divorce, a problem child, elderly parents who reside in your home, a hypercritical boss, unrealistic performance standards (at work or in social relationships), loneliness, or unrealistic health expectations (Benson, 1979). Frequently the stressors present as major life changes (Rahe, 1975) or multiple minor hassles or as chronic ambigious and ambivalent feelings that progressively elicit cumulative psychophysiological hyperarousal and sustained muscular bracing (Whatmore & Kohli, 1974). It is easy to feel ambivalent about an unhappy marriage that ends in a divorce that brings relief and sadness. These complex psychosocial problems cannot be remediated by primitive fight or flight mechanisms or alternatively by modern drugs or surgery. Beating your spouse and running away are not long-term solutions to these problems, nor are benzodiazepines and symptomatic surgery. Patients need to know that when they cannot fight or flee they can learn to "flow" with what cannot be changed. Skills like cognitive reframing and low arousal training (relaxation, etc.) can facilitate acceptance of the inevitable. Yet many patients continue to seek, and many physicians to offer, exclusively biomedical solutions (drugs and surgery) to these complex psychosocial problems (Cummings, 1979).

There are probably several reasons why patients continue to look for and why physicians continue to provide exclusively medical solutions to complex human problems.

1. The mass media and voluntary health care organizations (e.g., Heart Association, etc.) continue to dramatize the real achievements of modern medicine but also create unrealistic expectations. Organized medicine has, on the whole, encouraged the belief in the physician's omniscience. Hamburg and Brown (1978) stated, "It is probably true that expectations about the scope and abilities of medicine are out of line with reality." This propaganda needs to be moderated by a critical appreciation of the scope and limits of modern medical science. A critical appreciation of these factors includes knowledge of the base rates of pathological events, spontaneous remission rates, nonspecific effects, the distinction between palliation and cure, the role of the immune

system in recovery, and recognition that the etiology of poor health is often multifactorial (Frazier & Hiatt, 1978). Ingelfinger (1978) pointed out that

> organized medicine has on the whole encouraged a belief in the doctors omniscience rather than ignorance. The news media, whether printed or televised, compete with each other to broadcast the latest "breakthrough" with findings that are at best preliminary and at worst totally unfounded. But perhaps most culpable are the massive voluntary health groups. In one fearsome advertisement after another, these organizations suggest to the public that, if only a few more dollars were thrown in the research till, the major killer diseases would be contained. Tommy-rot. It is organizations such as these, along with medical societies, news media, and politicians that promise too much, that are in large part responsible for the fact that we are feeling worse though actually doing better. (pp. 944–945)

2. The strictly biomedical approach appears to get results in spite of ignoring psychosocial factors in dysfunction and disease. This is a tempting and seductive alternative. It does not inconveniently intrude on the patient's life-style or priorities, however maladaptive they may be to the patient's health from a long-term viewpoint. Patients would like to do all the conflicting, complex, and stressful things they do currently and insist that the "miracles of modern medicine" be prostituted to stifle the complaints (aches and pains) of their body. For example, a popular TV commercial suggests that ingesting a pill rather than reducing gluttony is the proper solution to the problem of indigestion. Medicine has clearly reached the limits of a strictly biological approach to illness, as demonstrated by the recent plea of a distinguished medical educator for a biopsychosocial model of illness (Engel, 1977).

3. The medical model appears to encourage a perception of the patient as a passive recipient of both illness and medical interventions. The patient does not appear in any way to need actively to participate in his own resistance to illness and its treatment. But, of course, this is an illusion because healing is in fact a function of the interaction of the body's own defenses against disease and trauma with the specific medical treatments. Also, psychological and behavioral reactions can potentiate or attenuate the effectiveness of medical management. There is now growing evidence that psychological and behavioral factors can increase or decrease vulnerability to physical illness and disease. For example, it has been shown that stress and depression may reduce the antibody response and that adult immunological responsivity may be related to childhood experiences (Rasmussen, 1969; Solomon, 1969; Solomon, Amkraut, & Kasper, 1974). There is preliminary evidence that psychological factors can influence the clinical course of human cancer (Krantz,

Grunberg, & Baum, 1985) and there is experimental evidence that Pavlovian conditioning can influence the immune system (Ader & Cohen,
1984). Several studies have shown that susceptibility to infectious disease is influenced by psychosocial factors (Jemmott & Locke, 1984). Retrospective and predictive studies show a strong relationship between a
certain type of behavior (Type A) and the incidence of heart disease
(Friedman & Rosenman, 1974; Review Panel on Coronary-Prone Behavior and Coronary Heart Disease, 1981).

An experimental study of young healthy volunteers who were exposed to experimental tularemia demonstrated that: (a) the onset of
psychological mood changes (during incubation) preceded the onset of
fever by at least 6 hours in 24 of 34 subjects (70.5%) who developed
fever. (b) Subjects who were psychologically more vulnerable (as defined by scores on a specific scale) before exposure to infection became
more severely physically ill on the average than nonvulnerable subjects
during the acute illness period. They also showed greater mood change
and more depressive moods during the incubation and acute illness
periods. Hence it appears that persons who are psychologically vulnerable are also biologically more vulnerable. (c) Mood changes appear to be
a sensitive indicator of impending changes in the biological state (Canter, 1972). In a study of 315 normal adults, significantly ($p<.001$) more of
the psychologically vulnerable subjects developed a hypersensitive reaction (erythema, induration, and/or edema at the site of the innoculation,
chills, fever, diarrhea, etc.) to innoculation than psychologically nonvulnerable subjects (Canter, Cluff, & Imboden, 1972). Retrospective and
now prospective studies have shown that the rate of recovery from
influenza, chronic brucellosis, and respiratory infections is predictable
from psychological data (Brodman, Mittelman, Wechsler, Weider, &
Wolff, 1947; Imboden, Canter, & Cluff, 1961) and a recent comprehensive review (Rogers, Dubey, & Reigh, 1979) of the evidence for the
influence of the mind and brain on immunity and disease susceptibility
leaves little doubt that such a functional relationship exists. But the
mechanisms of such interaction remains unclear.

The previously cited studies demonstrate that psychological variables can potentiate or attenuate a person's vulnerability to physical
disease. A psychologically vulnerable individual is likely to be also biologically vulnerable. Also, the vast literature on the placebo effect in
medicine demonstrates, albeit in a less systematic way, that even the
active ingredient in a drug can be attenuated, potentiated, or negated in
at least one-third of patients by psychological variables in patient and
therapist (Shapiro, 1971; Wickramasekera, 1985).

4. Psychological interventions are intrusive, complex, and time-

consuming. They frequently conflict with established life-styles and priorities and require that patients movilize their own resources toward the uncertain attainment of a goal. Medical interventions are typically circumscribed, nonintrusive of one's life-style, and require a minimum of a patient's time and effort. Hence, they are more likely to be popular with most patients.

5. The conventionally trained psychotherapist (M.D. or Ph.D.) is not eager to see these patients for several reasons. First, the "somatizing" patient's definition and perception of his or her own problem is the major obstacle. Psychotherapy for a migraine headache has zero face validity to the patient. This perception produces a skeptical, noncompliant patient with little or no commitment to conventional psychotherapy. Second, conventional psychotherapists have typically felt ineffective with these patients and hence there may be a tacit conspiracy of silence to discourage the patient's return. Third, many of these patients do not fit the widely recognized characteristics of the good psychotherapy candidate (who is bright, introspective, psychologically minded, middle class, etc.). In fact, it is very likely that psychotherapy is an essential but an insufficient condition for durable and effective intervention with these chronic-stress-related disorders.

6. Patients regard physical problems as totally involuntary and as making no reflection on their self-esteem, but they see psychological problems as voluntary and possibly implying a "weak" mind. The research on biofeedback demonstrates that even clearly physical problems like classic migraine are amenable to voluntary self-regulation, whereas the poor rate of response and high rate of recidivism for certain behavioral problems like obesity, smoking, and alcoholism, demonstrates the quasi-involuntary character of some chronic behavioral problems. The simplistic view that all behavioral problems are voluntary and that all medical problems are involuntary is no longer tenable.

In response to patient pressures (Barsky & Klerman, 1983; Orleans *et al.*, 1985), lack of physical information about efficacious psychobehavioral alternatives (Jencks, 1985; Orleans *et al.*, 1985), and perhaps in some cases because of financial incentives (Ingelfinger, 1978; Relman, 1980), some physicians continue to trot out the same old tired remedies such as tranquilizers, sleeping pills, pain pills, (Blackwell, 1975; Cummings, 1979), more hospitalization, and more diagnostic tests. For example, in 1985 the five most frequently prescribed drugs were Dyazide, Inderal, Lanoxin, Valium, and Tylenol with codeine (Pierson, 1985). All the drugs cited are prescribed for chronic-stress-related disorders and seldom for acute active infectious disease. A strictly biomedical approach to health care ignores the patient's potential coping skills, potential social supports, and personal but modifiable psychophysiological vulnerabilities. Drugs, hospitalization, and surgery alone are not adequate long-term remedies for the somatic symptoms that are the final common pathway for multiple complex psychosocial conflicts that mark complex industrial cultures and physical environments. In the Mumford, Schlesinger, Glass, Patrick, and Cuerdon (1984) review of 58 studies, 85% of the studies reviewed reported a decrease in medical utilization following psychotherapy. The fact that the reduction in medical utilization was most pronounced for inpatient medical costs (presumably more severely ill patients) and for persons over age 55 (who are generally regarded as less able to learn new skills and have more documented physical disease) is a powerful illustration of the inseparability of mind and body in health care. It is becoming clear that the mind–body dichotomy is *the* major obstacle to a cost-effective health care system.

Crocks and Quacks

Meanwhile the cost of health care continues to soar, from 4.6% of the G.N.P. in 1950 to 10.81% in 1986. The new medical-industrial complex (proprietary hospitals, proprietary nursing homes, home care services, laboratory, and other services, etc.) was estimated (Relman, 1980) to have a gross income of approximately 35 to 40 billion dollars in 1980. Dr. Relman, writing in the highly respected *New England Journal of Medicine*, which he edits, points out that physicians, because of "informational inequality," serve as trustees for their patients' medical expenditures and hence they should have no "pecuniary association" with the new medical-industrial complex. But in fact, as Dr. Relman points out, it is likely that many practicing physicians are heavily invested in the new health care industry. Third-party reimbursement policies continue to provide the patient and physician with financial incentives for somatic presentations of psychosocial distress. For example, tension headaches or chronic low back pain are more reimbursable diagnoses than anxiety and depression. These insurance reimbursement policies persist in spite of the growing evidence that the provision of psychotherapy reduces the utilization of medical services by at least 20% (Jones & Vischi, 1979) and the more recent evidence that this reduction is most marked for inpatient costs (hospital), and particularly for persons over age 55 (Mumford et al., 1984).

The cognitive and behavioral components of these physically presented disturbances are seldom systematically examined by a primary care physician. There is, in fact, often a tacit conspiracy of silence between patient and physician regarding psychosocial factors in the patient's illness. The busy medical practitioner often does not have the training, the time, or the inclination to sit down and explore the psychosocial origins or exacerbating factors in the chronic diseases these patients present (Jencks, 1985; Orleans et al., 1985). The physician would rather treat legitimate disease with clear physical findings, or acute medical emergencies (Ingelfinger, 1978). He treats legitimate disease, for which he was specifically trained, effectively, rapidly, and economically. But many of his patients, who are committed to a physical presentation (e.g., pain and insomnia) of psychosocial distress, insist that in spite of the negative physical findings on exam and lab studies, the physician do something medical for them immediately. Often the patient is also resistant to a psychosocial exploration, much less explanation, of his symptoms. The health insurance industry, through its reimbursement policies, reinforces physician and patient for the continued exploration of organic causes with expensive biomedical tests. Health insurance policies are much more likely to pay for expensive radical surgical interventions and extended hospitalizations than for more conservative psychosocial investigations and outpatient psychological therapy (Mumford et al., 1984; Orleans et al., 1985). The physician may be pressured by his patient into prescribing a psychotropic or analgesic medication, or perhaps into ordering a new series of expensive and sometimes even hazardous medical tests, plus hospitalization. Because of errors in medication administration, and exposure to pathogens, hospitalization per se is not without risk (Benson, 1979). The results of the new tests are frequently negative or inconclusive and merely serve to confirm the physician's original impression from history and physical examination (Frazier & Hiatt, 1978; Ingelfinger, 1978; Tancredi & Barondess, 1978). The patient is dissatisfied with these new inconclusive or negative diagnostic findings and new drug treatments because of his persisting subjective symptoms. He loses confidence in his physician and in his physician's investigations because no physical cause has been identified. The reality of his complaints is challenged. He may gradually come to regard the physician as an incompetent "quack." The frustrated but conscientious physician, in this atmosphere of failure, frustration, and hostility, may come to retaliate by privately regarding the patient as a "crock" (Barsky & Klerman, 1983). The patient's failure to respond to narrow biomedical investigations and therapy and his resistance to psychosocial investigations (Jencks, 1985; Orleans et al., 1985) leaves the physician feeling ineffective and uncomfortably impotent. Impotence is not a feeling many physicians like (Ingelfinger, 1978), and consequently the recalcitrant patient is labeled a "crock." After this often tacit and unproductive "crock–quack" interchange, the patient will often move on to another medical practitioner who is again pressured into repeating another set of laboratory test procedures and even escalating to exploratory surgery. As these frustrating and unpleasant transactions between physician and patient continue, the confidence of the patient in the general health care system slowly erodes, further reducing the probability of resolving the patient's problems.

Numerous double-blind studies have shown that patients' confidence in their physicians and other nonspecified therapeutic effects account for at least 33% of positive outcome effects in drug studies of physical illness (Beecher, 1959; Evans, 1974; Shapiro, 1971; Wickramasekera, 1977, 1980). These frustrating, credibility-dissolving and passive-aggressive contacts with physicians reduce the likelihood that the future application of even the most appropriate clinical judgment and active ingredients will easily resolve the patient's physical symptoms (Wickramasekera, 1980, 1985).

The patient's continued commitment to a somatic presentation and explanation of a largely or exclusively functional problem has several consequences. The cost of the health care system is inflated by excessive use of diagnostic tests (Culliton, 1978), and valuable and scarce medical and hospital resources are tied up in costly and ineffective evaluations and interventions (Barsky & Klerman, 1983) of these patients who remain committed to a physical presentation and a medical solution. Many of these patients end up personally demoralized, alienated from their social support systems (because of their chronic complaints), and are eventually chronically managed with tranquilizers, analgesics, and/or sleep medications. Chronic use of these medications can include hazards like tolerance, dependence, and negative physical and mental side effects (Blackwell, 1975; Cummings, 1979). Because of hazardous tests and inappropriate surgery, some develop iatrogenic complications. All of the previously cited conditions can create further psychosocial problems. This appearance of medical treatment that is directed at symptoms may postpone attention to the underlying psychosocial etiology or exacerbating factors.

A number of these patients require a biological-medical excuse to talk about psychosocial distress with their medical doctor. If the physician should suggest that the patient see a "shrink" (psychologist or psychiatrist), the probability of resolution is not significantly improved because of the low rate of patient compliance with such referrals. The patient does not believe that he is crazy or that the problem is all "in his head" and, in fact, his symptoms may have subtle and typically unrecognized (by standard medical tests) psychophysiological correlates

(Whatmore & Kohli, 1974). Most of these patients keep biological and psychological matters stringently separate. Their conviction of illness and commitment to a physical presentation of psychosocial distress is expressed in the decision to see a primary care medical doctor. It is estimated that 80% of the visits to emergency rooms in general hospitals are not strictly medical emergencies (Gibson, Bugbee, & Anderson, 1970; Knowles, 1973). Cummings (1977) and others (Mumford *et al.*, 1984) review the evidence that people with emotional and mental disorders overutilize medical services. Franz Ingelfinger (1978) stated that three-quarters of physician–patient contacts are occasioned by complaints that are either self-limited or for which medicine has no specific remedies. However, the skill, tact, and knowledge required to help a patient make the major transition from a biological to a psychological definition and presentation of their problem is often unappreciated by the naive and impatient mental health practitioner. Psychotherapists prefer to see patients who are already inclined to a psychological definition of their problem. But somatic packaging of psychosocial distress is even objectively preferable today. Because when somatically packaged, the symptoms are most reliably and completely reimbursable by insurance companies; additionally, somatic packaging has few or no aversive social, vocational, or political consequences for the patient.

The crux of the problem is that the patient defines his symptoms in strictly biological or physiological terms (a change in tissue structure or function) and is committed to a physical solution to his problem. The patient does not believe that physical symptoms can be the final common pathway for psychosocial stress. Even if there are several years of good rapport between a primary care physician and patient, it is unlikely, for several reasons, that the patient will accept a stress explanation of his symptoms. First, the patient may not currently, subjectively feel under stress; in both the psychological and physiological (e.g., muscle tension, etc.) domains the patient may feel subjectively relaxed except for his or her episodic, unpleasant physical symptoms. This is possible because people can be unaware of or habituate (become subjectively unaware) to chronically and abnormally elevated levels of, for example, muscle tension or elevated blood pressure, until these physiological elevations cross a threshold at which point the patient becomes clinically symptomatic (headache, backache, angina, stroke, myocardial infarction, etc.). This situation is commonly seen with muscle tension headache, vascular headache, and essential hypertension in which silent changes in physiology occur while the patient may be for several months or years subjectively symptom free. Second, the patient may be unable to identify or recognize any current psychological stress in his or her life and cannot see how past or impending stressors can be causing the present physical symptoms. This inability to recognize current psychological stressors could result from unconscious ego defense mechanisms, simple forgetting, or lack of systematic attention during the typical medical history to the review of stressors. Third, it may seem unlikely to the patient that psychological stress can account for physical symptoms as frequent and intense as those he is currently experiencing. The physician's word that psychological stress can alter biological functions is viewed skeptically. In fact, as recently as 15 years ago, an illustrious cardiologist stated that he could not see how psychosocial stress could occlude an artery. The crux of the problem is a credibility gap. The patient will not be treatable until he can be redirected credibly and cognitively from a strictly somatic definition of his problem to a psychophysiological definition of his problem.

I propose the following approach to the resolution of the problem. The physician should first do a complete physical investigation of the patient's physical symptoms, with appropriate medical tests that may previously have been omitted and occasionally even consultation with appropriate medical specialists. The single most important event that needs to occur next is a compelling psychophysiological demonstration that pierces the patient's skepticism about the mind's ability to influence somatic functions. This demonstration often requires a psychophysiological laboratory, and the patient should be referred to such a laboratory for a stress profile. The first specific purpose of a stress profile is to identify the nature, the number, the magnitude, and the "delay" in recovery of physiological changes induced in the individual patient by a standardized psychological stressor (e.g., mental arithmetic). The second purpose of the psychophysiological profile (Wickramasekera, 1979, 1983) is to identify any situational factors (major life change, etc.) and psychological features (hypnotic ability, catastrophisizing, coping skills, support systems, neuroticism) that are known to be able to amplify, attenuate, or buffer physiological reactivity. Because one of the major problems is that the patient does not recognize that he is currently psychophysiologically tense (he or she may have psychologically habituated to a chronic, physiologically abnormal, "red alert" state), it is crucial to confront the patient in the laboratory with this fact. This can be done, for example, by confronting the patient with the discrepancy between the patient's subjective estimate of muscle tension and the actual physiological measure. It is also important to show the patient in the laboratory that an innocuous psychological stressor (e.g., mental arithmetic) can dramatically alter blood flow, tissue temperature, muscle tension, heart rate, blood pressure, etc. This can be accomplished by showing the patient, from resting baseline to stress, his or her actual strip chart recordings and graphs, or the response meters and counters on the biomedical instruments in the laboratory. Specific methods of doing a compelling psychophysiological demonstration to erode the mind–body dichotomy for various patient types are described in Chapter 7 on the psychophysiological role induction. A psychophysiological report with specific therapy suggestions can bridge the mind–body dichotomy credibility gap for the referring primary care physician. A laboratory report with the graphs should be sent to the referring primary care physician identifying the patient's most reactive physiological system or systems ("window or windows of vulnerability") plus a recommendation about what type of low arousal training (which type of biofeedback, hypnosis, relaxation, etc.) and specific psychotherapy (desensitization, marriage counseling, sex therapy, etc.) would be most likely to enable the patient to close and keep closed his windows of physiological vulnerability.

Why Skills Taught by Psychotherapists May Be Promising Alternatives to Pills for Some Patients

Several studies have shown that including outpatient psychological services provided by psychotherapists to the health care system reduces the incidence of medical utilization and the length of hospitalization (Cummings, 1977; Mumford et al., 1984). The Kaiser Permenente Health Plan Study (Cummings, 1977) showed a sustained reduction in the use of medical services of 60% when psychological services were available to patients. The cost of psychological services were more than offset by the reduction in medical utilization (Cummings, 1977). These findings have been independently confirmed by Rosen and Wiens (1979) in different health care settings. A recent study (Mumford et al., 1984) reviewed 58 controlled studies of outpatient psychotherapy on subsequent medical care utilization and found that 85% of all these studies found a decrease in medical utilization following psychotherapy. The study found that the largest cost offset was a reduction in inpatient medical care and for older people. The finding is surprising because psychological services that are learning based are believed to be least likely to benefit the old (physically deteriorated) and the more seriously sick (hospitalized patients). The findings are a powerful challenge to the mind–body dichotomy that dominates health care today. The philosophical doctrine of the mind–body dichotomy that underlies the biomedical model is one of the major current obstacles to a cost-effective health care system. Studies like those of Cummings (1977) and Mumford et al. (1984) challenge the biomedical assumption of mind–body dichotomy in health care at a practical monetary level. Today depression, sustained states of hyper-arousal, eroding traditional support systems (family, church, neighborhood), maladaptive personal habits (smoking, gluttony, alcoholism, etc.), and life-styles feed the chronic diseases that kill and cripple most people. Concepts of disease and healing based on a narrow biomedical model, limited to verifiable changes in biological structure or function, lack heuristic value today. Psychosocial events as causes or potentiators of disease are typically excluded by the biomedical model from investigation; the biomedical model limits the scope of its research and intervention to verifiable alterations in biological function and structure induced only by physiochemical agents (germs, physical trauma, drugs, etc.). But there is, in fact, converging evidence that mind (brain) and body work together to protect health. The immune system, for example, is a surveillance system that protects us from disease-causing microorganisms. There is now evidence from three converging directions that the CNS and the endocrine system influence the immune system. First, there is evidence from studying hypothalamic lesions that the CNS influences the immune system. Second, stress research (Ader, 1981; Jemmott & Locke, 1984; Sklar & Anisman, 1981) also demonstrates that psychosocial stressors can reduce the number of lymphocytes, lower the level of interferon, and cause damage to the immunologically important tissue. Third, there is strong evidence for classical or Pavlovian conditioning of the immune system. Ader (1981) has shown that pairing a neutral stimulus (CS) with immunosuppressive drugs (UCS) results in an immunosuppressive response (CR) to the neutral stimulus (e.g., saccharin CS).

Basic and clinical biofeedback research has cogently demonstrated that ANS functions like tissue temperature, blood flow, heart rate, skin temperature, and blood pressure can be brought under voluntary (CNS) control, within biological limits, by at least some people. The mechanism of this control and the issue of placebo effects (nonspecified effects) still requires attention. In spite of the still incomplete resolution of the specific versus unspecified (Stroebel & Glueck, 1973; Wickramasekera, 1977, 1980, 1985) variables issue, the clinical efficacy of biofeedback procedures has forever challenged the security of the biomedical model by questioning two of its crucial assumptions. The practical efficacy of biofeedback has challenged the physiological doctrine of the dichotomy of the voluntary-involuntary nervous system, and the philosophical doctrine of the mind–body dichotomy. It is a curious irony of history that the potency of *psychological* factors as independent variables was most cogently demonstrated first on physical or *biological* dependent variables (e.g. EMG levels, vasospasms, skin temperature, medication reduction) and not on the typical "soft" psychological (Rorschach, MMPI) dependent variables of the psychotherapy research literature.

Previous challenges to the mind–body dichotomy doctrine from hypnosis, autogenic training, yoga, and meditation were ignored. However, Wickramasekera (1977, 1978) has stated that, in contrast, clinical biofeedback will be remembered not so much for any unique clinical efficacy over hypnosis, yoga, psychotherapy and/or autogenic training, but because it packaged the challenge to the mind–body dichotomy in the very language system and using the very tools (modern electronic and medical instruments) of the scientific-biomedical establishment. Further, this credibly packaged challenge has been successfully utilized in the therapy of those clinical disorders (chronic functional stress-related illness) where the biomedical model was therapeutically most inert and most vulnerable. Electronic biofeedback simply provided the rationale, the scientific tools (Wickramasekera, 1977), and the objective confirmatory evidence that motivated and mobilized western man to make consistent efforts to manipulate his physiology in ways he has always been able to do, but was barred from trying by the limitations of his own skeptical belief systems. Biofeedback merely used the methods and technology of science to validate a belief system (it is possible within limits to self-regulate the involuntary nervous system) that previously had been blockaded by skepticism. A skeptical belief system can be as limiting to self-mobilization as the absence of an arm or a leg (Wickramasekera, 1979).

Hypnosis is a technique without equal for creating belief and altering perception in very selective ways. For those people (approximately 15%) in the general population who have good hypnotic ability and who are motivated to use it, biofeedback training will simply slow down the rate of psychophysiological skill acquisition; instead, for those with good hypnotic ability and motivation, verbal instructions and a comfortable chair is enough.

Recent advances in the assessment of hypnotic susceptibility in the laboratory and clinical situation have significantly increased the practical utility of hypnotic procedures in the therapy of chronic stress. Hypnotic susceptibility has also stimulated basic research on the psychophysiological mechanisms underlying the transduction of psychological events into chemical and electrical changes associated with learning and conditioning. It is becoming clear that the brain transduces sensory signals into systems of meaning that can have biological consequences for disease or health. The study of people of high-hypnotic ability may provide the purest culture in which to learn how sensory signals are changed into meanings that have physiological consequences. Progress in defining the parameters of hypnotic behavior (Barber, 1969; Hilgard, 1965; Spanos & Barber, 1974) have provided a reliable set of experimentally established facts and principles on which clinical practices can be based. A recent model of psychophysiological disorders (Wickramasekera, 1979, 1983) implicates superior and very low hypnotic susceptibility as major risk factors in the development of psychophysiological disorders.

References

Ader, R. (Ed.) *Psychoneuroimmunology*. New York: Academic Press, 1981.

Ader, R., & Cohen, N. Behavior and the immune system. In W. D. Gentry (Ed.), *Handbook of behavioral medicine*. New York: Guilford Press, 1984.

Barber, T. X. *Hypnosis: A scientific approach*. New York: Van Nostrand Reinhold, 1969.

Barsky, A. J., & Klerman, G. L. Overview: Hypochondriasis, bodily complaints, and somatic styles. *American Journal of Psychiatry*, 1983, 140(3), 273–283.

Beecher, H. K. *Measurement of subjective responses: Quantitative effects of drugs*. New York: Oxford University Press, 1959.

Benson, H. *The mind/body effect*. New York: Simon & Schuster, 1979.

Blackwell, B. Minor tranquilizers: Use, misuse or overuse? *Psychosomatics*, 1975, 16, 28–31.

Brodman, K., Mittelmann, B., Wechsler, D., Weider, A., & Wolff, H. The relation of personality disturbances to duration of convalescence from acute respiratory infections. *Psychosomatic Medicine*, 1947, 9, 37–44.

Brown, J. W., Robertson, L. S., Kosa, J., & Alpert, J. J. A study of general practice in Massachusetts. *Journal of American Medical Association*, 1971, 216, 301–306.

Canter, A. Changes in mood during incubation of acute febrile disease and the effects of pre-exposure psychologic status. *Psychosomatic Medicine*, 1972, 34, 424–430.

Canter, A., Cluff, L. E., & Imboden, J. B. Hypersensitive reactions to immunization innoculations and antecedent psychological vulnerability. *Journal of Psychosomatic Research*, 1972, 16, 99–101.

Cohen, W. S. Health promotion in the workplace: A prescription for good health. *American Psychologist*, 1985, 40(2), 213–216.

Culliton, B. J. Health care economics: The high cost of getting well. *Science*, 1978, 200, 883–885.

Cummings, N. A. The anatomy of psychotherapy under national health insurance. *American Psychologist*, 1977, 32, 711–718.

Cummings, N. A. Turning bread into stones: Our modern antimiracle. *American Psychologist*, 1979, 34(12), 1119–1129.

DeLeon, P. H., & VandenBos, G. R. The new Federal Health Care frontiers: Cost containment and "wellness." *Psychotherapy in Private Practice*, 1983, 1(2), 17–32.

Engel, G. L. The need for a new medical model: A challenge for biomedicine. *Science*, 1977, 196, 129–136.

Evans, F. J. The placebo in pain reduction. In J. J. Bonica (Ed.), *Pain advances in neurology*. New York: Raven Press, 1974.

Fineberg, H. V. Paper presented at the Sun Valley National Forum, Sun Valley, Idaho, August 1977.

Frazier, H. S., & Hiatt, H. H. Evaluation of medical practices. *Science*, 1978, 875–878.

Friedman, M., & Rosenman, R. H. *Type A behavior and your heart.* New York: Knopf, 1974.

Garfield, S. R., Collen, M. F., Feldman, R., Soghikian, K., Richart, R. H., & Duncan, J. H. Evaluation of an ambulatory medical care delivery system. *New England Journal of Medicine,* 1976, *294,* 426–431.

Gibson, G., Bugbee, G., & Anderson, O. W. *Emergency medical services in the Chicago area.* Chicago: Center for Health Administration Studies, University of Chicago, 1970.

Goldberg, D. P. *Mental illness in the community.* London: Tavistock, 1980.

Hamburg, D. A., & Brown, S. S. The science base and social context of health maintenance: An overview. *Science,* 1978, *200,* 847–849.

Hilgard, E. R. *Hypnotic susceptibility.* New York: Harcourt, Brace & World, 1965.

Imboden, J. B., Canter, A., & Cluff, L. E. Convalescence from influenza. *Archives of Internal Medicine,* 1961, *108,* 393–399.

Ingelfinger, F. J. Medicine: Meritorious or meretricious. *Science,* 1978, *200,* 942–946.

Jemmott, J. B., & Locke, S. E. Psychosocial factors, immunologic mediation, and human susceptibility to infectious diseases: How much do we know? *Psychological Bulletin,* 1984, *95,* 52–77.

Jencks, S. F. Recognition of mental distress and diagnosis of mental disorder in primary care. *Journal of American Medical Association,* 1985, *253*(13), 1903–1906.

Jones, K. R., & Vischi, T. R. Impact of alcohol, drug abuse and mental health treatment on medical care utilization. *Medical Care,* 1979, *17,* 1–82.

Knowles, J. H. The hospital. *Scientific American,* 1973, *229,* 128–137.

Krantz, D. S., Grunberg, N. E., & Baum, A. Health psychology. *Annual Review of Psychology,* 1985, *36,* 349–385.

Lowy, F. H. Management of the persistent somatizer. *International Journal of Psychiatry Medicine,* 1975, *6,* 227–239.

Mumford, E., Schlesinger, H. J., Glass, G. V., Patrick, C., & Cuerdon, T. A new look at evidence about reduced cost of medical utilization following mental health treatment. *American Journal of Psychiatry,* 1984, *141*(10), 1145–1158.

Orleans, C. T., George, L. K., Houpt, J. L., & Brodie, H. K. H. How primary care physicians treat psychiatric disorders: A national survey of family practitioners. *American Journal of Psychiatry,* 1985, *142*(1), 52–57.

Pierson, R. Top 200 drugs of 1984: 2.1% increase in refills pushes 1984 RXs 1.7% ahead of 1983. *Pharmacy Times,* April, 1985, pp. 25–33.

Rahe, R. H. Life changes and near-future illness reports. In L. Levi (Ed.), *Emotions—Their parameters and measurement.* New York: Raven, 1975.

Rasmussen, A. J., Jr. Emotions and immunity. *Annals of the New York Academy of Sciences,* 1969, *164,* 458–461.

Regier, D. A., Goldberg, I. D., & Taube, C. A. The de facto U.S. Mental Health Services System. *Archives of General Psychiatry,* 1978, *35,* 685–693.

Relman, A. S. The new medical-industrial complex. *New England Journal of Medicine,* 1980, *303*(17), 963–970.

Review Panel on Coronary-Prone Behavior and Coronary Heart Disease. Coronary-prone behavior and coronary heart disease: A critical review. *Circulation,* 1981, *63,* 1199–1215.

Rogers, M. P., Dubey, D., & Reigh, P. The influence of the psyche and the brain on immunity and disease susceptibility: A critical review. *Psychosomatic Medicine,* 1979, *41,* 147–164.

Rosen, J. C., & Wiens, A. N. Changes in medical problems and use of medical services following psychological intervention. *American Psychologist,* 1979, *34,* 420–431.

Shapiro, A. Placebo effects in medicine, psychotherapy, and psychoanalysis. In A. E. Bergin & S. Garfield (Eds.), *Handbook of psychotherapy*. New York: Wiley, 1971.

Sklar, L. S., & Anisman, H. Stress and cancer. *Psychological Bulletin*, 1981, *89*, 369–406.

Solomon, G. F. Emotion, stress, and the central nervous system and immunity. *Annals of the New York Academy of Sciences*, 1969, *164*, 335–343.

Solomon, G. F., Amkraut, A. A., & Kasper, P. Immunity, emotions, and stress, with special references to the mechanisms of stress effects on the immune system. In H. Musaph (Ed.), *Mechanisms in symptom formation*. Basel, Switzerland: S. Karger, 1974.

Spanos, N. P., & Barber, T. X. Toward a convergence in hypnosis research. *American Psychologist*, 1974, *29*, 500–511.

Stroebel, C. F., & Glueck, B. C. Biofeedback treatment in medicine and psychiatry: An ultimate placebo? *Seminars in Psychiatry*, 1973, *5*, 379–393.

Tancredi, L. R., & Barondess, J. A. The problem of defensive medicine. *Science*, 1978, *200*(4344), 879–882.

Whatmore, G. B., & Kohli, D. R. *The physiopathology and treatment of functional disorders*. New York: Grune & Stratton, 1974.

Wickramasekera, I. The placebo effect and biofeedback for headache pain. *Proceedings of the San Diego Biomedical Symposium*. New York: Academic Press, 1977.

Wickramasekera, I. *A conditioned response model of the placebo effect*. Paper presented at symposium on Nonspecific Effects in Biofeedback, Biofeedback Society of America, Albuquerque, New Mexico, February, 1978.

Wickramasekera, I. *A model of the patient at high risk for chronic stress-related disorders: Do beliefs have biological consequences?* Paper presented at Annual Convention of the Biofeedback Society of America, San Diego, California, 1979.

Wickramasekera, I. A conditioned response model of the placebo effect: Predictions from the model. *Biofeedback and self-regulation*, 1980, *5*(1), 5–18.

Wickramasekera, I. *A model of people at high risk*. Paper presented at the International Stress and Tension Control Society, Brighton, England, August 1983.

Wickramasekera, I. The placebo as a conditioned response: With 17 predictions from the model. In L. White, B. Tursky, & G. E. Schwartz (Eds.), *Placebo: Clinical phenomena and new insights*. New York: Guilford Press, 1985.

5

WHAT IS THE PLACEBO EFFECT AND HOW DOES IT WORK?

*You should treat as many patients as possible with
the new drugs while they still have
the power to heal.*
—Trousseau (1854)

*What he [Bernheim] called suggestibility is
nothing else than the tendency to
transference . . . we have to admit that we have
only abandoned hypnosis in our methods to
discover suggestion again in
the shape of transference.*
—Freud (1938)

The Placebo Effect

Until the twentieth century, physicians had not much more than the placebo effect to offer their patients (Benson & Epstein, 1975). In spite of this situation and the fact that they subjected their patients to purging, leeching, puncturing, cutting, heating, and freezing, physicians generally occupied respected social positions. This paradox is accounted for by the potency of the placebo effect in the history of medicine. The

A preliminary version of this chapter was first presented at the San Diego Biomedical Symposium (invited paper), San Diego, California, November 1977. Later it was presented at a symposium on Non-Specific Effects in Biofeedback, Biofeedback Society of America, Albuquerque, New Mexico, February 1978. It has been published in abbreviated form in *Proceedings of the San Diego Biomedical Symposium*, New York: Academic Press, 1977, and the *Journal of Clinical Engineering*, 1977. Additionally, another version was published as a chapter in Leonard White, Bernard Tursky, and Gary E. Schwartz (Eds.), *Placebo: Theory Research and Mechanisms*.

disapproval of the placebo effect developed mainly with the start of controlled drug studies in the 1950s.

A placebo may be defined as a presumably inert, or neutral substance or procedure that elicits a therapeutic response (Beecher, 1959; Evans, 1974, 1977; Shapiro, 1971). Reviews of 26 double blind studies covering 1,991 patients found that approximately 35% of patients have severe clinical pain reduced by at least one half of its original intensity by an inert substance or placebo drug. The placebo rate. however, for experimentally induced laboratory pain is considerably lower (Evans, 1977). This discrepancy between the placebo rate in experimental and clinical pain strongly suggests that the psychological significance of the therapy situation is a major determinant of the magnitude of the placebo effect.

Placebo effects are not limited to chemical treatments, but may include surgical and psychological therapies. In a classic paper "Surgery as a Placebo," Beecher (1961) compared the results of enthusiastic and skeptical surgeons performing the once popular internal mammary-artery ligation for angina pectoris. Two independent skeptical teams (Cobb et al., 1959; Dimond, Kittle, & Crockett, 1958) using a single blind procedure performed a bilateral skin incision on all patients under local anesthesia and in randomly selected patients the internal mammary artery was ligated. Dimond found that 100% of the nonligated, and 76% of the ligated patients reported decreased need for nitroglycerin and increased exercise tolerance. All nonligated patients showed improvement for more than 6 weeks, and followed patients remained improved 6 to 8 months later. Neither the ligated nor the nonligated group showed any improvement on electrocardiography. The Cobb et al. (1959) team reported that 6 months after surgery five ligated and five nonligated patients reported more than 40% subjective improvement. Two nonligated patients showed dramatic improvement in exercise tolerance and one nonligated patient even showed improved electrocardiographic results after exercise. These studies demonstrated that ligation of the internal mammary artery was no better than a skin incision, and that *skin incision could generate a dramatic and sustained therapeutic effect.*

Placebo effects are not limited to the relief of acute pain. Placebos may be useful in the therapy of coughs, headaches, asthma, multiple sclerosis, the common cold, diabetes, ulcers, arthritis, emesis, seasickness, cancer, Parkinsonism, and so forth (Beecher, 1955; Haas, Fink, & Hartfelder, 1959; Horningfeld, 1964a, b; Wolf, 1950). Nor are placebo effects limited to chemical and surgical treatments; in fact Sox, Margulies, and Sox, (1981) reported that diagnostic tests (electrocardiogram and serum creatinine phosphokinase test) with no apparent diagnostic value affected the outcome care of patients with nonspecific chest pain. Fewer patients in the test group (20%) reported short-term disability after the test than patients in the non-test group (46%) ($P = 0.001$). A work site hypertension detection program found that workers who were told they were hypertensive had more disability days after diagnosis than before learning of their disease (Haynes et al., 1978). A review of controlled studies of psychological therapies like systematic desensitization (Kazdin & Wilcoxon, 1976) and a pioneering credible double blind study of clinical biofeedback (Cohen, Graham, Fotopoulas, & Cook, 1977) have also found equally high rates of placebo response. For example, in the Cohen et al. (1977) study, subjects who received false feedback (the placebo treatment) improved clinically as much as those who received true feedback under double blind conditions. In fact, an early study by Schwitzgebel and Traugott (1968) found that mechanical devices (like medical instruments) can also generate placebo effects, and Wickramasekera (1977b) discussed the placebo effect of medical instruments in biofeedback.

It has been found that a placebo can potentiate, attenuate, or negate the active ingredients in a drug (Shapiro, 1971). Suggestion can be used to reverse the active ingredients in a drug. Wolf (1950) reported two cases of severe nausea and vomiting in which one patient was given 10 cc syrup of ipecac by mouth and the other patient was given 10 cc syrup of epicac by Levine tube and both patients were told that the medication would inhibit nausea. Both patients reported relief of nausea and also the resumption of normal stomach contractions. Ipecac is known to induce nausea and vomiting and to inhibit stomach contractions. Placebos can also have powerful effects on organic illness and malignancies, and can even mimic the effects of active drugs (Shapiro, 1971). Studies have found that dose response and time-effect curves for an active drug and a placebo can be similar and that the side effects of an active drug and a placebo can also be similar (Evans, 1977).

The preceding review suggests that a therapeutic phenomena like the placebo that occurs across such a wide range of clinical treatment modalities (drugs, surgery, psychotherapies, biofeedback) and across such a wide range of physical and mental symptoms (pain, anxiety, edema, tachycardia, emesis, fever, vasoconstriction, phobias, depressions, etc.) to people who are physically or psychologically immobilized by symptoms or in a state of health deprivation must be a true general ingredient in all clinical situations.

A review of the placebo literature leads to several conclusions. First, a subset of patients show a significant therapeutic response to presumably inert or placebo substances, procedures, and objects in any clinical study. Second, no reliable procedure exists to date to identify, in advance, the previously cited subset of patients. Third, the same subset may not reliably respond to placebos. Fourth, any object or procedure offered with therapeutic intent can, under the right conditions, generate placebo effects. Fifth, the mechanism of the effect is unknown and all the right conditions are unclear.

Clearly, we are dealing with a real effect that has been regarded as a nuisance for several reasons previously discussed (Wickramasekera, 1976b, 1977a, b) and summarized as follows: (a) its action is not logically related to the known etiology (theory of cause) of the disease or condition; (b) the mechanism of its action is unknown; (c) the effect to date is unreliable; (d) the effect may not be durable; (e) it is an effect that can occur in any therapeutic situation.

The effect has been called nonspecific because our ignorance of its parameters has limited our ability to manipulate the effect systematically. One purpose of the present chapter is to contribute toward the specification of what is now nonspecific, and toward the specific ways in which the effect might be manipulated. Eventually, perhaps, some placebo effects can be attenuated or negated in laboratory studies, and systematically manipulated to potentiate other specific effects in clinical studies. Such a psychological technology can increase the reliability of positive clinical outcome when other clearly specified active ingredients are used in routine clinical practice.

Theories of the Placebo

Many hypotheses have been advanced to explain the mechanism of the placebo response. Shapiro (1971) and T. X. Barber (1959) appear to favor a suggestion hypothesis, and Evans (1977) appears to favor a trait anxiety reduction hypothesis. Frank (1973) and Stroebel and Glueck (1973) have stressed the role of expectancy in potentiating therapeutic response. In fact, Stroebel and Glueck (1973) proposed a clinically useful way of approaching and quantifying expectancy. For reasons of brevity these analyses will not be presented here and are discussed elsewhere (Wickramasekera, 1976a, 1977a, b). The present chapter offers a new[1,2]

---

[1]After this article was written and submitted for a journal publication, one of the reviewers drew my attention to a relevant paper by Gleidman, Gantt, and Teitelbaum, (1957). I located and read this paper in July 1979. It was very exciting to note that Gleidman et al. advanced one of the central components of the present theory over 20 years ago. Their brief, excellent paper "summarizes some experiences in conditional reflex studies in dogs

model of the placebo, traces the predictions and postdictions from this model, and presents the relevant subject, therapist, and procedural variables. This analysis points out that intrinsic to all unconditioned stimuli (UCS) or reliably effective interventions or events (physicochemical, behavioral-psychological, or surgical) is the potential for Pavlovian conditioning (Pavlov, 1927) and therefore placebo learning.

This suggests that reliable mechanisms of pathophysiology that have clearly and sharply defined onsets and offsets can operate as UCSs. Chemicals and procedures that reliably and clearly turn on or off such pathophysiology can also operate as UCSs. Hence, reliable and visible mechanisms of disease and healing may not be insulated from conditioning effects. The unconditioned response (UCR) is a function not only of the UCS, but also of an associated CS. The symptomatically immobilized and expectant-dependent patient in a state of health deprivation (not unlike food deprivation) is an ideal candidate for conditioning. Counterintuitively, this theory predicts that therapists who use active ingredients (UCS) will get stronger placebo effects than those who use only inert (CS) ingredients. The model also paradoxically predicts that progress in isolating active ingredients (UCS) will inevitably lead to more and stronger placebo effects.

There is no systematic human evidence to support this model. But there is some strong controlled animal evidence (Ader, 1981; Drawbraugh & Lal, 1974; Goldberg & Schuster, 1967, 1970; Schuster & Thompson, 1969; Siegel, 1978; Wilker & Pesor, 1970) that supports the view that neutral stimuli can elicit complex biological and biochemical changes as postulated by the conditioned response model of the placebo.

---

that relate placebo reactivity to established learning concepts" (Gleidman et al., 1957). The observations are cited in informal-anecdotal style and deal with three groups of "unpublished" studies. The first group of studies "demonstrates that the effect of a person" can be conditioned. The second series stresses the importance of "central excitatory states" in conditioning. The third group of studies is "a miscellaneous one," which pertains to the general state of the organism and the general setting with respect to placebo effects. Their thoughts with respect to the first point are almost identical to mine and with respect to points two and three, there is substantial implicit agreement. But there is no elaboration with respect to hypnotizability, brain lateralization, and the possibility that the UCS can be nonchemical behavioral events.

[2]After this article was written and accepted for journal publication, the editor of *Biofeedback and Self-Regulation*, Dr. J. Stoyva, drew my attention (on October 29, 1979) to a study by R. J. Herrnstein (1962). In this controlled study of the disruptive effects of scopolamine hydrobromide on lever pressing in the rat, physiological saline is shown to mimic the effects of scopolamine hydrobromide. Based on this study, Herrnstein infers that the placebo effects appears to be an instance of simple Pavlovian conditioning.

Origins of the Conditioned-Response Model

Early in 1970, during clinical electromyograph (EMG) feedback therapy (Wickramasekera 1972a, 1973a) with patients with diagnosed chronic and continuous muscle contraction headaches of over 20 years duration, I made some puzzling observations. A subset of these patients reported relief of headache pain with startling rapidity. Often this occurred after no more than one or two sessions of EMG feedback therapy and several sessions before they demonstrated any measurable ability to reduce the muscle tension levels (EMG) in their head and neck. Because the etiology and mechanisms of muscle contraction headache pain are presumed to involve sustained contraction of muscles of the head and neck, changes in the verbal report of the intensity and frequency of headache pain should correlate with or follow, not precede, a drop in frontal EMG levels.

I wondered if this very short latency therapeutic response was not a placebo response to the impressive medical and highly credible biofeedback instruments in anticipation of actual healing. It is well known that CRs mediated by the central nervous system (CNS) can have a shorter latency than a UCR, or in this case, the actual reduction in peripheral muscle tension levels in the head and neck. I conceptualized the positive short latency therapeutic response of this subset of patients as a type of fractional anticipatory goal response (Hull, 1952) or conditioned response to the impressive electronic medical instruments used in this therapy (Wickramasekera, 1977b). This rapid therapeutic response (CR) to the sight of the biofeedback instruments (CS) was like conditioned salivation (CR), a fractional component of actual eating of food (UCR) that occurs in anticipation of food (UCS). The rapidity of this response reminded me of the well-known clinical observation that ingestion of aspirin often relieves the headache long before its pharmacological effect could occur. The response by the placebo group suggests that respondent or Pavlovian conditioning was one factor that could account for a portion of the positive therapeutic outcome in EMG feedback therapy for headache. In those early years of EMG feedback, the mechanism of therapeutic response in EMG feedback therapy for headaches was considered to be exclusively operant or Skinnerian conditioning of reduced frontal EMG.

The Clinical Situation and Conditioning Phenomena

This analysis predicts that (a) psychological responses (CRs) that were previously relegated to the realm of nonspecific factors can come reliably to attenuate or potentiate health and illness; (b) that initially neutral stimuli (CSs) can come either directly or indirectly to influence the underlying physicochemical and cellular mechanism (pathophysiology) of health and illness; and (c) that theoretically, the influence of such variables on the symptom and mechanism of disease can be demonstrated in appropriately controlled double blind studies in which the UCS (e.g., active chemical ingredient) is withheld.

Until as recently as the first two decades of this century, physicians had only a few active ingredients or UCSs (e.g., digitalis, opium) with which they could reliably control certain disease or disorder mechanisms. Yet, for centuries, physicians have inspired confidence in patients, and individual physicians have enjoyed high credibility and high social status. Physicians occupied positions of confidence long before they could reliably and effectively control pathophysiological mechanisms (UCRs) in any significant number of disorders. The conditioned response model of the placebo can illuminate at least a part of this historical paradox. The perceived potency of a healer can stem not only from his or her ability to control pathophysiological mechanisms but also from his or her ability accurately and precisely to predict the time course, the specific sequence of changing physical symptoms, and the antecedents of disease. The ability to predict or prophesy requires only careful observation, recognition of the descriptive features of symptoms, access to medical records of prior observations, a knowledge of the base rates of certain deviant biological events, and a lawful disease process.

It is likely that patients frightened by the eruption of unfamiliar symptoms on their bodies and uncertain about their future were not prone to think analytically about their physicians' behavior. Consequently, they confused the ability accurately to predict biological symptoms with the ability to control disease mechanisms. They attributed therapeutic potency to the physician who reduced their fear and uncertainty by identifying and labeling their disease and accurately predicting its symptomatic course. A physician's predictive knowledge replaces disorganizing fear and uncertainty with a sense of familiarity, illusory control, and security. For centuries, physicians have carefully observed, recorded, and labeled multiple common diseases and disorders. They were often also knowledgeable about the likely antecedents (e.g., hereditary or familial antecedents, dietary and environmental antecedents) of some of these disorders. A learned physician could easily recognize the specific symptoms a patient was currently experiencing, and could predict the specific symptoms the patient would develop within 12 to 48 hours, and the sequence of symptomatic changes that would occur as the disease progressed. For example, in the case of a disease like small pox (*Variola major*), the following sequenced predictions can be made:

Incubation: 12 to 14 days
Prodrome: Abrupt headaches, chills, aches, and fever rapidly as high as 106, sometimes followed by vomiting, drowsiness, convulsions and coma.
Day 1 and 2: Transient rash that disappears on Day 3 or 4; widespread rash usually heralds severe infection.
Day 3 and 4: "Raised measles" over face, changing to papules that change to vesicles in 24 hours and then to pustules on Day 5 or 6. The early appearance of this rash signals severity of infection.
Day 9: Crusts form.

Such a physician also knew the death rate and sometimes the rate of spontaneous remission for the disease. This enabled the knowledgeable practitioner, after a brief physical examination, to make to the patient and his or her family uncannily accurate predictions about the patient's current and future experiences with the disease. As a specific disease (e.g., gonorrhea) progressed and the physician's prior predictions about the symptoms were verified, the physician's credibility escalated in the patient's and the community's perception. In addition, a knowledge of the likely antecedents of a disease or disorder (diet, hereditary factors, environmental exposure or trauma) could not only enable the physician to predict the future, but also to reveal to the patient the precursors of his or her illness stemming from his or her past. In short, accurate prediction (future) and postdiction (past) can be the basis of great perceived therapeutic potency and the basis of the illusion of physician control over the disease process. In the field of clinical practice, a physician is never asked to reinstate a cured disease ("do that again") to demonstrate his or her control over the mechanisms of disease. Clinical practice, unlike laboratory research, never requires experimental replication of unpleasant illness.

The conditioning analysis of the historical health care situation demonstrates how perceived therapeutic potency can be acquired by simply being a good observer and accurate record keeper, and having a detailed knowledge of the sequence of onset of specific symptoms of common diseases. The ability to recognize that one has confused prediction and description with the control of pathophysiological mechanisms requires a level of critical-analytic thought that is unlikely in a fearful and dysfunctional patient.

These speculations lead to the more general notion that all stimuli in the clinical therapeutic situation (the therapist and his or her behavior, the staff, the tools and procedures, the physical environment and furnishings, etc.) can be conveniently divided into two classes of events: (a) UCSs and (b) CSs or discriminative stimuli. This analysis assumes that all people who are sick because of disease, injury, or dysfunction or some other life-threatening predicament are in a state of health deprivation that selectively sensitizes their attentional process to stimuli (UCSs and CSs) labeled therapeutic by their culture. The disruptive, uncomfortable, and perhaps life-threatening predicament of patients focuses their attention on stimuli that *in vivo* or vicarious social learning has shown to reduce the unpleasant drive stimuli associated with illness.

Unconditioned Stimuli

UCSs (physiological/chemical or behavioral/psychological) are a class of events that reliably elicit or increase the probability of therapeutic responses (UCRs) by altering the mechanisms of pathophysiology. For example, digitalis (UCS) is known to increase the contractions of myocardial fibers (UCR) and the lack of such contractions is associated with congestive heart failure. Another example of such stimuli would be behavioral responses (UCSs) that reduce the elevated frontal EMG levels that are presumed (Ostfeld, 1962; Wolff, 1963) to be etiologic to muscle contraction headache pain. Theoretically, the definitive feature of UCSs in this analysis is their ability reliably (within the limits of adaptation at the receptor or reflex level) to alter the underlying response mechanism (sustained contraction of muscles of head and neck, or UCR) of disease, injury, or dysfunction and eventually its observable physical and/or behavioral symptoms. Some UCRs (e.g., emesis, eye blink) can be triggered by multiple physical stimuli (UCSs). For example, a puff of air and a loud noise may elicit an eye blink. Emesis may be elicited by ipecac and mechanical methods like fingers in the throat.

However, other UCRs may be elicited only by a narrow class of UCSs. For example, some acute infectious diseases are activated only by pneumococci (UCS) and are deactivated by penicillin. Most modern chronic diseases (e.g., cardiovascular disease, respiratory disease) are reliably responsive only to a combination of several interventions (UCSs), such as diet, medication, exercise, and life-style change (e.g., smoking cessation, alcohol ingestion cessation, etc.). The onset or offset of many chronic diseases appear to be determined by multiple UCSs. Some UCSs, or reliable elicitors or reinforcers of the mechanisms of disease or dysfunction, are easier to see and specify in medicine than in psychology—for example, the effect of appropriate doses of insulin (UCS) on the glucose metabolism response (UCR) of diabetic, or the effects of morphine (UCS) on the pain response (UCR) of the postsurgical patient, or the effects of penicillin (UCS) on pneumococcal pneumonia. Such UCSs (morphine, penicillin, insulin, etc.) are believed to operate directly or indirectly on the theoretical mechanism (etiology) of the illness or its pathophysiology.

In the original Pavlovian laboratory analogue, which is not obscured by presumed theoretical etiologic mechanism, the UCS, food in the mouth or the sight of food, will reliably elicit salivation (UCR), particularly if the animal is hungry (selectively sensitized to certain classes of stimuli by food deprivation). Similarly the sight of a socially sanctioned healer (doctor, swami, or shaman) will reliably elicit hope, particularly if the patient is health deprived. Health deprivation is a general state of reduced physical and psychological functioning and mobility and consequent dependency, induced in sick people by the eruption of unpleasant, painful, and unfamiliar physical symptoms (e.g., changes in skin color, edema, fever, pain on movement, boils and pus, respiratory distress, etc.). This state of health deprivation selectively sensitizes the patient to a class of stimuli (the healer, his or her substances, tools, and rituals) that have previously reduced or been reported to reduce unpleasant and unfamiliar symptoms. A state of health deprivation appears to be an important precondition for the learned component (CR) of disease or dysfunction.

Conditioned Stimuli

CSs are certain neutral stimuli that initially do not elicit a UCR (e.g., change in glucose metabolism, emesis) but that, as a function of repeated association with an appropriate UCS (insulin, ipecac), can come to inhibit (placebo) or disinhibit (nocebo) even temporarily the symptoms and/or underlying mechanism of the disease. The neutral CS (e.g., the sight of a syringe), as a function of contiguity with the UCS, can now elicit a fractional anticipatory component of the UCR. Neutral stimuli (CSs) may also be associated with the onset of the underlying mechanisms or symptoms of disease or injury (UCSs). Immersion in such CSs may actually potentiate the disease or illness. CSs are ineffective with vertebrates if the UCR is elicited by a route other than the central nervous system (Hilgard & Marquis, 1961). CSs may alter some disease mechanisms indirectly by modifying, for example, neuroendocrine or other CNS mechanisms that can inhibit immunocompetence (Ader, 1981; Ader & Cohen, 1982; Bowbjerg, Ader, & Cohen, 1982), or that can theoretically disinhibit or potentiate immunocompetence. If, on the other hand, the UCR (depression, anxiety, pain, etc.) is elicited directly through CNS activity, then CSs may act directly on the presumed mechanism of the disorder (e.g. excessive sympathetic activation, depletion of norepinephrine, or activation of endorphins, etc.) and rapidly cause a positive clinical outcome. For example, the ingestion of a tablet of aspirin is frequently reported to relieve headache pain long before the active ingredient (pharmacological effect) working peripherally can alter pain.

CSs may also operate as safety signals (Mowrer, 1960) to potentiate healing. Mowrer (1960) demonstrated that neutral stimuli associated with the offset of pain or fear can be termed safety signals because they are associated with the reduction of anxiety or equivalently with the arousal of hope. They (CSs) indicate that the period of suffering is over. Neutral stimuli (CSs) in the health care situation can become conditioned by their association with either the onset of the mechanisms and symptoms of health or the offset of the symptoms and mechanisms of disease. Certain CSs or discriminative stimuli in the medical situation are repeatedly associated with onset of potent UCS (morphine, digitalis, antibiotics, insulin). For example, CSs like syringes, stethoscopes, white coats, and behavioral procedures like cleaning the skin and physical examinations are routinely paired with potent UCSs like morphine, insulin, and antibiotics. Also, culture-specific cognitive verbal labels for places ("hospital," "laboratory," "emergency room," "clinic"), procedures ("medical," "scientific," "graphing," "measuring") and persons ("medical," "professor," "doctor"), can also be associated with potent UCSs or active ingredients, and come to acquire conditioned properties. CSs reliably associated with the offset of aversive stimuli (electric shock, childbirth, ugly skin eruptions, headache, painful injury, etc.) can acquire conditioned positive reinforcing properties (Mowrer, 1960). In other words, these CSs come to operate like safety signals (Mowrer, 1960). These phenomena are well established in the laboratory (Kimble, 1961) and are discussed in the following sections.

The Placebo as a Conditioned Response

I propose that a variety of inert, neutral, or nonspecific substances, procedures, persons, or places can come to function as CSs (Pavlov, 1927) or discriminative stimuli (Skinner, 1953) for the alleviation of anxiety, pain, dysfunction, trauma, and disease if such CSs or discriminative stimuli have been repeatedly associated with the onset (see Footnote 2) of powerful UCSs (like penicillin, nitroglycerin, insulin, morphine, etc.)

that reliably relieve the mechanisms and overt symptoms of illness (e.g., pneumococcal pneumonia, angina pectoris, diabetes, and postsurgical pain).

Mowrer's (1960) analysis of secondary reinforcement based on negative primary reinforcement points to other ways in which neutral stimuli can come to acquire nocebo and placebo effects. Unfamiliar reactions (skin eruptions, pus discharges, etc.) and other unpleasant symptoms (fever, pain, insomnia, etc.) are naturally occurring aversive reactions (UCRs) that are triggered by some underlying disease process, injury, or dysfunction (UCS). Neutral stimuli (CSs) associated with the onset and course of the disease (UCRs) may become negative CSs. These CSs may elicit CRs that potentiate the UCRs or disease process, by either directly or indirectly inhibiting mechanisms of immunocompetence (Ader, 1981). Such conditioned stimuli can be termed *nocebos* and the learned response to them, a nocebo response. In fact, it is sometimes observed that simply changing the patient's physical environment (deleting those negative CS or nocebos) will potentiate spontaneous remission of symptoms, when other variables (medication ingestion, degree of environmental structure, etc.) are held constant. This phenomenon is most often observed with the hospitalization of mental patients.

Neutral stimuli associated with the offset (because of spontaneous remission or delivery of an active drug) and diminution of unpleasant symptoms and/or painful disease processes (UCSs) may come to acquire positive conditioned properties for healing, anxiety reduction, and operate as safety signals as discussed earlier. Instances of such neutral stimuli may be the arrival of the physician/therapist, the physical examination, the prescription of medication, and the rituals of medication ingestion.

Hence, CSs for pain reduction and healing can be produced in at least two ways: (a) by association with the onset of an active ingredient for healing (like morphine, insulin, nitroglycerin, penicillin); (b) by association with the offset of the symptoms (UCRs) of an unfamiliar, unpleasant, and painful disease or injury. Finally, neutral stimuli associated with the onset of the symptoms of a painful and unfamiliar disease process may come to elicit conditioned anxiety and/or a fractional anticipatory disease response components, and may be called nocebos.

In view of the preceding analysis, the labels *inert* and *nonspecific* appear to be less heuristic today. Because this analysis suggests that a variety of neutral substances or procedures that are initially inert or do not reliably alter the underlying presumed mechanisms of disease can, if repeatedly associated with appropriate unconditioned stimuli, come either to attenuate or potentiate the disease process and pathophysiology based on conditioning mechanisms.[3] This analysis predicts (a) that psychological responses (CRs) that were previously relegated to the realm of nonspecific factors can come reliably to attenuate or potentiate health and illness, (b) that initially neutral stimuli (CSs) can come either directly or indirectly to influence the underlying physiochemical and cellular mechanisms (pathophysiology) of health and illness, and (c) that, theoretically, the influence of such variables on the symptom and mechanism of disease can be demonstrated in appropriately controlled double blind studies in which the UCS (active chemical ingredient) is withheld.

The notion of active ingredients in a drug or procedure has generally been that which the relevant therapeutic theory singled out as specifically remedial for the condition. For example, penicillin is the active ingredient according to therapeutic theory for pneumococcal pneumonia because the disease is caused by pneumococcus, which is sensitive to penicillin. The notion of specific activity (Wickramasekera, 1977a, b, 1980) in medicine has traditionally meant (a) that the therapeutic mechanism of action was exclusively a physiochemical one, (b) that the action of the active ingredient was logically related to the presumed etiology (pathophysiology) of the disease, (c) that the therapeutic effect was reliable, and (d) that the therapeutic effect was durable.

Clearly the earlier CR analysis of the placebo effect and the new psychobiological models (Engel, 1977; Lipowski, 1977; Weiner, 1977) of disease and dysfunction make the notion of specific activity outmoded. On theoretical and empirical grounds it is clear that most modern chronic illness is multiply determined and the present analysis points out that every disease process (UCR) may have a CR component and is therefore psychophysiological in nature. The Pavlovian concept of a UCS (physiochemical or psychological) as an independent variable may be more heuristic today than the notion of specific activity. As this analysis points out, illness and disease mechanisms are not insulated from conditioning effects. The UCR is a function not only of the UCS (specific ingredient) but also of any associated CS. This learning or conditioning effect is inevitable given an intact, complex CNS. The present analysis indicates that intrinsic to all effective interventions or events (chemical, surgical, psychological or psychophysiological) is the potential for learning or Pavlovian conditioning in conscious organisms. Learning that is initially electrical in nature, and later physiochemical in character can lead to neuroendocrine and neuroimmunologic changes that alter bio-

---

[3]There are some exceptional instances in which the CR and the UCR move in opposite directions (e.g., the UCR to atropine is a dry mouth and the CR is salivation. The UCR to small doses of insulin is hypoglycemia but the CR is hyperglycemia).

logical structures. Current models of disease (Engel, 1977; Weiner, 1977) suggest that changes in the dependent variable, or health (UCR) can be accounted for by several specifiable independent variables (UCSs) operating either directly or indirectly on the UCR, and that some of these independent variables (CSs) may be learned.

The literature of respondent conditioning clearly demonstrates that the response to a UCS (e.g., nitroglycerin) will inevitably involve two components. The first component will be an unconditioned response (nonplacebo response) elicited by the active ingredient or UCS (e.g., nitroglycerin). The second component is a CR or learned fractional component of the UCR, elicited by neutral events surrounding the delivery of the drug. The latency and magnitude of these two response components may be different. The CR will have a shorter latency because it is centrally mediated. The CR would also be of smaller magnitude than the UCR. Hence, the UCS inevitably elicits two response components, a CR and a UCR.

This analysis saliently points out that intrinsic to all effective interventions (physiochemical, surgical, or behavioral) is the potential for Pavlovian conditioning (Pavlov, 1927) and therefore for placebo learning. Counterintuitively, it predicts that therapists who use UCSs or active ingredients will get stronger placebo effects than those who use only CSs or neutral ingredients because regular UCS–CS association strengthens the CR. This model also paradoxically predicts that progress in isolating UCSs or active physiochemical, surgical, or behavioral procedures will inevitably lead to more and stronger placebo effects. Thus, therapists who routinely use UCS or active ingredients will eventually enjoy escalating placebo effects and may be perceived as miracle workers, when in fact only a part of their "miracles" can be directly traced to their use of UCSs or active pharmacological or surgical techniques. In this analysis, then, medical science emerges as a uniquely human historical endeavor to isolate UCSs or reliably effective ingredients (nitroglycerin, digitalis, etc.). But the potential for respondent conditioning exists in all human situations (not just medical ones) in which UCSs are used or in which reliably effective events occur.

Components of the Conditioned Placebo Response

The nature of the conditioned placebo response in healing is unknown today. It is probably a complex patterned psychophysiological response (Schwartz, 1976) that for purposes of analysis can be regarded as a composite of (a) cognitive-verbal, (b) motor, and (c) physiochemical responses.

The Cognitive-Verbal Component

The cognitive-verbal component may be recognized subjectively as an emotion like hope (Frank, 1973; Mowrer, 1960). But not all cognitive and emotional information processing is explicitly verbally mediated or conscious. There is now evidence from several converging experimental and empirical sources that a salient amount of cognitive and emotional information processing continues in the absence of conscious awareness (Davidson, 1980; Dixon, 1971; Kihlstrom, 1987; Nisbett & Wilson, 1977; Shevrin & Dickman, 1980). In fact, in the case of overlearned behaviors that are critical to survival or where channel space for conscious information processing is limited, unconsciousness and automaticity in response may be very adaptive features of behavior.

Mowrer (1956) proposed that neutral stimuli associated with the onset of pain (e.g., a common symptom of disease, dysfunction, or injury) will acquire drive (e.g., anxiety) properties, and that stimuli associated with the offset (cessation) of pain will acquire reinforcing properties (hope) or operate as safety signals. CSs (cognitions, visual impressions, tactile-kinesthetic sensations) associated with the onset of the injury or unpleasant symptoms of disease (UCS) will come to elicit conditioned anxiety. The visit to the doctor, the prescription and ingestion of medication, and the like are neutral events (safety signals) that have previously (in health care history) been associated with active pharmacological agents or UCSs and the offset or reduction of pain and discomfort. Hence, these safety signals (CSs) may have acquired anxiety- and/or uncertainty-reducing properties or even fractional anticipatory healing properties (the physiochemical correlates of which remain unspecified today). Neutral events like the visit to the doctor and the prescription can operate as conditioned safety signals that can inhibit the aversive conditioned anxiety (CR) from cognitions (CSs) and sensations (CSs) associated with the disease onset and maintenance. Safety signals like a white coat (CS), and a prescription (CS) can indicate that the period of pain, uncertainty, fear, and depression is over, and that the period of relief and healing is here. The safety signals can inhibit anxiety and disinhibit the subjective emotion of hope.

The Motor Component

The motor component of the placebo response is probably strongly controlled by the patient's mood (emotions) and current environmental reinforcement contingencies. Current reinforcement contingencies may sometimes be able temporarily to override mood and alter motor behavior prior to stable and positive changes in emotion. But generally, as the patient's mood starts to improve and as the inhibition of motor activity by emotions like pain and depression recede, the patient may expand his behavioral repertoire by resuming normal activities like eating, copulating, and returning to work. These adaptive activities then recruit the temporal and behavioral vacuums that were previously occupied by maladaptive uncertainty, fear, pain, and depressive cognitive-affective ruminations (CS or nocebos). These conditioned aversive cognitive-affective ruminations (occurring consciously and unconsciously) probably potentiated the unconditioned components (UCRs) of the disease or injury. This analysis may be particularly relevant to chronic diseases and functional disorders (e.g., low back pain, diabetes, cardiovascular disorders, musculoskeletal disorders, cancer, etc.) where the long-term and intermittent reinforcement nature of the UCSs (disease process, injury, or dysfunction) enhances the probability of conditioning effects. It is a well-established fact that intermittent reinforcement by the UCS will make a maladaptive cognitive, motor, or affective habit maximally resistant to extinction. The chronic intermittent activation of the disease mechanism by the UCS (physicochemical cause) may lead to increasingly pervasive aversive anticipatory cognitive and affective responses, markedly resistant to extinction and that inhibit the motor system even when the UCS is dormant or inactive in chronic diseases.

The Physicochemical Component

The physicochemical component of the placebo response probably involves at least two subcomponents: psychoneuroendocrine and psychoneuroimmunological components.

The Psychoneuroendocrine System. It now appears that there are descending pain inhibitory pathways from the medial brain stem to the dorsal horn of the spinal cord (Cannon, Liebeskind, and Frank, 1978; Mayer, Wolfe, Akil, Carder, & Liebeskind, 1971). These pathways may involve opiate and nonopiate mechanisms. The opiate mechanisms can be activated by endogenous morphinelike substances termed endorphins, and apparently also by electrical stimulation of certain brain sites (e.g., periaqueductal gray matter, etc.). Whether certain types of state-specific cognitive-affective (e.g., hypnotic analgesia) activity can stimulate these brain sites is not known. It appears that the opiate mechanism can be activated within seconds of CNS stimulation; that the analgesic effects extend beyond the period of stimulation; and that the stimulation is particularly effective with clinical as opposed to experimental pain. It appears that there are other rapidly activated nonopiate pain inhibitory systems (e.g., hypnotic analgesia) that are not blocked by naloxone (Barber & Mayer, 1977; Goldstein & Hilgard, 1975; Mayer, Prince, Barber, & Rafii, 1976). A recent study (Levine, Gordon, & Fields, 1978) and two extensive literature reviews (Basbaum & Fields, 1978; Verebey, Volavka, & Clouet, 1978) suggest that the activation of the endorphin system may be one of the primary chemical mechanisms of pain reduction in the placebo response. However, other cognitively initiated (hypnotic analgesia), but chemically mediated psychoneuroendocrine pain inhibitory systems may also exist (Sternbach, 1982).

There is good evidence that depression potentiates chronic clinical pain (Merskey & Hester, 1972; Taub & Collins, 1974) and it has been suggested that decreased functional activity in the endogenous opioid system may be linked to the pathophysiology of depression (Gold, Pottash, Sweeny, Martin, & Extein, 1982). Pain sensitivity and deficits in pleasure (depression susceptibility) may be mediated through the catecholamines, serotonin, norepinephrine, and dopamine, which are known to alter opiate action. Hence, one rapidly activated psychoneuroendocrine mechanism through which a placebo stimulus may reduce depression and pain sensitivity is through the recruitment of the endorphin system.

The Psychoneuroimmunological System. There is now evidence that the immune system, the primary mechanism of healing, is not totally independent of the CNS and the psychosocial environment. At least three lines of evidence (hypothalamic lesions, adrenocorticotropic hormone (ACTH) and the adrenal cortical axis, and classical conditioning) suggest that CNS events can potentially and reliably alter the immune response (Ader, 1981; Hirsch, 1982). More specifically, there is now evidence that anxiety and depression can inhibit the immune system (Rogers, Dubey, & Reich, 1979). There is also good experimental evidence that Pavlovian or respondent conditioning procedures can modestly but reliably reduce immunocompetence (Ader, 1981). Theoretically, respondent conditioning procedures may also be able to significantly potentiate immunocompetence, but this remains to be experimentally demonstrated. The clinical implications of this prediction are quite profound. Hence, through such CNS mechanisms as emotion and expectancy learning (Pavlovian conditioning), even the immune system may be influenced by placebo stimuli (CSs).

In summary, the placebo response is probably a composite of patterned interacting verbal-subjective, motor, neuroendocrine, and neuroimmunological response systems that can attenuate or potentiate the underlying mechanisms of pathophysiology and overt clinical symptoms.

Developmental Aspects of Conditioned Placebo Response

Historical Aspects

Developmentally, the child or immature organism, in a stage of dependency and deprivation, is the ideal candidate for conditioning or placebo learning. The reliable delivery of food, clothing, and shelter to dependent immature organisms is, in the final analysis, associated with the strength and intelligence of the adult parent. In the developmental history of the immature organism, the effective and reliable satisfaction of needs may be associated with certain neutral (CS) features, of persons (height, weight, color), response styles (authoritarian, permissive), and places. The ability of an adult caretaker to intervene effectively and reliably to reduce discomfort, uncertainty, fear, and pain, or to produce specific changes (pain, fear) in the individual, the tribe, or the physical environment, is the original basis of the notion of active ingredients or UCSs. For example, a dominant adult baboon who loses his teeth (UCS) or a political leader who loses his or her wits (UCS) because of senility, both likely to be eventually pushed aside by younger, stronger, and more intelligent members of the group who can more reliably and effectively consequate (punish or reward) the older, weaker, and less intelligent group members. Both the dominant baboon and the leader will eventually encounter "placebo sag" (Wickramasekera, 1977b, c) or credibility extinction as their active ingredient or UCS (teeth, muscles, claws, IQ) fade with senility. The potency of their packaging or neutral features (CSs) cannot be sustained without at least intermittent demonstrations of strength and intelligence (UCSs).

From this analysis, general intelligence, a UCS, emerges as a potent and highly generalizable new (on the evolutionary scale) behavioral UCS. A complex active ingredient or UCS like general intelligence can produce specific and reliable changes in physiochemical and psychological domains. General intelligence, when coupled with pertinent information, can be a potent behavioral UCS, on par with other active ingredients (e.g., physiochemical) and capable of producing respondent conditioning effects. *High credibility* in this analysis is a quality of any behaviors (stimulus events) that reliably produce precise and potent physical, biological, and/or psychological changes in the environment for one's own benefit or the benefit of others. Hence, baboons, leaders, and therapists who come to lean increasingly on their CS or packaging (neutral features) will inevitably encounter placebo sag as their active ingredients (muscles, teeth, IQ) or UCSs fade. They will be discovered to be impostors and historically identified as "quacks." On the other hand, those who use primarily UCS or active ingredients will get stronger placebo effects than quacks, will enjoy escalating credibility, and will be seen as miracle workers, when, in fact, only half of their miracles can be traced to their active ingredients or UCSs. The other half will be a function of the subject's anticipatory response (CRs) elicited by neutral features (CSs) of the "miracle workers." Science, in this analysis, emerges as a uniquely human quest to identify, isolate, and manipulate UCSs, so that our physical, biological, and psychosocial environments may be rendered more predictable, more reliably controllable, and more nearly explainable.

Acquisition Phase

A dependent organism is a prerequisite for effective conditioning. The physical and psychological immobilization of the organism by health deprivation (injury, infection, tissue damage, high fever, disorientation, unpleasant and unusual symptoms, fear and depression) creates the prerequisite dependent patient role (Mechanic, 1972) and the opportunity for conditioning.

Fear, anxiety, and uncertainty can be inhibited and the attentional process brought to focus in expectant arousal, when parents or caretaker surrogates (doctors, priests, etc.) enter the health deprived person's environment. The focusing of the attentional mechanism on the physician and the inhibition of anxiety and fear by a psychophysiological attitude of expectant arousal (hope) are based on prior primitive and infantile social learning (operant, respondent, vicarious), in which parental entry and intervention are associated with the reliable offset of aversive events (danger and deprivation) and the onset of reinforcing events (food, protection from danger and pain, etc.). Parental figures have acquired the properties of safety signals (Mowrer, 1960) that inhibit fear and anxiety and disinhibit an attitude of expectant arousal (hope).

During the acquisition or credibility formation phase, the placebo stimulus and response to be conditioned probably involve (a) awareness of the CS-UCS and the response reinforcement contingency, (b) implicit or explicit verbal mediation of this contingency, and (c) conscious awareness of several culture-specific, socially learned, credible safety signals (discriminative stimuli). These culture-specific, credible safety signals (e.g., rattles, syringes, pills, potions, wands, stethoscopes, etc.) may or may not be verbally encoded as safety signals. The CSs or safety signals can inhibit worry, doubt, and skepticism. Worry can interfere with the operation of natural homeostatic healing mechanisms. For example, worry and doubt can cause sleep onset or psychophysiological insomnia, thereby inhibiting sleep onset and its healing neuroendocrine consequences. It is clear that the bulk of insomnia is psychophysiological and is caused by cognitive or physiological hyperactivity (Association of Sleep Disorders Centers, 1979) stimulated by anxiety and worry that is conscious or unconscious. There is also growing evidence that anxiety can inhibit the immune system (Rogers *et al.*, 1979).

The inhibition of worry and doubt by conditioned safety signals (e.g., a placebo pill or an ointment) can make the patient more receptive to healing or instructional suggestions given by a physician or therapist. Safety signals may potentiate the instructional signal by inhibiting noise or worry, and improving reception of therapeutic messages. For example, the migraine patient may be given suggestions to constrict cerebral arteries in the second (pain) phase of the disorder by relaxing and reducing sympathetic outflow. The patient with asthma may be given suggestions for bronchodilation. A study by Luparello, Leist, Lourie, and Sweet (1970), in fact, demonstrated that the pharmacological action of a bronchodilating drug (UCS) could be doubled on a measure of airway resistance, if bronchodilating suggestions (CSs) were associated with the delivery of the drug (UCS). Hence, safety signals may also potentiate the action of active pharmacological agents (UCS) by inhibiting noise or cognitions of uncertainty and doubt. Cognitions of uncertainty and doubt may operate as negative CSs that attenuate the effects of a UCS (active drug).

These discriminative stimuli or CSs may also influence the rate of acquisition of the placebo response by potentiating attentional and arousal mechanisms. These credible signals may be quite diverse: (a) the labeling of the therapist (e.g. doctor, swami, professor, etc.) can influence his or her attention and arousal stimulus value in a given culture. (b) The credibility of the therapeutic setting (emergency room of a hospital, temple, university medical center, park bench) can also influence the above mechanisms of learning. The university medical center in North American culture is the new temple of healing. (c) The credibility of the placebo *per se* (e.g., size, shape, color, taste) and (d) the credibility of the administration ritual (e.g., oral versus injection, a single dramatic or startling episode like surgery) can also influence attention and arousal conditions. (e) Finally, and very saliently, the nature of the interpersonal relationship between the patient and the therapist (e.g. accurate empathy, confidence, warmth, authoritarianism) can influence the attention and arousal properties of these events. The attention and arousal value of these CSs can be directly related to the extent to which they have previously been reliably associated with specific and effective interventions on behalf of the patient when he or she was an immature and dependent organism.

In the acquisition of most new concepts (e.g., math) or tasks (driving a car), it is likely that the specification of component responses facilitates conditioning. The sequential specification of the emission or elicitation of these component responses and the accurate verbal mediation of these component responses will reduce errors in the acquisition phase of learning. During this first phase, large individual differences in pertinent subject characteristics (autonomic nervous system lability, hypnotizability, general intelligence), a subject's history of reinforcement and punishment, and the culture-specific context of learning can influence placebo learning through the determination of attentional and arousal mechanisms and the specification of what is a credible CS for a given subject.

Consolidation Phase

After the placebo response is well established through repeated association with potent UCSs or active ingredients, the CR probably (a) becomes increasingly abbreviated, (b) involves minimal or no awareness, (c) becomes involuntary, (d) involves a bypass of the verbal or dominant hemisphere, and (e) preferentially involves the minor hemisphere. Hypnosis, like the consolidated placebo response, also appears preferentially to involve the nondominant hemisphere. Indeed, the conditioned placebo response may be potentiated or attenuated by some of the same variables that determine hypnotic responsivity; these variables will be specified later. The importance of bypassing the dominant hemisphere is that the lack of verbal mediation, and very rapid, automatic elicitation of the placebo response make it relatively independent of the critical, skeptical, analytic mode of information processing that is typical of the dominant hemisphere. Hence, the short-latency placebo response occurs before doubt and skepticism (noise) can inhibit or attenuate the message or signal. Stimulus events can directly elicit physiochemical or visceral changes without the interference of the critical, skeptical filtering mode of information processing that is typical of the dominant hemisphere. This may be similar to the profound visceral and neuroendocrine changes that can occur in response to a CNS event (e.g., being charged by a lion in a dream) when there is an inhibition of critical-analytic brain functions during sleep.

Developmentally, the placebo response may begin as what Spence and Taylor (1951) and others (Cerekwicki, Grant, & Porter, 1968; Grant, 1972) called a V form of classical conditioning, but it can develop into a C form of conditioning. The basis of this distinction is the degree of verbal mediation and volition involved in the conditioned response. The mechanism of placebo responding is probably most effective when, in the C or second stage, it is increasingly automatic and involves a bypass of the dominant verbal hemisphere's critical-analytic mode of information processing. In the C phase it is probably a short latency, automatic response that can be labeled an unconscious response. Currently, the bulk of experimental evidence from several fields of empirical research (selective attention, cortical evoked potentials, subliminal perception) supports the position that the registration of perceptual stimulation can occur outside of conscious awareness (Dixon, 1971; Erdelyi, 1974; Kahneman, 1973; Nisbett & Wilson, 1977; Shevrin & Dickman, 1980) and may be consciously recognized only as a change in behavior or a subjective change in mood or feeling. There is also evidence unrelated to psychodynamic speculation that many of the determinants of social behavior are not open to conscious inspection or specification (Nisbett & Wilson, 1977) and that a large part of cognitive and emotional activity occurs without conscious awareness (Davidson, 1980). It appears that overlearned and less conscious information processing is preferentially localized in the nondominant hemisphere (Luria & Simernitskaya, 1977) and that the frontal lobes are preferentially involved in emotional arousal.

Placebo Responding

Health Deprivation, Anxiety, Dependency, the "Core Conditions," and Placebo Responding

The eruption of strange physical symptoms on the patient's body, pain, and discomfort all induce uncertainty and anxiety, from which the patient craves relief. This situation of physical and psychological immobilization (health deprivation) by symptoms like pain and fear reactivates earlier or regressive dependent attitudes that increase patient receptivity to directions from caretaker figures or credible healers. In other words, health deprivation makes the patient particularly dependent and receptive to direction from others. Effective conditioning requires a deprived, anxious, and dependent subject. Anxiety has been shown (Evans, 1974; Thorn, 1962) to be reliably related to placebo responding.

The clinical situation (doctor-patient) reactivates the dependency of the original parent-child relationship (transference) increasing the probability of regression into dependency and enhanced vulnerability to social influence and learning. The "core conditions" (Rogers 1951, Truax and Carkhuff 1965) or accurate empathy, warmth, positive unconditional regard, and so on, are probably pure forms of the ideal parent–child relationship. These interpersonal conditions are probably the ideal preconditions for all complex human social learning. Their use by the therapist will further potentiate placebo responding by *separate* mechanisms that will inhibit the critical analytic-skeptical mode of information processing in the clinical situation. If the patient perceives accurate empathy, warmth, positive unconditional regard, etc. in the therapist, his level of skepticism and suspicion in the relationship will be inhibited and his hypnotic susceptibility will be increased at least modestly (2–3 points or more on the Harvard Scale). So that the social learning component of placebo responding will be motivated not only by the need to *escape* from negative affect (fear, uncertainty, deprivation, etc.) but also the desire to *approach* a trustworthy, attractive parental figure who is positively reinforcing and validating of the patient's worth.

The acquiescence tendency or the tendency to agree ("yea saying") has also been reliably, but modestly and positively correlated with both placebo-responding (Jospe, 1978) and hypnotizability (Hilgard, 1965). Hence, the results of multiple theoretical and empirical studies point to the role of anxiety, dependency, the "core conditions," and the non-analytic, nonskeptical mode (nondominant hemisphere or hypnotic mode) of information processing in placebo responding.

Placebo Responding and Hypnotizability

Shapiro (1971) pointed out that laboratory tests of hypnotic susceptibility show an unreliable relationship to placebo responding. Several other analyses have also cast doubt on the existence of a reliable relationship between hypnotizability and the placebo response (Evans, 1969; Katz, Kao, Spiegel, & Katz, 1974; Moore & Berk, 1976; Thorn, 1962). It is possible that the previously mentioned unreliability results from the activity of other moderating variables (e.g., low credibility, accurate empathy, authoritarianism, levels of attention and arousal, potency of instructional signals) that were not systematically manipulated in the studies relating hypnotic susceptibility and placebo responding. The observation of reliable and orderly relationships between complex events in the empirical world awaits attention to all the relevant variables.

The strongest evidence to date showing a lack of relationship between hypnotizability and placebo responding is a laboratory-experimental pain study by McGlashan, Evans, and Orne (1969). This study found the degree of hypnotizability to be unrelated to the magnitude of the placebo response. However, there are several problems with making inferences and generalizing to a clinical situation from this laboratory study, and therefore, any conclusion may be premature. The McGlashan *et al.* study was a study of experimental pain, and in several areas the parameters of experimental and clinical pain do not overlap (Melzack, 1973). Caution is necessary in generalizing from this otherwise excellent study to the phenomena of clinical pain. In the McGlashan *et al.* study, there was a failure to use strong, extended, and specific instructions of dominant arm analgesia fully to mobilize the potential of the highly hypnotizable subjects in the placebo-analgesia session. The presentation of a rationale for a drug (placebo) can cognitively mobilize the hypnotic ability of the patient and can function as a hypnotic induction (Wickramasekera, 1976b). A study by Glass and Barber (1961) found that a placebo administered as a hypnosis-inducing drug was as effective as an actual trance induction in eliciting enhanced suggestibility. A more recent study of experimental pain by Knox and Gekoski (1981) contradicted the McGlashan *et al.* (1969) study, showing clearly that a subject's level of hypnotizability is related to the placebo response (see Figure 12). Evans (1967) reviewed two nonpatient and five patient studies of the relationship between suggestibility and placebo responding. In neither of the nonpatient studies, and in all but one of the patient (clinical) studies there was a positive relationship between suggestibility and placebo responding.

I predict that with increased attention to those variables (e.g., anxiety, core conditions, dependency and deprivation, etc.) mentioned earlier that moderate the relationship between hypnotizability and placebo responding, more reliable and stronger relationships between suggestibility and placebo responding will emerge in clinical studies.

If the mechanism of the placebo response is conditioning, and if conditioning is enhanced by the degree of bypass of dominant-hemisphere functions (Saltz, 1973), then it is clear why good placebo responders, like good hypnotic subjects, inhibit the critical-analytic mode of information processing that is characteristic of the dominant verbal hemisphere. Good placebo responders will tend to be individuals who are prone to see conceptual or other relationships between events that seem randomly distributed to others. They will inhibit the interfering

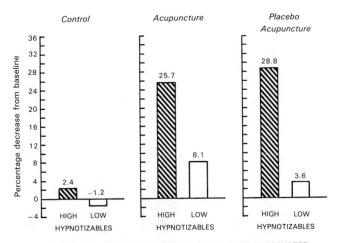

Figure 12. In a series of carefully controlled studies using electroacupuncture both before and during pain stimulation, Knox and Gekoski (1981) demonstrated that high hypnotizables show a greater response to the placebo aspects of a treatment procedure than low hypnotizables. The study consisted of a treatment control group, a placebo (false acupuncture point) acupuncture group, and an acupuncture group.

signals of doubt and skepticism, which are a consequence of the more analytic mode of information processing typical of the dominant (left) hemisphere. Like good hypnotic subjects, good placebo responders are likely covertly to embroider or elaborate on the given stimulus properties of a drug, potentiating it out of their own rich subjective repertoires. Alternatively, they may negate or attenuate the effects of a UCS (drug) through negative attributions or elaborations.

Shapiro (1971) described placebo nonresponders as "rigid and stereotypic and not psychologically minded." There is a striking similarity between such a description and that of a poorly hypnotizable subject. There is increasing evidence (Bakan, 1969; Graham & Pernicano, 1976; Gur & Gur, 1974; Lachman & Goode, 1976) that hypnotizability or suggestibility is predominantly a right-hemisphere (nondominant or minor hemisphere) function for right-handed people. Minor-hemisphere functions include holistic and imaginative mentation with diffuse, relational, and simultaneous processing of information (Ornstein, 1973; Sperry, 1964); the tendency to see some relationship or meaning in data, however randomly generated (e.g., like a Rorschach inkblot), would appear to be an aspect of creative mentation that is posited to be a property of the nondominant hemisphere. This explanation can account for the common features of good placebo responders and good hypnotic subjects.

In the second phase (the consolidation phase) of placebo learning, the placebo response may become regnant in the right hemisphere, which appears to be the hemisphere mainly involved in the hypnotic or suggestible mode of information processing. I hypothesize that, at this stage, the same variables that can influence hypnotic responding can also influence placebo responding. I predict that the placebo response can be potentiated through strong implicit or explicit verbal instructions (Wickramasekera, 1976b), if the following hypnosis-potentiating conditions are also systematically manipulated: (a) low arousal states or training procedures that induce low arousal (e.g., meditation, biofeedback) appear temporarily to increase hypnotic responsivity (Arons, 1976; Engstrom, 1976; Schacter, 1976; Wickramasekera, 1971, 1973b, 1977c), (b) procedures that induce high arousal appear to increase hypnotic responsivity temporarily (Gur, 1974; Wickramasekera, 1972b, 1976b), (c) sensory deprivation procedures also appear to increase hypnotic responsivity temporarily (Pena, 1963; Sanders & Reyher, 1969; Wickramasekera, 1969, 1970), (d) the subject's level of attention to relevant stimuli appears to influence hypnotic responsivity (Graham & Evans, 1977; Krippner & Bindler, 1974; Mitchell, 1967; Van Nuys, 1973), and (e) the baseline suggestibility or hypnotizability of the individual subject (Barber, 1969; Hilgard, 1965) has a profound effect on hypnotic responsivity.

Parameters of Placebo Learning

The Interstimulus Interval (CS–UCS). Contemporary research (Kimble, 1973) on conditioning and learning clearly demonstrates that interstimulus (CS–UCS) intervals are not immutable, particularly with human subjects, and that they can exceed .5 milliseconds. A positive UCS in the health care situation can be defined as a stimulus that reliably elicits a set of specific therapeutic changes (UCRs) in the verbal-subjective, physiochemical, and motor response systems of a human subject. The UCS can alter not only the overt symptoms but also the pathophysiology of the disease or disorder. The CSs are initially neutral features of the physician, the context, and the procedures. There are several ways in which the CS–UCS association can occur in the health care situation.

Simultaneous Conditioning. If the onset and offset of the CS and UCS occur simultaneously, the procedure is called simultaneous conditioning. This situation is unlikely to occur except perhaps in the association of a neutral CS with the relief of acute pain with a powerful fast-acting analgesic (UCS).

Delayed Conditioning. Delayed conditioning is a procedure in which CS onset occurs prior to the UCS and lasts at least until the UCS appears. Historically, an example of this would be the arrival of the physician (CS) prior to the onset of spontaneous remission and his or her departure timed to occur with the onset of the physiochemical events (UCSs) that precede or correlate with symptomatic improvement. This is not unlikely, because for hundreds of years physicians had observed and tracked the natural invariable symptomatic course of several common diseases; therefore, they could predict or prophesy the sequential progression and resolution of symptoms long before they could control these symptomatic events. It is probable that sagacious physicians timed their arrivals and departures to coincide with visible symptomatic changes in the patient. For example, physicians who were good observers and knowledgeable about the progression and timing of symptoms could time the delivery of their rituals (CSs) to coincide clearly and dramatically with the onset of the spontaneous remission of obvious symptoms. On a simple correlational basis, this could be a dramatic demonstration of therapeutic power. But prediction and correlation are not control. It would be control if they could turn the disease process on and off again at will. Fortunately, early physicians were not told, "Do that again."

Trace Conditioning. Trace conditioning occurs when the CS comes on briefly and goes off before the onset of the UCS. A physician with a very detailed and confident knowledge of the course of an illness could arrive late, stay briefly, and leave long before the onset of spontaneous remission, accurately prophesying the course of the patient's symptoms even in his or her absence. Before leaving, the physician might order the performance of some inert rituals and leave, confidently predicting a cure within a specified time interval.

Backward Conditioning. Backward conditioning occurs when the CS follows the UCS, or the physician (CS) arrives after the recovery (UCR) has started. It is unlikely that too many smart early physicians used this conditioning procedure. It is now known to lead to weak and unreliable conditioning.

Temporal Conditioning. Temporal conditioning is a situation in which a specific time interval functions as a CS. A UCS occurs or is presented at regular time intervals and during the test period the UCS is omitted on a portion of the trials. Under these conditions, a CR will occur at the time the UCS typically occurs. This form of conditioning may occur with some chronic diseases that have a fairly reliable intermittent onset. For example, primary dysmenorrhea may be caused part of the time by physiochemical (endocrine) stimuli (UCSs) of varying magnitude. But the chronic maintenance of severe clinical symptoms of unvarying or increasing intensity may be in part related to psychoneuroendocrine events (CSs), such as temporarily conditioned anticipatory dysmenorrhea responses (e.g., irritability, depression, pain, etc.).

Phenomena of Conditioning

Adaptation. Repeated presentations of even potent UCSs can lead to the failure to evoke the UCR and to an absent or extinguishing CR. This phenomena is particularly likely to occur in the treatment of chronic functional problems treated symptomatically. In this instance, even initially potent but nonspecific drugs, such as Valium given for classic migraine headaches, can become less effective over time and the physician and most aspects of his or her practice can lose the ability to elicit conditioned therapeutic responses. The physician has encountered placebo sag and becomes a quack in the eyes of his or her patient. Hence, even a careful CS-UCS analysis of the therapy situation would focus attention on the clear and urgent need for therapeutic stimuli to be targeted on the known or presumed etiology of the disorder and not simply on peripheral symptoms.

Summation. When two or more CSs are presented together, the strength of the CR will be stronger than to either stimulus alone. This implies that the presence of several safety signals or CSs will lead to a stronger placebo response (e.g., not 36% but perhaps 60%). The humane use of high dollar diagnostic medical technology (CAT scan) (CSs) and efficacious drugs (UCSs) and/or surgical procedures (UCSs) may inflate the size of the placebo component in healing. When high technology and irrelevant (nonspecific) state-of-the-art diagnostic and therapy procedures are used without sacrificing humane patient care by practitioners even with minimal UCSs, a large placebo component will be found. This situation probably prevails in large and prestigious tertiary care medical centers to which many patients with chronic functional disorders journey over long distances, as if on a pilgrimage to temples of healing.

Two-Component Response. A UCS will always elicit two components, a CR and UCR. This is predicted because it is probably impossible to deliver a pure UCS isolated from a CS to a conscious vertebrate.

Response Generalization. A person who has learned to respond therapeutically to Physician A or Procedure A has also learned to respond therapeutically to almost equivalent stimuli (e.g. Physician B and Procedure B). This phenomena is often clearly observable in the medical management of acute illness. Acute illness is effectively treated by the health care system, and psychosocial factors seldom have enough time to interfere with healing. In the case of chronic illness, we often observe attentuated therapeutic effects, even to active therapeutic ingredients (UCSs), because of generalization of negative CRs from previous illness episodes or ineffective therapy.

Generalization of Extinction. When physicians use ineffective UCSs to treat chronic conditions, we often observe not only extinction of the placebo response to the original primary care physician, but to all subsequent physicians. This extinction of the placebo component to even an effective UCS may jeopardize even a rational and effective treatment program, because it has been found that the placebo response may not only potentiate or attenuate a UCS (active drug) but may also negate its effects.

The Impact of Explicit or Implicit Verbal Instructions and Information on Conditioned Responses. There is good evidence that awareness of contingency can potentiate the acquisition of CRs (Bandura, 1969). The patient's conscious recognition of the association between his physician and efficacious UCSs (e.g., penicillin) will enhance the acquisition of placebo responses. Also, information about the physician's credentials, reputation among colleagues, and therapeutic record, can potentiate or attenuate the placebo component of the healing. There is a large, well-established experimentally based literature documenting the fact that instructions and information can potently influence both respondent and operant conditioning procedures (Bandura, 1969).

Predictions from the Model

The following predictions appear consistent with the CR model of the placebo, and empirical data disconfirming any of these predictions will cast doubt on the theory.

1. Therapists who routinely use active ingredients (UCSs) will get stronger placebo effects (CRs) than those who do not. This procedure associates and reinforces the CS–UCS relationship that optimizes the conditions for hope (Frank, 1973). Intrinsic to all interventions with

active ingredients (UCSs) is the potential for Pavlovian conditioning, and therefore placebo learning. Hence, the stronger the active ingredient (UCS) or drug used, the stronger the placebo effect; the weaker the active ingredient or UCS intensity, the weaker the placebo response.

2. The response to any active ingredient (UCS) will come to include two components (CR + UCR): a placebo (CR) and an active component (UCR). In other words, a fraction of the response to a UCS will always include a CR—for example, the response to the sight of the syringe (CS) or the ingestion *per se* (CS) of the pill. In fact, it is very likely that the fractional anticipatory response (CR) will have a shorter latency than the response (UCR) to the UCS (e.g., morphine). The shorter latency of the CR will result from the posited central mediation of conditioning effects as opposed to the initial peripheral mediation of some drug effects.

3. Therapists who frequently use inert or placebo medication or procedures (CSs) will get weaker placebo responses over time. This is an extinction procedure because withdrawal of the UCSs (active ingredient) will eventually lead to extinction of the CR, or placebo sag. Therapists who have the right packaging (CS) but who lack a science or truly efficacious UCSs will eventually collapse under the weight of their own incompetence.

4. Numerous repeated presentations of the UCS in drug therapy can lead to temporary tolerance or habituation. But temporary withdrawal of the UCS will abolish placebo sag. CSs alone will not reliably show this recovery feature.

5. Dose-response and time-effect curves for a placebo and an active medication will be similar but not identical. Literature review by Evans (1974a) supports this prediction. The response to CS is like the response to UCS but of shorter latency.

6. Patients higher on trait anxiety will be stronger placebo responders. It is known that trait anxiety is related to the rate of acquisition and magnitude of CRs (Spence & Taylor, 1951). This model can comfortably embrace the anxiety reduction data reviewed by Evans (1974).

7. The placebo response is predicted to be stronger under modified double blind conditions. This implies that neither patient nor therapist should know that an inert or CS procedures is being used. In fact, they should both be told that only an active ingredient or UCS is used. In general, there will be less inhibition of the expectancy mechanism when this modified double blind procedure is used. Credibility will be optimal with this modified double blind. Orne (1974) and Frank (1973) have stressed the role of expectancy and credibility in their analyses of the placebo.

8. The use of several placebo (inert or neutral) stimuli (CS_1, CS_2, CS_3) can lead to a stronger placebo response (higher than typical 35% rate) than the use of one placebo (CS_1) stimulus. It is known that when two ($CS_1 + CS_2$) or more CS are presented together, the strength of the CR is often greater than to either stimulus alone. This phenomenon is called summation (Kimble, 1961).

9. In the final analysis, there can be no CRs without UCSs (active ingredients). Paradoxically, progress in isolating and manipulating active ingredients (UCS) will inevitably lead to more and stronger placebo effects (CR). In other words, faith will grow with progress in science and it may be increasingly difficult to separate out the effects of CS and UCS.

10. If the baseline suggestibility of the patient is mobilized with specific explicit or implicit instructions, then the CR can be potentiated or attenuated.

11. Children, highly hypnotizable adults, and early adolescents can be stronger placebo responders because of their inherently higher baseline suggestibility (Hilgard, 1965).

12. Treatment procedures that use systematic (a) attentional manipulations, (b) induction of low or high arousal, and (c) sensory restriction can potentiate placebo components (CSs) plus any active ingredients (UCSs) in a procedure or substance.

13. Neutral persons, places, and procedures can operate as positive or negative CSs. This may explain iatrogenic illness and suggest ways of arranging the conditions for iatrogenic health. Nocebo effects can arise out of associating neutral stimuli with negative UCSs.

14. Patients whose childhood histories combine firm discipline with warm and effective relief of needs, plus an ability to entertain themselves alone, as children, will be the best placebo responders. Whereas children who have few or no instances of predictable, reliable, and effective (positive or negative) interventions in the child's environment or on the child's behalf will demonstrate weak placebo responses to culture-specific, socially sanctioned health rituals. For example, schizophrenics and autistic children will be poor placebo responders.

15. Skeptical critical-analytic modes of thinking or information processing (typical of the dominant hemisphere) will attenuate or negate placebo responding (CR).

16. The placebo response will not occur if the healing ritual involves bypass of consciousness and the central nervous system.

17. The placebo response will occur maximally under conditions of strong motivation or real personal health deprivation (e.g., escape from life-threatening illness, pain, or fear). In clinical situations with sick patients, the threat to well-being is real, intense, cross-situational, and

of unknown duration, whereas with nonpatients in experimental studies, the threat to well-being is superficial, situation-specific, reversible, and of known duration. The magnitude of the placebo response will generally be weaker with nonpatients. In general, the placebo response will be most potent in life-threatening medical situations, and not in personally trivial social-psychological experiments in university laboratories.

18. The placebo response will generally be stronger in countries where acute unifactorial diseases that respond to a single specific remedy are common (e.g., India), and weaker in countries where chronic multifactorial diseases predominate (e.g., United States).

Testing the Model

Conditioned stimuli for human subjects are not equally neutral because of preexisting belief systems (Wickramasekera, 1977b,c). For example, for patients with scientific training, calibrated quantitative instruments will be more effective placebos. But for patients with more humanistic education or training, a wider range of stimuli (feathers, roses, meters, etc.) will be effective. The model must be tested under conditions of ecological validity. Ecological validity refers to the extent to which we may generalize from controlled laboratory studies of a phenomena to similar phenomena in nonexperimental situations (clinical or natural environments). For example, it is well known that the parameters of clinical and experimental pain are different (Melzack, 1973; Sternbach, 1978). For example, the placebo rate in double blind experimental pain studies is small and ranges between 9% and 16% (Evans, 1974), whereas the average placebo rate in double blind clinical pain (postsurgical) studies is 36%, and thus substantially larger (Beecher, 1959). A sick or health-deprived person is in several psychological and physical respects different from a well person in an experimental study. A sick person is often immobilized by his symptoms cross-situationally. An experimental subject is only immobilized by experimental pain in a situation-specific (laboratory) sense. An experimental subject exposed to a physical stressor (radiant heat, ischemic pain, etc.) is a voluntary subject involved in an episodic and reversible stressful event that does not intrude on the rest of the subject's life. A sick person is immobilized cross-situationally in an involuntary situation, whose outcome is uncertain and that intrudes on all social, personal, and vocational aspects of his or her life. Uncertainty about the consequences of diagnosis and therapy, dependency on others, and lost mobility cause loss of self-esteem over the erosion of important social roles (income provider, caretaker, adult). Sometimes the impatience and progressive withdrawal of loved ones from the patient causes frustration, anger, and depression. These psychological reactions are often superimposed on the pain and physical discomfort caused by the physiological disease process. Therefore, physically and psychologically a sick person is not like a typical experimental laboratory subject. The CR model has been developed to predict behavior in a clinical situation and should be tested on sick patients in therapy.

Conclusion

Because this model of the placebo effect is formulated in terms of experimental psychology and learning, it may have some heuristic value in that it may lead us to design experiments that raise different questions about treatment and may lead us to interpret the responses in unexpected ways. This model makes several specific counterintuitive and paradoxical predictions that may be worth testing empirically. A large body of precise and empirically validated principles from learning theory can now be related to the nebulous field of the placebo. This conceptual translation may stimulate new, sharper, and more focused thought and empirical investigation into this neglected psychobiological realm.

This realm includes psychological effects that are powerful but unreliable, rapid but not always durable, and clearly worthy today of investigation in their own right. It may even turn out that this realm includes the only therapeutic effects that are primarily psychological. It is perhaps time that we settled down to the systematic business of making these nonspecific effects specific by isolating, explicating, and specifying the subject, the therapist, and the situational and procedural conditions under which these effects can be negated, attenuated, or potentiated. It seems unlikely that all the phenomena lumped under the label *placebo effects* can be comprehended within the present CR model. But we can no longer continue to dismiss these effects with impatience and embarrassment as nonspecific, placebo, or plain nuisance effects. It appears to me that these effects reside at and regulate the intersections of all psychobiological actions and transactions.

References

Ader, R. (Ed.). *Psychoneuroimmunology*. New York: Academic Press, 1981.

Ader, R., & Cohen, N. Behaviorally conditioned immunosuppression and murine systemic lupus erythematosus. *Science*, 1982, *215*, 1534–1536.

Arons, L. Sleep assisted instructions. *Psychological Bulletin*, 1976, *83*, 1–40.

Association of Sleep Disorders Centers. Diagnostic clarification of sleep and arousal disorders. *Sleep*, 1979, *2*, 1–137.

Bakan, P. Hypnotizability, laterality of eye movements and functional brain asymmetry. *Perceptual and Motor Skills*, 1969, *28*, 927–932.

Bandura, A. *Principles of behavior modification*. New York: Holt, Reinhart & Winston, 1969.

Barber, J., & Mayer, D. Evaluation of the efficacy and neural mechanism of a hypnotic analgesia procedure and experimental and clinical dental pain. *Pain*, 1977, *4*, 41–48.

Barber, T. X. Toward a theory of pain: Relief of chronic pain by prefrontal leucotomy, opiates, placebos, and hypnosis. *Psychological Bulletin*, 1959, *56*, 430.

Barber, T. X. *Hypnosis: A scientific approach*. New York: Van Nostrand Reinhold, 1969.

Basbaum, A. I., & Fields, H. L. Endogenous pain control mechanisms: Review and hypothesis. *Annals of Neurology*, 1978, *4*(5), 451–462.

Beecher, H. K. The powerful placebo. *Journal of the American Medical Association*, 1955, *159*, 1602–1606.

Beecher, H. K. *Measurement of subjective responses: Quantitative effects of drugs*. New York: Oxford University Press, 1959.

Beecher, H. K. Surgery as a placebo. *Journal of the American Medical Association*, 1961, *176*, 1102–1107.

Benson, H., & Epstein, M. The placebo effect: A neglected asset in the care of patients. *Journal of the American Medical Association*, 1975, *232*, 1225–1227.

Bowbjerg, D., Ader, R., & Cohen, N. Behaviorally conditioned suppression of a graft-versus-host response. *Proceedings of the National Academy of Sciences USA*, 1982, *79*, 583–585.

Cannon, J. T., Liebeskind, J. C., & Frank, H. Neural and neurochemical mechanisms of pain inhibition. In R. A. Sternbach (Ed.), *The psychology of pain*. New York: Raven Press, 1978.

Cerekwicki, L. E., Grant, D., & Porter, E. C. The effect of number and relatedness of verbal discriminanda upon differential eyelid conditioning. *Journal of Verbal Learning and Verbal Behavior*, 1968, *7*, 847–853.

Cobb, L. A., Thomas, G. I., Dillard, D. H., Merendino, K. A., & Bruce, R. A. An evaluation of internal-mammary-artery ligation by a double blind technic. *New England Journal of Medicine*, 1959, *260*, 1115–1118.

Cohen, H. D., Graham, C., Fotopoulos, S. S., & Cook, M. R. A double-blind methodology for biofeedback research. *Psychophysiology*, 1977, *14*, 603–608.

Davidson, R. J. Consciousness and information processing: A biocognitive perspective. In J. M. Davidson & R. J. Davidson (Eds.), *The psychobiology of consciousness*. New York: Plenum Press, 1980.

Dimond, E. G., Kittle, C. F., & Crockett, J. E. Evaluation of internal mammary artery ligation and sham procedure in angina pectoris. *Circulation*, 1958, *18*, 712–713.

Dixon, N. F. *Subliminal perception: The nature of a controversy*. London: McGraw-Hill, 1971.

Drawbraugh, R., & Lal, H. Reversal by narcotic antagonist of a narcotic action elicited by a conditioning simulus. *Nature*, 1974, *247*, 65–67.

Engel, G. L. The need for a new medical model: A challenge for biomedicine. *Science*, 1977, *196*, 129–136.

Engstrom, D. R. Hypnotic susceptibility, EEG-alpha and self-regulation. In G. E. Schwartz & D. Shapiro (Eds.), *Consciousness and self-regulation*. New York: Plenum Press, 1976.

Erdelyi, M. H. A new look at the new look: Perceptual defense and vigilance. *Psychological Review*, 1974, *81*, 1–25.

Evans, F. J. Suggestibility in the normal waking state. *Psychological Bulletin*, 1967, *67*(2), 114–129.

Evans, F. J. Placebo response: Relationship to suggestibility and hypnotizability. *Proceedings of the 77th Annual Convention of the American Psychological Association*, 1969, *4*, 889–890.

Evans, F. J. The power of a sugar pill. *Psychology Today*, April 1974, p. 32.

Evans, F. J. The placebo response in pain reduction. In J. J. Bonica (Ed.), *Advances in neurology: Vol. 4. Pain*. New York: Raven Press, 1977.

Frank, J. D. *Persuasion and healing: A comparative study of psychotherapy*. Baltimore: Johns Hopkins University Press, 1973.

Freud, S. *A general introduction to psychoanalysis*. New York: Garden City, 1938.

Glass, L. B., & Barber, T. X. A note on hypnotic behavior, the definition of the situation and the placebo effect. *Journal of Nervous and Mental Disease*, 1961, *132*, 539–541.

Gleidman, L. H., Gantt, W. H., & Teitelbaum, H. A. Some implications of conditional reflex studies for placebo research. *American Journal of Psychiatry*, 1957, *113*, 1103–1107.

Gold, M. S., Pottash, A. C., Sweeney, D., Martin, D., & Extein, I. Antimanic, antidepressant and anti-panic effects of opiates: Clinical, neuroanatomical and biochemical evidence. In K. Verebey (Ed.), *Opioids in mental illness*. New York: New York Academy of Sciences, 1982.

Goldberg, S. R., & Schuster, C. R. Conditioned suppression by a stimulus associated with nalorphine in morphine dependent monkeys. *Journal of the Experimental Analysis of Behavior*, 1967, *10*, 235–242.

Goldberg, S. R., & Schuster, C. R. Conditioned nalorphine induced abstinence changes: Persistence in post-morphine dependent monkeys. *Journal of the Experimental Analysis of Behavior*, 1970, *14*, 33–46.

Goldstein, A., & Hilgard, E. R. Failure of the opiate antagonist naloxone to modify hypnotic analgesia. *Proceedings of the National Academy of Sciences USA*, 1975, *72*, 2041–2043.

Graham, C., & Evans, F. Hypnotizability and the development of waking attention. *Journal of Abnormal Psychology*, 1977, *86*, 631–638.

Graham, K., & Pernicano, K. *Laterality, hypnosis and the autokinetic effect*. Paper presented at the meeting of the American Psychological Association, Washington, D.C., 1976.

Grant, D. A. A preliminary model for processing information conveyed by verbal conditioned stimuli in classical conditioning. In A. Black & W. Prokasy (Eds.), *Classical conditioning: II. Current research and theory*. New York: Meredith, 1972.

Gur, R. C. An attention-controlled operant procedure for enhancing hypnotic susceptibility. *Journal of Abnormal Psychology*, 1974, *83*, 644–650.

Gur, R. C., & Gur, R. E. Handedness, sex, eyedness, and moderating variables in relation to hypnotic susceptibility and functional brain symmetry. *Journal of Abnormal Psychology*, 1974, *83*, 635–643.

Haas, H., Fink, H., & Hartfelder, G. Das Placeboproblem. *Fortschritte der Arzneimittelforschung*, 1959, *1*, 279–454.

Haynes, R. B., Sackett, D. L., & Taylor, D. W., Gibson, E. S., & Johnson, A. L. Increased absenteeism from work after detection and labelling of hypertensive patients. *New England Journal of Medicine*, 1978, *299*, 741–744.

Herrnstein, R. J. Placebo effect in the rat. *Science*, 1962, *138*, 677–678.

Hilgard, E. R., & Marquis, D. G. *Conditioning and learning*. New York: Appleton, 1961.

Hilgard, E. R. *Hypnotic susceptibility*. New York: Harcourt, Brace, 1965.

Hirsch, J. Current state of research in psychoneuroimmunology and cancer. In J. Holland (Ed.), *Current concepts in psychosocial oncology*. New York: Sloan-Kettering Memorial Cancer Center, 1982.

Horningfeld, G. Nonspecific factors in treatment: I. Review of placebo reactions and placebo reactors. *Diseases of the Nervous System*, 1964, *25*, 145–156. (a)

Horningfeld, G. Nonspecific factors in treatment: II. Review of social-psychological factors. *Diseases of the Nervous System*, 1964, *25*, 225–239. (b)

Hull, C. L. *A behavioral system*. New Haven: Yale University Press, 1952.

Jospe, M. *The placebo effect in healing*. Lexington, MA: Lexington Books, 1978.

Kahneman, D. *Attention and effort*. Englewood Cliffs: Prentice-Hall, 1973.

Katz, R. L., Kao, C. Y., Spiegel, H., & Katz, G. J. Pain, acupuncture, hypnosis. In J. J. Bonica (Ed.), *Advances in neurology: Vol. 4. Pain*. New York: Raven Press, 1974.

Kazdin, A. E., & Wilcoxon, L. A. Systematic desensitization and nonspecific treatment effects: A methodological evaluation. *Psychological Bulletin*, 1976, *83*(5), 729–758.

Kihlstrom, J. F. The cognitive unconscious. *Science*, 1987, *237*, 1445–1452.

Kimble, G. *Conditioning and learning*. New York: Appleton-Century-Crofts, 1961.

Kimble, G. Scientific psychology in transition. In F. McGuigan & D. Lumsdan (Eds.), *Contemporary approaches to conditioning and learning*. New York: Wiley, 1973.

Knox, V. J., & Gekoski, W. L. *Analgesic effect of acupuncture in high and low hypnotizables*. Paper presented at the meeting of the Society for Clinical and Experimental Hypnosis, Portland, Oregon, October 1981.

Krippner, S., & Bindler, P. R. Hypnosis and attention: A review. *American Journal of Clinical Hypnosis*, 1974, *16*, 166–177.

Lachman, S., & Goode, W. J. *Hemispheric dominance and variables to hypnotic susceptibility*. Paper presented at the meeting of the American Pyschological Association, Washington, D.C., 1976.

Levine, J. D., Gordon, N. C., & Fields, H. L. The mechanism of placebo analgesia. *Lancet*, 1978, *2*, 654–657.

Lipowski, Z. J. Psychosomatic medicine in the seventies: An overview. *American Journal of Psychiatry*, 1977, *134*, 233–244.

Luparello, T. J., Leist, N., Lourie, C. H., & Sweet, P. The interaction of psychologic stimuli and pharmacologic agents reactivity in asthematic subjects. *Psychosomatic Medicine*, 1970, *32*, 509–513.

Luria, A. R., & Simernitsakaya, E. G. Interhemispheric relations and functions of the minor hemisphere. *Neuropsychologia*, 1977, *15*, 175–178.

Mayer, D. J., Wolfe, T. L., Akil, H., Carder, B., & Liebeskind, J. C. Analgesia from electric stimulation in the brainstem of the rat. *Science*, 1971, *174*, 1351–1354.

Mayer, D. J., Prince, D. D., Barber, J., & Rafii, A. Acupuncture analgesia: Evidence for activation of a pain inhibitory system as a mechanism of action. In J. J. Bonica & D. Albe-Fessard (Eds.), *Advances in pain research and therapy* (Vol. 1). New York: Raven Press, 1976.

McGlashan, T. H., Evans, F. J., & Orne, M. T. The nature of hypnotic analgesia and placebo response to experimental pain. *Psychosomatic Medicine*, 1969, *31*, 227–246.

Mechanic, D. Social psychological factors affecting the presentation of bodily complaints, *New England Journal of Medicine*, 1972, *286*, 1132–1139.

Melzack, R. *Puzzle of pain*. New York: Basic Books, 1973.

Merskey, H., & Hester, R. A. The treatment of chronic pain with psychotropic drugs. *Postgraduate Medicine Journal*, 1972, *48*, 594–598.

Mitchell, M. G. *Hypnotic susceptibility and response to distraction*. Unpublished doctoral dissertation, Claremont Graduate School, 1967.

Moore, M. E., & Berk, S. M. Acupuncture for chronic shoulder pain: An experimental study with attention to the role of placebo and hypnotic susceptibility. *Annals of Internal Medicine*, 1976, *84*, 381–384.

Mowrer, O. H. Two factor learning theory reconsidered, with special reference to secondary reinforcement and the concept of habit. *Psychological Review*, 1956, *63*, 114–128.

Mowrer, O. H. *Learning theory and behavior*. New York: Wiley, 1960.

Nisbett, R. E., & Wilson, T. D. Telling more than we can know: Verbal reports on mental processes. *Psychological Review*, 1977, *84*, 231–259.

Orne, M. T. Pain suppression by hypnosis and related phenomena. In J. J. Bonica (Ed.), *Advances in neurology: Vol. 4. Pain.* New York: Raven Press, 1974.

Ornstein, R. *The psychology of consciousness.* New York: Viking, 1973.

Ostfeld, A. M. *The common headache syndromes: Biochemistry, pathophysiology, therapy.* New York: Grune & Stratton. 1962.

Pavlov, I. P. *Conditioned reflexes* (G. V. Anrep, Trans.). London: Oxford University Press, 1927.

Pena, F. *Perceptual isolation and hypnotic susceptibility.* Unpublished doctoral dissertation, Washington State University, 1963.

Rogers, C. R. *Client-centered therapy.* Boston: Houghton Mifflin Co., 1951.

Rogers, M. P., Dubey, D., & Reich, P. The influence of the psyche and the brain on immunity and disease susceptibility: A critical review. *Psychosomatic Medicine*, 1979, *41*(2), 147–164.

Saltz, E. Higher mental processes as the bases for the laws of conditioning. In F. McGuigan & D. Lumsden (Eds.), *Contemporary approaches to conditioning and learning.* New York: Wiley, 1973.

Sanders, S., & Reyher, J. Sensory deprivation and the enhancement of hypnotic susceptibility. *Journal of Abnormal Psychology*, 1969, *74*, 375–381.

Schacter, D. L. The hypnogogic state: A critical review of the literature. *Psychological Bulletin*, 1976, *83*, 452–481.

Schuster, C., & Thompson, T. Self administration of and behavioral dependence on drugs. *Annual Review of Pharmacology*, 1969, *9*, 483–502.

Schwartz, G. E. Self-regulation of response patterning: Implications for psychophysiological research and therapy. *Biofeedback and Self-Regulation*, 1976, *1*, 7–30.

Schwitzgebel, R., & Traugott, M. Initial note on the placebo effect of machines. *Behavioral Science*, 1968, *13*, 267–273.

Shapiro, A. Placebo effects in medicine, psychotherapy and psychoanalysis. In A. Bergin & S. Garfield (Eds.), *Handbook of psychotherapy and behavior change.* New York: Wiley, 1971.

Shevrin, H., & Dickman, S. The psychological unconscious. *American Psychologist*, 1980, *35*(5), 421–434.

Siegel, S. A Pavlovian conditioning analysis of morphine tolerance. In N. A. Krasnegor (Ed.), *Behavioral tolerance: Research and treatment implications* (National Institute on Drug Abuse Monograph No. 18: U.S. DHEW Publ. No. ADM 78-551). Washington, D.C.: U.S. Government Printing Office, 1978.

Skinner, B. F. *Science and human behavior.* New York: Macmillan, 1953.

Sox, H. C., Margulies, I., & Sox, C. H. Psychologically mediated effects of diagnostic tests. *Annals of Internal Medicine*, 1981, *95*, 680–685.

Spence, K., & Taylor, J. A. Anxiety and the strength of the UCS as determiners of the amount of eyelid conditioning. *Journal of Experimental Psychology*, 1951, *42*, 183–188.

Sperry, R. The great cerebral commissure. *Scientific American*, 1964, *210*, 42–52.

Sternbach, R. A. *The psychology of pain.* New York: Raven Press, 1978.

Sternbach, R. A. On strategies for identifying neurochemical correlates of hypnotic analgesia. *International Journal of Clinical and Experimental Hypnosis.* 1982, *30*(3), 251–256.

Stroebel, C. F., & Glueck, B. C. Biofeedback treatment in medicine and psychiatry: An ultimate placebo. In L. Birk (Ed.), *Biofeedback: Behavior medicine*, 1973, *30*(3), 251–256.

Taub, A., & Collins, W. F., Jr. Observations on the treatment of denerveral dysthesia with psychotropic drugs: Posttherapeutic neuralgia, anesthesia dolorosa, and peripheral neuropathy. In J. J. Bonica (Ed.), *Advances in neurology: Vol. 4. Pain.* New York: Raven Press, 1974.

Thorn, W. F. The placebo reactor. *Australian Journal of Pharmacy*, 1962, *43*, 1035–1037.

Traux, C. B., & Carkhuff, R. R. *Toward effective counseling and psychotherapy: Training and practice.* Chicago: Aldine, 1967.

Trousseau, A., cited in M. S. Straus (Ed.), *Familiar medical quotations.* Boston: Little, Brown & Company, 1968.

Van Nuys, D. Meditation, attention, and hypnotic susceptibility: A correlational study. *International Journal of Clinical and Experimental Hypnosis*, 1973, *21*, 59–69.

Verebey, K., Volavka, J., & Clouet, D. Endorphins in psychiatry. *Archives of General Psychiatry*, 1978, *35*, 877–888.

Weiner, H. *Psychobiology and human disease.* New York: Elsevier/North-Holland, 1977.

Wickramasekera, I. The effects of sensory restriction on susceptibility to hypnosis: A hypothesis and some preliminary data. *International Journal of Clinical and Experimental Hypnosis*, 1969, *17*, 217–224.

Wickramasekera, I. Effects of sensory restriction on susceptibility to hypnosis: more data. *Journal of Abnormal Psychology*, 1970, *76*, 69–75.

Wickramasekera, I. Effects of EMG feedback training on susceptibility to hypnosis: Preliminary observations. In J. Stoyva, T. Barber, L. V. DiCara, J. Kamiya, N. E. Miller, & D. Shapiro (Eds.), *Biofeedback and self-control.* Chicago: Aldine, 1971.

Wickramasekera, I. EMG feedback training and tension headache: Preliminary observations. *American Journal of Clinical Hypnosis*, 1972, *15*(2), 83–85. (a)

Wickramasekera, I. A technique for controlling a certain type of sexual exhibitionism. *Psychotherapy: Theory, research and practice*, 1972, *9*, 207–210. (b)

Wickramasekera, I. The application of verbal instructions and EMG feedback training to the management of tension headache. *Headache*, 1973, *13*(2), 74–76. (a)

Wickramasekera, I. The effects of EMG feedback on susceptibility to hypnosis. *Journal of Abnormal Psychology*, 1973, *82*, 174–177. (b)

Wickramasekera, I. Aversive behavior rehearsal for sexual exhibitionism. *Behavior Therapy*, 1976, *7*, 167–176. (a)

Wickramasekera, I. (Ed.). *Biofeedback, behavior therapy and hypnosis.* Chicago: Nelson-Hall, 1976. (b)

Wickramasekera, I. On attempts to modify hypnotic susceptibility: Some psychophysiological procedures and promising directions. *Annals of the New York Academy of Sciences.* 1977, *296*, 143–153. (a)

Wickramasekera, I. The placebo effect and biofeedback for headache pain. In *Proceedings of the San Diego Biomedical Symposium.* New York: Academic Press, 1977. (b)

Wickramasekera, I. The placebo effect and medical instruments in biofeedback. *Journal of Clinical Engineering*, 1977, *2*, 227–230. (c)

Wickramasekera, I. A conditioned response model of the placebo effect: Predictions from the model. *Biofeedback and Self-Regulation*, 1980, *5*, 5–18.

Wilker, A., & Pesor, F. T. Persistence of relapse tendencies of rats previously made physically dependent on morphine. *Psychopharmacologia*, 1970, *16*, 375–384.

Wolf, S. Effects of suggestion and conditioning on the action of chemical agents in human subjects: The pharmacology of placebos. *Journal of Clinical Investigation*, 1950, *29*, 100–109.

Wolff, H. G. *Headache and other pain.* New York, Oxford University Press, 1963.

6

INITIAL PATIENT INTERVIEW

Why Patients Come to See Us

Patients may be referred to a behavioral medicine practitioner for a variety of reasons. Generally, the bulk of these referrals come from physicians with patients who present chronic physical complaints in the absence, on repeated investigations, of physical findings. Alternatively, they are patients whose somatic complaints have been unresponsive to multiple, conventional chemical and/or surgical interventions. Often the referrals are poorly made. Without rapid and effective patient reorientation by the behavioral medicine practitioner, these patients are unlikely to make or keep an appointment, or if they come in, to return after the first visit.

Such situations can be reduced to several subtypes of referral. First, a physician may refer a patient who has been unresponsive to a variety of chemical and surgical interventions simply to be rid of a nuisance. These "dumped" patients, if they follow through on the referral and are still fighting for their health, are frequently defensive, skeptical, pessimistic, and angry in the initial interview. They are intimidated and immobilized by their symptoms and have spent large amounts of money, time, and energy in an elusive quest for a medical solution to their problem. The referral to the psychologist or psychiatrist who is a behavioral medicine practitioner is seen by the patient as a challenge to the authenticity of his or her symptoms. These patients require rapid reorientation. Their need to validate the authenticity of their physical symptoms must be rapidly defused by accepting up front the reality of their complaints. They should be allowed to present their impressive medical credentials (a folder with a record of numerous medical tests, surgeries, and prescriptions, etc.). The practitioner should then empathetically reflect their feelings of frustration, disappointment, anger, and hopelessness about the failure to resolve their somatic symptoms.

Second, some patients are referred because they cannot tolerate the side effects of the drugs they are on or because they have habituated to their medications (e.g., sleep medications, minor tranquilizers and analgesics, etc.) These patients are frequently demoralized, chronically depressed spectators of life, and have settled into a constricted, uneventful, or destructive life-style in which their chronic patient role alienates them from their families and other natural support systems. These patients are the hardest to mobilize, and they require small but consistent experiences of hope at each therapy session. Hope can be revived by judicious use of procedures ranging from a covert gain adjustment[1] during feedback training to guarantee progress, to cognitive reframing of an old and unproductive perception of a problem.

Third, another subset of patients is referred because the patient is either unresponsive or unwilling to continue medical management and may request referral to a behavioral medicine practitioner because of information in the mass media. Such patients often have unrealistically high expectations (Stroebel & Glueck, 1973) that require recalibration during the initial evaluation process. Fourth, another group of patients is referred because a careful medical work-up identifies no clear physical findings and consequently, by exclusion, the referring physician assumes there will be positive psychological or behavioral findings. It is seldom that this type of referral is accompanied by a letter from a physician requesting confirmation of his suspicion that positive psychological or behavioral findings could explain the presenting physical complaints. Even though the physician may have concluded that no physical basis for the symptoms exists, it is possible in this case that the appropriate or adequately sensitive medical test was not done, particularly if we fail to identify positive psychophysiological findings (Wickramasekera 1979, 1984).

Fifth, a small number of patients may be referred by previous patients who are pleased with the positive outcome of their own therapy. It is critical in such a case to determine if there has been a prior and adequate medical investigation of the patient's problems before accepting him or her for treatment. Finally, there are a small number of patients who are referred from major tertiary care medical centers where they have already been medically and psychologically evaluated by sophisticated clinicians who often do a good job of educating and orienting the patient prior to referral. These patients have been told that there are

---

[1]Clinically, I have observed that this covert gain adjustment or placebo procedure will, in fact often produce an actual change in the absolute frontal EMG measure. There is at least one controlled study supporting this clinical observation.

new behavioral and psychophysiological techniques that are cost-effective, efficacious, and have none or fewer side effects than the standard medical treatments. The patient is told that they should be tried first before escalating to more radical and risky medical interventions.

In conclusion, the manner in which the referring physician prepares the patient's mind with respect to mind–body interaction issues can powerfully influence the patient's decision to follow through on a referral to a behavioral medicine practitioner. It can also influence the patient's decision actively to participate in the initial assessment and therapy process.

Priorities and Procedures

Even before the patient comes in for the initial interview it is important that he or she have some specific expectations regarding your competencies, skills, and reputation for dealing with his specific problem. The source of these expectations may be your published work, previous patients, or the mass media. It is in the first two or three sessions that your social-psychological influence with the patient will be maximal, after that your credibility will start to sag unless your stated observations and interventions impact the patient's distress and symptoms at a direct experiential level. These initial sessions provide a window of opportunity. It is critical that you "get your foot in the patient's head" before the window closes.

It is the first priority of the initial evaluation, from the therapist's viewpoint, to determine what the patient perceives to be the primary problem that requires attention and resolution. Encouraging the patient to describe the symptoms and reactions to the symptoms can provide an opportunity for the patient to temporarily relate regressively to the therapist. This creates an altered state of consciousness that briefly reinstates the original parent–child relationship. Second, it is extremely important to attempt to identify what the patient believes is causing his or her problem or what factors the patient believes are associated with the onset and the eventual solution of the problem. Whether these patient speculations are valid or not is a separate issue. Clinically, it is important to identify these patient speculations and to confront the patient with what he believes about his problem. This provides the first step in engagement or bonding between therapist and patient.

In addition, there are frequently unverbalized, underlying fantasies that the patient may have regarding a symptom that he or she is embarrassed about or considers so ridiculous that they are unwilling to talk about them. The therapist needs to give the patient permission to talk about them, and even to imply that the therapist suspects what they are, though they exist only in the shadows of his or her mind. This can be done by looking directly into the patient's eyes in an inquiring and accepting way, during episodes of pregnant silence in an atmosphere of focused ambiguity. During these regressive episodes the patient may blurt out a "confession" of some personal mythology. For example, the patient may believe he or she is suffering from an undiagnosed catastrophic disease or is being punished for his or her sins or parents' sins or for some previous transgression of a moral or legal code. For example, the patient may hold such beliefs as "I am no good," a "black sheep," or a "victim" of events, or conversely, "it is my destiny to rescue and care for others" or "I am good only when I am compulsively helping others." These unverbalized fantasies are extremely important to elicit in the early sessions of therapy, because verbalizing them to another person can be therapeutic in and of itself. Additionally, the patient's eventual recognition and disclosure of this unconscious personal belief increases the patient's vulnerability to social influence, and will build a bond of closeness between the patient and therapist. Confronting the patient with these hitherto unverbalized fantasies is the second step in therapist–patient engagement. This bonding is important because the patient can now subjectively feel that he or she is not alone, but with a powerful and wise person when the exploration proceeds to even darker and more shadowy aspects of functioning and the self. It is crucial rapidly to develop this type of patient perception, which is the authoritative aspect of the transference, regardless of how unreal the perception is. It gives the patient the support and courage for further self-exploration.

It is important to identify the objective and subjective antecedents or conditions that are associated with the onset of changes in the frequency or intensity of the presenting symptoms. It is also important to identify what conditions (interpersonal, intrapsychic, or environmental) are associated with the offset or the tapering down of the symptoms. For example, can the onset of a more serious problem or crisis occurring in the patient's life or a recurring dream change the frequency or intensity of a presenting symptom? What is the role of environmental change? For example, what happens to the symptoms on weekends and vacations? How does a change in the patient's daily schedule affect his symptom? These inquiries should be made in a direct and active way that both leads and follows the patient into activity. The therapist should be sensitive to verbal and nonverbal feedback cues elicited by prior questions and be willing to branch out into apparently unrelated but pregnant areas. One should never stick rigidly to a predetermined format in the initial sessions unless there is a very good reason to do so.

The second priority from the therapist's viewpoint is to get some estimate of the patient's commitment to change as behaviorally demonstrated by a willingness to put therapy and one's self on the front burner and other less essential activities on the back burner at least for the duration of the engagement. This means reserving the choicest portions of a day to be devoted to doing therapy homework. This also implies being punctual for sessions and not cancelling sessions except for emergencies. Without commitment of time and effort to therapy, complex and salient changes are unlikely to occur soon enough for the patient to see progress. Significant change is painful, and can be slow. An important part of the evaluation of the patient's candidacy for therapy includes evaluating his or her commitment to therapeutic work. The patient is explicitly told that we are evaluating his or her candidacy for therapy, and that "I will seldom ask you to do anything that is easy" or "I am, in a sense, looking for a few good people who can learn to substitute skills for pills." The therapeutic work-pain starts with a commitment to complete honesty and vulnerability. I will often say to the new patient, "since I don't read minds, you have to make yourself vulnerable in this protected setting if I am going to help you find the key to your problem." The patient is plainly told that lies by commission or omission delay and destroy therapeutic work; not making a decision to talk about a salient topic is a decision. "Lack of honesty wastes my time and your money. You can tell when you are doing good therapeutic work because it will always hurt most when it counts."

The third priority from the therapist's viewpoint, is to induce an aggressive attitude in the patient toward his symptoms and problem. "Once I know what your dragons are, I will be asking you to go after your dragons and not to wait for them to come looking for you." Our goal is self-exploration, self-mastery, and eventually, the ability to practice at the "scene of the crime," the time and place where the patient has been previously symptomatically immobilized. "People do not change, grow, and rise above their symptoms from merely doing easy things, nor do they change until they *have* to; and if change was easy, you would not be here today sitting in front of me." It is very important for the patient to remember that at times you will have to be hard on him or her but that there can be a lot of love even in a psychosurgical knife. Caring has to involve firmness and discipline. It may be unpleasant for the therapist to implement this discipline, but that is precisely what the healthy portion of the patient's personality expects and is paying you to do. Therapy in the final analysis is not terminating symptoms but learning flexible conceptual, affective, and motor skills that can be widely used in high-stress interpersonal situations. Reducing symptoms is only a temporary goal on the road to increasing interpersonal competencies.

Commitment to change is also behaviorally demonstrated by following through on specific self-monitoring activities and homework assignments (e.g., assigned reading, relaxation practice with tape, practice at the "scene of the crime," etc.) These data are essential to enable the patient to do adequate self-exploration, self-diagnosis, and microanalysis of contingencies between environmental events, emotional and cognitive events, and behavioral responses at work or home. Self-monitoring of target symptoms (e.g., anxiety episodes, pain reports, depressive thoughts, urges to smoke, etc.) makes the patient a keener observer of his own overt and covert behaviors and more analytic about emotions and beliefs. This is important for the *high* hypnotizables, who tend to have too many global impressions, and for the low hypnotizables, who tend to have no impressions at all from psychological self-analysis. Awareness of contingencies between symptoms and emotions and environmental events reduces the probability of reflex behavioral responding (CS-CR) and interposes delays that makes possible conscious (attended) behavioral choices of new coping techniques. In starting self-monitoring, it is good to start with something that has high face validity or something the patient has already noticed informally to be relevant to the problem. Self-monitoring is contracted initially for a week. As the patient begins this process of self-monitoring of overt or covert behaviors, he or she may also notice other relationships between these behaviors and apparently unrelated events. When these diary and self-monitoring materials are brought in it is very important that time be allocated during therapy, preferably up front, carefully to discuss the fruits of the patient's labors during the week and the patient's associations, thoughts, and elaborations about the data he or she has collected. This communicates to the patient that you consider this activity important and that you respect the patient's curiosity about discovering contingencies between behaviors and intrapsychic or social-psychological events in his or her environment. Through all these activities the patient is explicitly told and helped to recognize that he or she is becoming an active participant in his or her own self-diagnosis, self-assessment, and rehabilitation planning. In the process of self-evaluation the patient may participate and request tasks that you might want to assign later, and when he or she does you warmly congratulate the patient for being ahead of you, on track, and on target. The therapy model is explicitly one of a self-education or self-investigation and not the medical one in which the patient is the passive recipient of interventions. This model raises the patient's self-esteem.

It is most important to point out somewhere in the initial three sessions of therapy that there will be numerous symptomatic ups and downs, particularly in the early course of therapy, and that initially the patient may have to get worse before getting better. The ability to hold a therapeutic work course across time, when no progress seems to occur or when in fact things are getting episodically worse, is explicitly stated to be the mark of courage and of a "winner." "Failures can be the pillars of success." The patient should be shown the individual learning curve, which is marked by numerous ups and downs in acquisition and only gradual elevation of the baseline. It is often necessary to take one step backward to take two steps forward. Transitional points in therapy tasks are particularly vulnerable to regressions and relapses. For example, the patient with an obesity problem should be shown a graph of a previous patient losing weight. You should draw particular attention to the times of plateaus when discouragement often leads to relapses. Point out to the patient that it is decisions made at these nodal points in therapy, (e.g., no weight loss despite diet and exercise, pain getting episodically worse for no apparent reason, etc.) that determine the outcome of therapy in the long run. Plateaus are often pregnant with salient changes but require patience and holding a work course, in spite of apparent inertia. Transition points in therapy are particularly vulnerable because of uncertainty. Staying the course during psychic storms is crucial. Advanced organizers (Ausubel, 1963) such as "no gain without pain" cognitively immunizes the patient against the inevitable relapses that occur in the course of therapy. Because you have predicted relapses before they occur, they will not be as catastrophic when they arrive.

It is also important in this initial interview to get some informal estimate of the patient's hypnotic talent. This may be elicited by observation of the patient's conjugate lateral eye movements during reflective thought during the clinical interview, or with a paper-and-pencil test like the WAT.

In conclusion, it is important to point out to the patient that the goal of psychophysiological therapy is self-mastery, coping, and self-control, not cure in a medical sense. At some future time the patient may want again to experiment with the patient role but at that time he or she will have acquired skills to keep from getting stuck in that role. The goal is the substitution of skills for pills. Even after extended periods of symptomatic freedom, it is important to tell the patient that it is possible to have intense breakthrough symptoms that will test the patient's sense of self-efficacy, and analytic and psychophysiological skills. When confronted with situations the patient cannot change or fight, or from which he cannot flee, he or she has to learn to flow. Long-term follow-up is particularly important for these types of symptoms and therapy, to prevent the patient from getting stuck in relapses. Containment of breakthrough chronic symptoms that test psychophysiological skills requires practice and conviction, the time and money invested in acquiring these skills needs to be protected by long-term follow-up sessions in which these conceptual and motor skills are checked out periodically. At termination of the active phase of therapy, the patient is phased out over 5 years rather than terminated.

After the initial interview it is important that the patient find himself or herself thinking about what you have said and what has been discussed in the session after leaving the consulting room. The patient should carry some central or even peripheral aspects of the clinical interview outside the consulting room into his or her natural habitat and use them (in sleep or in the waking state) to reframe the experience of his or her distress in the course of the coming week. It is also important that the new patient look forward to the next session perhaps with mild or moderate anxiety, and preferably have a list of specific topics to discuss. The therapist should make time available up front for the patient to lead discussion of these materials. As the patient leads such a discussion, the therapist should listen intently and briefly comment in a way that captures the essence of the patient's comments. These brief comments or questions should cast some fresh light on the topic or enable the patient to see it from some unsuspected or fresh perspective. All of these operations are intended to communicate to the patient that contact with the therapist will recast the problem in a new light and that resolution of the problem can come from a hitherto unsuspected direction.

The purpose of the initial interview is to convey to the patient, in general, what long, hard, and painful therapeutic work needs to be done and what help and hope is available.

References

Ausubel, D. P. *The psychology of meaningful verbal learning.* New York: Grune & Stratton, 1963.

Stroebel, C. F., & Glueck, B. C. Biofeedback treatment in medicine and psychiatry: An ultimate placebo? *Seminars in Psychiatry,* 1973, *5,* 379–393.

Wickramasekera, I. *A model of the patient at high risk for chronic stress-related disorders. Do beliefs have biological consequences?* Paper presented at Annual Convention of the Biofeedback Society of America, San Diego 1979.

Wickramasekera, I. A model of people at risk to develop chronic stress related disorders. In F. J. McGuigan, W. E. Sime, & J. M. Wallace (Eds.), *Stress and tension control.* New York: Plenum Press, 1984.

7

PSYCHOPHYSIOLOGICAL ROLE
INDUCTION
OR THE TROJAN HORSE
PROCEDURE

It is absolutely essential immediately to move the patient presenting physical complaints without physical findings toward a psychophysiological model and away from a biomedical model (mind–body dichotomy model) of one's presenting complaints. The psychophysiological model is implemented through a role induction which should be administered within the first three sessions of patient contact, before the window of hope and opportunity, temporarily opened by a new therapy context, closes in the patient's head. The psychophysiological role induction is an effort to challenge and change the patient's perception of the possible origins of one's somatic complaint. This is done by challenging the patient's prior beliefs about the extent to which one's thoughts can influence or do in fact inaccurately reflect one's biological functions. This is accomplished through a psychophysiological role induction, which uses what I call a Trojan Horse Procedure. This procedure has at least four components, which start on the outside with somatic symptoms and work their way upward into the patient's head. (See Table 7.)

For the patient who presents somatic complaints without physical findings and who is skeptical about a referral to a psychologist, the initial interview can be conducted in the psychophysiological laboratory rather than in a consulting room. The psychologist should meet the patient in a white laboratory coat and confine his initial questions to very objective and quantitative questions. For example, "What physical complaints do you have today? When did these symptoms start and how long do they last, etc., etc.?" When the psychologist knows the nature, location, duration, and intensity of the patient's physical symptoms he

Table 7. Example of Physiological Role Induction

Session	Session activity	Time (hours)
1	Initial interview to evaluate candidacy for therapy	
2	Testing	
	Paper-and-pencil tests	1
	Harvard Hypnotic Scale	1
	Psychophysiological stress profile	1
	Behavioral EEG	1½
3	Feedback on interview and test results	
4	Therapy formally begins	

or she is ready to proceed to component one (psychophysiological demonstration) of the Trojan Horse Procedure.

Psychophysiological Demonstrations

The first component is in essence a high credibility psychophysiological demonstration of the mind–body interaction model. Three types of psychophysiological demonstrations obviously challenge the mind–body dichotomy. The first psychophysiological demonstration works by directly demonstrating on the patient's own physical body that cognitions can alter biological functions. If prior hypnotic testing indicates that the patient has good hypnotic ability (e.g., Harvard score 9–12), then a reversible anesthesia, a catalepsy, a muscular inhibition, or an involuntary movement can be induced in an area of the patient's body unrelated to his presenting symptom. This procedure, because it is counterexpectational, startles the patient and captures his or her attention for several weeks.

A second psychophysiological demonstration is appropriate for the patient of moderate-hypnotic ability. If the patient has only moderate- or low-hypnotic ability (Harvard score 7–0), one or more of several other psychophysiological demonstrations can be arranged to induce faith in mind–body interactions. For example, a variety of physiological functions can be monitored (e.g., heart rate, blood pressure, EMG, skin conductance, temperature, EEG-alpha density) under conditions of habituation. At the end of the habituation period the patient should be shown the stable baselines. Next, the patient should be unexpectedly and briefly (one minute) stressed with perhaps mental arithmetic or personally sensitive questions. Immediately after the cognitive stress period, the patient's attention should be drawn to his or her physiological reactivity tracked on the strip chart. The patient's attention should particularly be focused on that physiological system that is most reactive (either in terms of increased elevation or variability) and the one that takes the longest to return to the prior baseline after the brief cognitive stressor is terminated. The patient should be encouraged to ponder these physiological tracings and their implications for how the patient responds to transient psychosocial stressors in everyday life. The patient has now seen that a particular biological system in his or her own body is particularly reactive to psychological stress. The patient has seen that certain biological systems go on red-alert too easily and stay there long after the cognitive stressor is removed. The patient should recognize that chronic intermittent triggering of the red-alert system by transient or enduring psychosocial conflicts (e.g., a problem child, an unhappy marriage) has something to do with why the patient is in your office today. This little psychophysiological stress demonstration provides a credible face-saving biological rationale for the patient's physical complaints and demonstrates that psychosocial stress can profoundly alter biological functions. It should be noted that chronic functional activation may eventually lead to structural breakdown or erosion of organ systems and clinical complaints.

A third cogent method of demonstrating the inaccuracy or incompleteness of the patient's awareness of mind–body interaction is through a strip chart recording of a 10-minute baseline of frontal EMG. This strip chart can be used cogently to demonstrate how incomplete and/or inaccurate a patient's verbal-subjective estimate of muscle tension is when compared to an objective quantitative baseline EMG measure of muscle tension. For example, before a frontal EMG baseline is made the patient can be asked to estimate the extent of his or her muscle tension in the upper portion of the body, on a subjectively anchored scale (SUD scale, or subjective units of disturbance) ranging from zero (totally relaxed muscles) to 50 (extremely tense, an unbearable level of muscle tension requiring escape from laboratory setting and therapist) on the strip chart. Typically, even the anxious patient underestimates the level of EMG with, for example, a verbal rating of 25 or 30 on the chart. A 10-minute frontal EMG baseline recording is then made (5 minutes eyes open, 5 minutes eyes closed). Nearly always the objective measure of EMG is much higher than the subjective estimate and is often around 35 or 50 on the chart. The patient is directly and clearly confronted with the discrepancy between his verbal-subjective estimate and the objective EMG recording. This discrepancy is usually so large that the patient is startled and taken aback by the extent of insensitivity

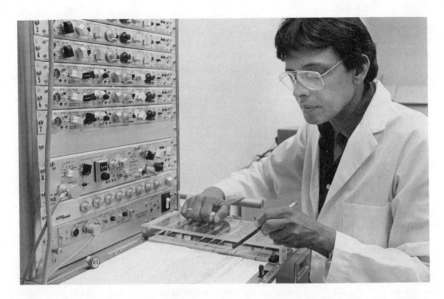

Figure 13a. The patient is shown the discrepancy between his SUDS scale and the objective EMG measure.

to his or her own body. In high hypnotizables one must dilute this demonstration and use it cautiously lest it trigger an exacerbation of the pain by suggesting that the patient should be having more pain than the patient is currently reporting. The patient is told that he or she has psychologically habituated to an abnormal physiological state of muscular bracing and that as progress occurs in psychophysiological therapy, the recognition of the level of muscle tension will become less blunted and more accurate. This increased sensitivity will enable the patient to identify early and defuse acute episodes of muscular bracing. Hypertension is another example of a psychologically silent, but physiologically important, change that has health consequences. I have found that this verbal-subjective versus EMG (frontal) discrepancy is nearly always quite large in patients with chronic functional disorders. (See Figures 13a, 13b.)

The procedures cited usually have a startling and credibility-building effect on the patient. It often induces a shift in the manner in which the patient perceives physical symptoms that is similar to opening an entirely new sunroof in the patient's head. It also provides a credible face-saving biological rationale for the physical symptoms that may, in fact, be the final common pathway for multiple psychosocial conflicts in the patient's life.

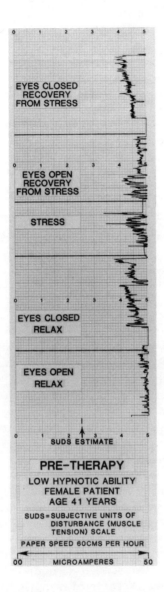

Figure 13b. Pretherapy low-hypnotic-ability (female patient, age 41 years).

Educational Model

The second component of the role induction is the shaping of the patient's cognitions into an educational model of illness, as opposed to a biomedical model in which the patient is the passive recipient of treatments. The psychophysiological demonstration is essentially a learning, or educational experience, about personal mind–body interaction. There are at least three important events that need to occur during this shift in perception of the therapy process from the passive patient role in biomedicine to the active participating student role in health education.

The first event is that the patient should not be pressured to give up the symptoms but rather to track, measure, and monitor them daily for educational and scientific purposes (i.e., the patient will collect baseline data on the frequency and intensity of his or her own symptoms). This psychologically turns the tables on the patient who, for the first time in the course of therapy, is paradoxically told not only to keep the symptoms for a while longer but also to monitor and record their frequency and intensity before they fade. Psychologically, this defuses a weapon the patient could have used to intimidate the therapist. There is also the confident, implicit suggestion that the symptom will fade in intensity. Under these conditions of reduced pressure to stop using or experimenting with the role of sickness (Parsons, 1965), some patients improve dramatically, at least temporarily. This invitation to the patient to continue to experiment for a while longer with the role of sickness occupies the patient's ground, forcing the patient out of a well-practiced and entrenched turf. This procedure is called "spitting in the patient's soup," making it distasteful for consumption. The second event is that the patient is told that his or her candidacy for entrance into the therapy program is being carefully evaluated, based on the patient's performance on a battery of tests (see Chapter 1 on the high-risk model). Because of the large behavioral component in chronic diseases or disorders (unlike acute active disease), the patient has to earn admission to therapy. The patient needs to take these tests in order to be evaluated for therapy at our clinic. The patient is told that we have limited resources, skills, and time, and that we cannot help everybody. We are looking for a few good patients who are willing to work hard in therapy to improve their symptoms. We believe that only those who will work hard deserve our help, because only they will improve fairly soon. The initiation rites involve taking a tedious battery of seven tests in our office that will consume about two sessions (3 hours) of patient contact time. This battery of tests is like a set of hurdles that forces the patient up front to make a decision to mobilize, and it operates as a screen for patient-generated motivation. Successful completion of each consecutive hurdle on the course increases the probability of admission to what may appear to the patient to be an exclusive private school or club. The fact is that this empirical procedure, for whatever private reasons, appears to motivate over 90% of the new intakes, and promotes a commitment up front to unpleasant and hard therapeutic work. It is rare to have a patient drop out after the admission procedure is outlined and even more rare after the test battery and role induction is completed. A third event in shifting to an educational model is to disable secondary gain or the rewards of the "sick role" and physical symptoms. To begin with, commitment to therapeutic work and rehabilitation makes acceptance of the rewards of the patient role ego-alien. Secondary gain also can be reduced by instructing significant others to withdraw attention, sympathy, etc., from the patient whenever the patient is expressing complaints and to be very alert, attentive, and gradually more empathic with the patient at the slightest indication that the patient's complaints or symptoms are reducing in frequency or intensity. Significant others are also told to inform the patient that they will gradually be escalating their expectations about what the patient can do for him or herself and others. Pain and other minor psychotropic medications are shifted from a PRN schedule to a fixed interval schedule during phase out.

Co-Investigator

The third component in the psychophysiological role induction is to move the patient from an educational model of the therapy process in which the role of student passes into that of co-investigator. The patient now graduates into an analytic, objective, scientific co-investigator of his or her own symptoms. This third component of the Trojan Horse procedure begins as usual on the periphery of the patient's body, and specifically with a focus on the symptoms. This can occur only after the patient can feel some self-control over the symptoms (frequency and intensity are reduced), which can tremendously increase the patient's self-esteem. I may enter the patient's body at the point of his low backache but eventually I need to work my way into his head and his central processes. This symptomatic focus is not without risk because as the patient starts to collect objective and quantitative (frequency or intensity counts) data on the symptoms, the patient could temporarily get worse even for some reason unrelated to data collection, and the personal data will make that relapse abundantly clear. The patient is prepared for these relapses by being shown up front the normal, individual learning curve, which is marked by erratic and slow acquisition. This means that first the patient may have to get worse before he or she can get better. Because the patient has to take risks and experiment with more effective coping behaviors, the course of learning real control of symptoms is not a short, positively accelerating course for which there is a "quick fix." Rather, it is an uneven course with gradual elevation interrupted by regression as physiological self-regulatory competencies develop.

He is shown that regressions are particularly likely during transition points in therapy as new tasks are encountered. Often this self-analytic, self-monitoring approach identifies some maintaining causative factors, in the environment or in the patient, that are associated with at least a temporary reduction in frequency or intensity of symptoms. Instructing the patient to practice an audio tape of deep muscle relaxation laced with positive, ego-strengthening suggestions increases the probability of at least temporary clinical improvement. Temporary placebo effects can also be generated by the quantitative scientific approach, the use of biomedical monitoring instruments in therapy (Wickramasekera, 1977b), and the verbal suggestions on the tape. It is important reliably to get this short-term, temporary reduction in clinical symptoms early in therapy, because it increases the patient's confidence in the therapist and makes the patient more willing later to risk exploring deeper underlying causes and more complex psychosocial issues maintaining the symptoms. Hence, our short-term goal is to put out the fire first, and to reserve looking for the matches until we have fully entered the patient's head through his or her backache or headache.

During this Trojan Horse phase of therapy, while the patient collects data on the symptoms, the patient may serendipitously stumble over or discover several subtle contingencies between thoughts, attitudes, and environmental events and symptoms. These discoveries can increase the patient's curiosity about larger issues in his or her life. It is very important to reinforce and support this curiosity. These findings are discussed analytically in therapy and can be used by the patient to expand a sense of self-regulation, within the limits of the symptoms. This early sense of even sporadic and modest self-control of previously immobilizing symptoms increases the patient's self-esteem, further motivating the patient to continue the painful process of exploration of self, as it interfaces with the interpersonal and physical environment.

Out of the Closet—The Psychotherapy Candidate

The fourth and final component in the psychophysiological role induction is directly and openly to investigate the psychosocial antecedents and consequences of the patient's symptoms. Now that the patient is no longer an imposter, he or she is out of the closet and is a psychotherapy candidate. The patient can now be approached just as one would do in traditional intensive psychotherapy with a patient presenting psychological symptoms (e.g., anxiety, guilt, depression, etc.) The difference is that there is often concurrent physiological monitoring (heart rate, EMG, blood pressure, skin conductance, peripheral skin temperature, etc.) to explore, identify, or confirm suspected sensitive topics. This physiological information is shared concurrently with the patient, so that the patient becomes a co-investigator in the exploration of the head-waters of the disorders and symptoms. At this fourth step, the patient's symptoms have typically shifted from predominantly somatic (pain, dizziness, etc.) to predominately psychological complaints (e.g., phobias, anxiety, depression, etc.) The polygraph is used in these sessions as a truth detector because the patient's body may be closer to the patient's unconscious mind. Often the most significant personal beliefs or mythologies are unconscious or "unattended" (Bowers, 1984) and need to be identified, examined, and then reframed or falsified.

The patient now shares with the therapist the sense of excitement of a co-investigator using all available tools to narrow down and corner the prey (dysfunctional beliefs or perceptions). The patient's body now has become a good friend and ally, who deserves more respectful attention because it is a mirror that is less easily distorted by ego defenses like denial, projection, repression, etc. This attitudinal shift often leads to important and durable life-style choices and changes (decisions to stop smoking, lose weight, do regular physical exercise, etc.) intended to protect and enhance one's body. These are a reflection of the growing recognition by the patient that, as one might put it, "this is the only body I will ever have." This body deserves care and respect, because although one can change one's home or residence, one is stuck with the same physical body.

If the unconscious perceptions, fantasies, and beliefs that cause and sustain physical symptoms have not been identified by psychophysiological monitoring during psychotherapy, then a variety of procedures that inhibit critical-analytic brain functions (ego defenses) and enable the patient to access and process present, past, or future information in a fresh way, may be used. For example, techniques that range from live role playing, the gestalt empty-chair technique, to *in vitro* or *in vivo* desensitization, can be used to access new perspectives on old problems. These techniques enable the patient to look at chronic problematic areas from multiple viewpoints that have been previously unattended but are potentially within the sphere of consciousness. In using these techniques, it is important also to emphasize the physiological habituation or extinction value of these procedures and to use concurrent physiological monitoring to give the patient highly credible sources of information (biomedical instruments) that extinction of fear and avoidance is occurring. In using these procedures, it is equally important to attend to any fresh information or new ways in which old problems can be conceptually represented in consciousness with new labels or frames. This reframing in language can have new physiological and behavioral consequences for the ways in which old problems are viewed and approached. For example, a patient may recognize that when he cannot fight or flee from a problematic situation, he can creatively search for new ways to flow with the situation until a more satisfactory remedy is available.

Hetero- or self-hypnosis is another technique of accessing a fresh perspective on old problems. A procedure like low arousal physiological training or self-hypnosis can often enable a patient to view an existing life problem from a fresh perspective. There is some evidence that the mind is more creative in the low arousal or self-hypnotic state (Bowers & Bowers, 1979; Fromm *et al.*, 1981). Also, in the low arousal state the patient may be more responsive to new information and fresh ways of looking at old problems that the therapist might suggest (heterohypnosis). These fresh reformulations of old problems can be repeatedly rehearsed for desensitization in the low arousal state with posthypnotic suggestions for more confident implementation and creative problem solving in the waking pedestrian world. The low arousal state and sensory deprivation have been shown (Wickramasekera, 1977a) temporarily to increase even the suggestibility of people of moderate- or low-hypnotic ability (Harvard 0–8). It may be possible to use these conditions to enhance suggestions that the patient will have night dreams that will clarify or resolve the meaning of waking conflicts.

The enhanced suggestibility of the low arousal state and the growing positive transference situation can be used to challenge the patient's dysfunctional attributions ("My pain is due to something I ate"; "It is important to look for scapegoats.") and irrational beliefs, and to encourage the patient to act experimentally (take a risk) on new assumptions or hypotheses about human relationships, etc. It is crucial on this final step explicitly to encourage risk taking that may involve confronting the prospect of failure, pain, and defeat. New and more effective coping strategies can then be developed even in the face of anticipated fear and pain, and new support systems (friends, social groups, church, athletic clubs, professional groups, etc.) can be found.

In the final analysis, it is the patient's growing personal competencies that will provide the best defense against further symptomatic regressions, and not a mere freedom from symptoms. All of the previously cited procedures will amplify the placebo effect (CR), which is known (Wickramasekera, 1980) to be stronger with intermittent reinforcement from active ingredients (UCS). These procedures also access central conscious or unconscious processes. These central changes increase the probability of transferring coping skills learned in the psychophysiological laboratory to the natural habitat. By teaching analytic problem solving, interpersonal risk taking, and assertiveness skills, and by increasing role flexibiity, we immunize the patient against symptomatic relapses and future sensitization. Preparation for more effective conflict resolution reduces symptomatic relapses by increasing personal competencies. In this final stage of therapy, the psychophysiological therapist is earmarked as a new kind of psychotherapist, who with the patient's permission encourages one to open the city gates to new sources of information (dreams, day dreams, fantasies, role playing, etc.) that would previously have been suspected and rejected as alien invaders at the city walls. Therefore the patient, rather than escaping from psychological pain through defenses like somatization, nomadism or acting out, accepts the responsibility of dealing with psychological conflicts at the appropriate level by using appropriate psychological mechanisms like insight, abreaction, desensitization, reframing, and the like. At this point of psychological maturation the incidence of somatic presentation reduces and the incidence of psychological presentations (anxiety, depression, fear, loneliness, etc.) increase in therapy. The patient is no longer a closet psychotherapy case or a medical imposter and is less likely to be able successfully to use somatization as a method of transducing psychological conflicts into physical presentations in the future.

Data on the Effects of the Psychophysiological Role Induction

The following are data from two equal (5-month) periods (A + B) in which the role induction was used to orient patients to the services of the Behavioral Medicine Clinic and Psychophysiology Laboratory (see Figure 14). Period A represents a phase when the role induction procedure was used nonsystematically by the present therapist in the early years of the clinic and laboratory. Period B is based on a recent patient sample when the present therapist was systematically using the role induction procedure. The number and type of patients (age, sex, diagnosis, chronicity, presenting problems, etc.) was very comparable in Periods A and B. The present author did the role induction in both cases, A and B.

During Period A ($N=20$), 60% of the referrals were retained after the psychophysiological role induction and 40% of the referrals dropped out. This 40% dropout rate is based on those patients who dropped out after the initial interview, after testing, and who did not come back for therapy after the feedback session. The feedback session presents the results of the clinical interview and all the psychological and psychophysiological tests. In this session the patient is essentially told the results of his or her application for candidacy for psychophysiological therapy. Sixty percent of the initial patient pool survived the evaluation procedure and started therapy. Based on a survey of 600 community

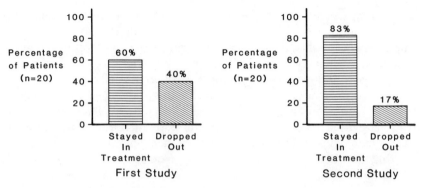

Figure 14. Retention rate after completed role induction (3 sessions).

mental health centers, Phillips (1985) concluded that of those patients who present themselves for psychotherapy only 50% return after the initial interview. It is well known that the dropout rate is much higher for the patient who presents somatic complaints without physical findings.

During Period B the role induction was used systematically with all patients screened. Eighty-three percent of the patients returned for therapy after the feedback session and 17% of the patients had dropped out after the feedback session. This dropout rate of 17% is particularly impressive because included in it are patients who the evaluation indicated were inappropriate for our services and who were referred elsewhere.

References

Bowers, K. S. On being unconsciously influenced and informed. In K. S. Bowers & D. Meichenbaum (Eds.), *The unconscious reconsidered.* New York: Wiley-Interscience, 1984.

Bowers, P. E., & Bowers, K. S. Hypnosis and creativity. In E. Fromm & R. E. Shor (Eds.), *Hypnosis: Development in research and new perspectives.* New York: Aldine, 1979.

Fromm, E., Brown, D. P., Hurt, S. W., Oberlander, J. Z., Boxer, A. M., & Pfeifer, G. The phenomena and characteristics of self-hypnosis. *The International Journal of Clinical and Experimental Hypnosis,* 1981, *29* (3), 189–246.

Parsons, T. *Social structure and personality.* New York: Free Press, 1965.

Phillips, E. L. *A guide for therapists and patients to short term psychotherapy.* Springfield: Charles C Thomas, 1985.

Wickramasekera, I. On attempts to modify hypnotic susceptibility: Some psychophysiological procedures and promising directions. *Annals of the New York Academy of Sciences,* 1977, *296,* 143–153. (a)

Wickramasekera, I. The placebo effect and biofeedback for headache pain. *Proceedings of the San Diego Biomedical Symposium.* New York: Academic Press, 1977. (b)

Wickramasekera, I. A conditioned response model of the placebo: Predictions from the model. *Journal of Biofeedback and Self-Regulation,* 1980, *5*(1), 5–18.

8

THE DIAGNOSIS AND PSYCHOPHYSIOLOGICAL MANAGEMENT OF CHRONIC PAIN AND ANXIETY

In many patients, chronic pain, I suspect, is an illness generated by interpersonal or social factors and is only distantly related to acute pain. It should not surprise us, then, that those therapies most effective for acute pain, such as rest or narcotics or neuro-muscular relaxants, are, in fact, detrimental to the chronic pain patient.
. . . I believe that the problems of chronic pain can only be solved if an approach to human illness broader than the biomedical model is developed by both researchers and clinicians.
—John D. Loeser, M.D.
Professor of Neurosurgery
University of Washington, 1980

Pain syndrome patients, in their desperate search for the elusive cure, often chase "windmills" and convince their doctors to perform a myriad of invasive tests and procedures. As a result of their pain behaviors, many experience iatrogenic complications, suffering, and disability.
—Gerald M. Aronoff, M.D.
Editor, *The Clinical Journal of Pain*, 1985

Acute and Chronic Pain

There is a growing awareness that the parameters of acute and chronic pain vary widely. Acute pain is easy to localize and recognize, and may, in fact, be mediated through different pathways from chronic pain (Sweet, 1981). These pathways include the (a) dorsal-column post synaptic system (DCPS), (b) spinocervical tract (SCT) and (c) neospinothalamic tract (NSTT), which are all rapidly conducting systems suited to convey phasic information (Melzack & Dennis, 1978). Acute pain is marked by an increase in mytonia, heart rate, blood pressure, skin conductance, and peripheral vasoconstriction together with other indicators of sympathetic activation. From a psychological or behavioral viewpoint we are seeing the same signs that indicate fear or anxiety. Chronic pain has been defined as any pain that has persisted for over 6 months and has not responded to standard medical management, including drugs, physical therapy, and surgery (Sternbach, 1974). Bonica, a pioneer in the study and therapy of chronic pain, defines it as "pain which persists beyond the usual course of an acute disease or a reasonable time for an injury to heal, or it recurs at intervals of months or years (Bonica, 1980). Studies by Johnson (1978) and Barton, Haight, Marsland, and Temple (1976) reveal that 75% of patients who complain of recent onset back pain experience spontaneous remission within 3 months. Chronic back pain is one of the most common types of chronic pain, and 80% of the population is affected by back pain at some point in their lives (Flor & Turk, 1984). Johnson (1978) found that more than one half of the 25% of patients who became chronic pain cases were ultimately medically judged to have permanent disability (total or partial). In the case of the permanently disabled people the incidence of clear physical findings was low. If disc disease is included as a physical finding, nearly 78.3% of the cases had no physical finding. If disc disease is excluded, 93.1% of the cases had no physical findings. Fordyce (1976) and others (Flor & Turk, 1984) concluded from the study cited that the relationship between chronic pain complaints and physical findings is "loose virtually to the point of obscurity." Radiographic imaging techniques can document a degenerative process in the spine, but it is recognized that the correlation between clinical symptomatology and degenerative changes is low. For example, a recent study (Wiesel, Feffer, & Tsoarnas, 1984) showed that 50% of asymptomatic subjects over the age of 40 have positive CAT scans, suggesting the need for surgical intervention. Schmorl and Junghanns (1932), in classic autopsy studies ($N = 4,353$), showed that degenerative changes in the spine are present in 50% of the population by age 50, 70% by age 60, and in 90% by age 70 years. Hult

(1954) confirmed these figures with radiological studies. Disc degeneration appears to be a natural aging process that occurs in everyone but is not necessarily associated with the complaint of low back pain.

Bonica (1980) estimated that one-third of the population have persistent or recurrent chronic pain and that chronic pain costs $60 billion annually because of health care costs, payments for compensation, litigation, lost workdays, and quackery. This figure of $60 billion was 10% of the national budget in 1980, but pain research was awarded only .02% of the N.I.H. research budget in 1980.

Chronic headache and chronic low back pain account for over 50% of all chronic pain patients but chronic pain syndromes also include phantom limb pain, neuralgia, causalgia, etc. In chronic pain most of the signs of sympathetic activation have adapted out and the primary signs of chronic pain are insomnia, loss of appetite, loss of libido, irritability, constriction of range of interests, inhibition of activity, and feelings of helplessness and hopelessness. From a psychological viewpoint these are the symptoms of depression. Hence, any approach to the chronic pain patient has to confront the patient's depressive affect, which can potentiate pain. Experimental research on chronic pain is fragmentary, mainly because there are no good animal models of chronic pain (Sweet, 1981). Chronic pain appears to be mediated through slow conductive fibers in the paleospinothalamic tract (PSTT) and the spinoreticular tract (SRT) and are poorly discriminated and poorly localized pain systems (Melzack & Dennis, 1978).

There has been salient progress made in the measurement of pain in the last 25 years. It is recognized now that pain is a complex perception and not a simple sensation. The role of the brain in modulating this sensory input is well established. The measurement of pain should focus on multiple response measures, namely, motor performance, subjective intensity, and physiological measures (Chapman et al., 1985). There is no reliable relationship between the amount of tissue damage and the intensity or frequency of pain complaints (Levine, 1984). This is true for acute and chronic pain. It is likely that this variability in pain intensity reported by patients with similar injuries is a function of psychological and physiological variables operating through descending inhibitory and endogenous analgesia circuits (Levine, 1984). Acute pain is associated with noxious or tissue damaging stimulation caused by disease or injury. Psychological factors (hypnosis, the placebo effect, distraction, etc.) can be used powerfully to control acute pain but psychopathology is very seldom the cause of acute pain. The pathophysiology of acute pain is fairly well established, diagnosis is reliable, and healing and therapy are effective 90% of the time. Hence, because of effective therapy or the self-limiting nature of the disease, acute pain remits within days or weeks. Most research knowledge of pain is based on acute, experimentally induced pain in man or in animals. Acute pain of disease, injury, or trauma has the survival value of warning the person that something is wrong that requires rest, healing, and medical counsel.

The adequacy of conventional medical methods of dealing with chronic benign pain has become increasingly doubtful (Bonica, 1980; Pagni & Maspes, 1974; White & Sweet, 1969). Typical surgical procedures and analgesic drugs appear to have limited effectiveness. They tend either to exacerbate the patient's pain problem and/or create new problems of drug tolerance and dependence which may, in fact, increase pain. It is the chronicity of these pain problems that makes analgesic drug management an unsatisfactory long-term solution. In fact, the response to most neurosurgical procedures is unreliable and the pain returns in 6 to 18 months (Crue, 1985; Kerr, 1980; White & Sweet, 1969). Benjamin Crue, professor of neurosurgery at the University of Southern California School of Medicine, stated:

> Neurosurgeons have a tremendous repertoire of surgical procedures aimed at pain relief. However, it is time for the neurosurgeon, as well as the anesthesiologists who rely on nerve blocks, to admit that, when it comes to treating patients with chronic pain . . . they are bankrupt. Anesthesiological peripheral nerve blocks as well as neurosurgical rhizotomies, chordotomies, and tractotomies have just not worked in a sufficient percentage of such patients, when they have been followed postoperatively over an adequate course of time, to be considered any longer as an acceptable treatment. This conclusion is reached with considerable sadness, not only because the writer is a neurosurgeon but because experience has shown that the statement may be misunderstood. (Crue, 1985, p. 34)

The same conclusion was reached by Frederick Kerr, professor of neurosurgery at the Mayo Clinic, who stated

> From a pragmatic point of view, this widespread distribution of nociception renders surgical control of pain difficult and unpredictable. Spinal cord transection of the anterolateral quadrant gives relief of pain for months but rarely for years, while at the thalamic level, stereotaxic lesions for pain limited to ventrolateral or to intralaminar areas have, with some exceptions, been disappointing. Neuroanatomical and neurophysiological investigation of the nociceptive pathways have, to a considerable degree, explained why surgical attempts to relieve pain have met with limited success. However, they have not as yet identified a site at which a lesion can be placed which abolishes chronic pain in an enduring manner and do so without unacceptable side effects. Whether such a site can ever be found seems very doubtful. (Kerr, 1980, p. 59)

Loeser, another neurosurgeon stated:

We all search for ways we can apply our skills to the patient; both ego and account book work against telling the patient we have nothing to offer. The patient often demands therapy even if the risks are high and the potential relief is small. Far too many surgical procedures are performed on patients with chronic pain due to benign diseases. (Loeser, 1977, p. 883)

Many physicians use aggressive interventions to get chronic pain complaints off their hands. They prescribe drugs that become addictive and perform surgeries that do more harm than good. Third-party reimbursements will pay for aggressive and radical physical interventions but are reluctant to pay for more conservative psychological or behavioral interventions. Hiring and firing policies in industry discriminate against the disabled. The system of worker's compensation in this country (Karron, DeGoode, & Tait, 1985) provides financial incentive to remain laid off and employers are reluctant to phase convalescents back to work with temporarily reduced work schedules.

It is likely that most of the problems with the conventional medical management of pain, particularly chronic pain, result from two factors: (a) the failure to distinguish between acute and chronic pain, and to recognize that the parameters of these two types of pain are very different, and (b) the failure to recognize the large psychological and behavioral components in acute and chronic pain and particularly the failure to recognize the onset of the "illness behavior syndrome" (Brena, 1983) in chronic pain patients. The features of this illness behavior syndrome will be discussed presently.

Illness Behavior Syndrome and Chronic Pain

In chronic pain patients a distinct behavioral and psychophysiological syndrome develops that becomes superimposed on and interwoven into any organic pathophysiology and that can persist long after the pathophysiology has cleared up. This illness behavior syndrome (Blackwell, 1981; Brena, 1983; Fordyce, 1976; Sternbach, 1974) has been variously described by several authors. Essentially it consists of the patient assuming a social role that is, in fact, reinforced by a health care system that responds to chronic pain as if it were an acute medical problem. The five components of this role are the (a) dramatization of complaints, (b) progressive dysfunction, (c) drug misuse, (d) progressive dependency and (e) income disability. The patient's dramatization of diffuse and *metastasizing* pain complaints often produces unnecessary and unproductive medical interventions (surgery, drugs, invasive tests, etc.) that further complicate the pain problem. Progressive dysfunction is often a consequence of low levels of physical activity and postural habits that cause contractures, myofibrositis, osteoporosis, obesity, circulatory and respiratory disorders, etc. (Brena, 1983). Chronic misuse or dependency on drugs that are prescribed for acute pain and acute anxiety conditions may occur (Turner, Calsyn, Fordyce, & Ready, 1982). This includes narcotic drugs and psychotropics. There is a tendency for patients to abdicate self-reliance and permit their complaints and their environment to control their lives. These patients float miserably and angrily from one physician to another with episodic visits to attorneys and insurance companies. They experience a growing dependency on income that continues to flow only if they continue to have pain and disability complaints. (See Figure 15.)

A Theory of the Acquisition of Chronic Pain and Anxiety

It appears that during any life-threatening situation (e.g., natural disaster, auto or industrial accident, mine disaster, near death experi-

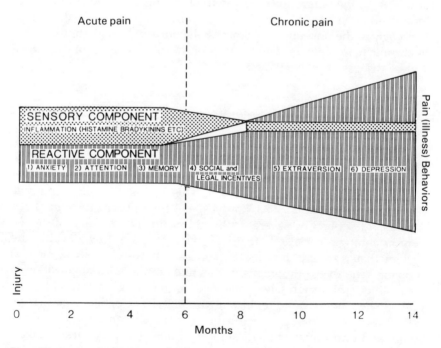

Figure 15. Acute pain changes to chronic pain as the reactive component in pain expands.

ences in warfare, etc.) it is likely that people will learn and retain memories that can unconsciously (Bowers & Meichenbaum, 1984; Kihlstrom, 1987; Lewicki, 1986) sustain peripheral physiological mobilization (autonomic vascular and/or muscular) or bracing (Whatmore & Kohli, 1974) that can continue outside of awareness for months or years after the objective threat has passed. This pattern of peripheral physiological mobilization is often associated with chronic pain and/or anxiety and vigilance, and is centrally sustained by unconscious motor memory circuits in the brain. The degree of peripheral physiological activation at any given time will vary as a function of the consciously or unconsciously (Forster & Govier, 1978) recognized similarity of the current place, topic, and time, to the original traumatic conditioning situation or event (e.g., the auto accident, etc.) based on stimulus and response generalization (Kimble, 1961). Similarly, aversive mental events occurring in dreams during sleep can activate or potentiate the learned chronic pain circuit. Further, at least three personality features (a) baseline hypnotic ability (Hilgard, 1965; Wilson & Barber, 1982), (b) neuroticism (Eysenck, 1983) or negative affectivity (Costa & McCrae, 1985; Watson & Clark, 1984; Watson & Tellegen, 1985), and (c) catastrophizing, increase the probability that certain people are more likely to acquire through conditioning this chronic pain and/or anxiety syndrome during life-threatening situations. A fourth factor that determines if somatic pain or psychological anxiety is learned is the number of familial pain models in the person's social environment. Several retrospective studies have shown a relationship between abdominal pain, dental pain, lower back pain, headaches, and family pain models (Edwards, Zeichner, Kuczmierzyk, & Boczkowski, 1985; Payne & Norfleet, 1986). The complaint of pain can be learned by observing a parent or significant relative.

Hypnotic Ability

It appears that very high or very low levels of autonomic arousal will temporarily increase hypnotic ability (see Figure 16) (Wickramasekera, 1977b). This means that sensory information is temporarily processed through a system marked by expanded personal or voluntary control of perception, memory, and mood. This means that during trauma (very high levels of sympathetic arousal), a more primitive (Jaynes, 1977) form of information processing is disinhibited and that environmentally constrained verbal-rational, sequential-analytic methods of information processing characteristic of the left hemisphere are inhibited. This means that during a life-threatening trauma people are more likely spontaneously and temporarily to enter a trance state. It is known that

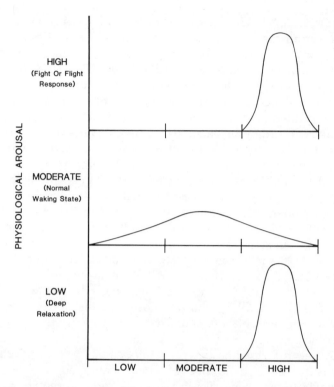

Figure 16. Hypothesized hypnotic ability in the general population as a function of the level of physiological arousal.

in the hypnotic state (mode of information processing) the verbal instructions of the hypnotist and/or the personal conscious or unconscious (Shevrin & Dickman, 1980) instructions of the subject acquire expanded control of perception (vision, smell, hearing, taste, etc.) memory and mood (Hilgard, 1965; Kihlstrom, 1985). In other words, unconscious factors (Shevrin & Dickman, 1980) that can distort perception, memory, and mood are more likely to influence behavior in this state and people are more likely to inhibit in the waking state traumatic memories (Hilgard, 1965) acquired in the hypnotic state. It is also known that systematic distortions of up to 40% (St. Jean & Mcleod, 1983) of clock time can occur in the hypnotic state. What was only a minute of trauma may seem like an hour of agony. During a life-threatening trauma, the subjective perception of time is very often expanded and slowed down relative to clock time. This subjective expansion of time may permit a larger degree of physiological (sympathetic) mobilization that typically could occur only in twice the amount of clock time. In other words, stress hormone production may be expanded in subjective time to twice that which would occur in clock time. This physiological bracing in peripheral body areas (neck, back, stomach, shoulders, etc.) can be maintained by unconscious memory circuits in the motor area after the trauma is over. Experimental phenomena like blind sight illustrate the role of unconscious factors in perception and they demonstrate the fact that detection and recognition in vision, for example, are mediated by different cortical regions (Robinson, 1984).

Negative Affectivity

Another personality feature that can increase the probability of acquiring a chronic pain and/or anxiety syndrome is high neuroticism (Eysenck, 1983) or negative affectivity (Watson & Clark, 1984; Watson & Tellegen, 1985). Reviews of numerous controlled studies demonstrate that neuroticism or negative affectivity (NA) is a cross-culturally and cross-situationally stable and universal human trait. People high on NA, independent of culture or language. are more likely to report discomfort at more times across more situations, even in the absence of objective trauma (Watson & Clark, 1984; Watson & Tellegen 1985). People high on NA are more self-reflective, tend to ruminate on their own negative features or the negative features of their environment, and they tend to report more somatic complaints (Costa & McCrae, 1985). It is likely that the biological basis for NA is excessive sympathetic reactivity (Eysenck, 1983). Individuals high on NA are more likely to be hyperattentive to and to remember threatening internal and external cues and physiological and psychological responses (pain, anxiety, fear, guilt, etc.) learned during a trauma. It is known that anxiety, up to a point, increases the probability of conditioning or learning (Kimble, 1961). This enhanced awareness of negative affect (NA) may increase the probability of inadvertently learning and retaining false or superstitious (Skinner, 1953) contingencies associated with muscular bracing, etc.

Catastrophizing

Catastrophizing is a learned tendency perceptually to amplify sensory stimuli by cognitively rehearsing a wide range of anticipated or remembered negative antecedents or consequences. It is likely that this overlearned response occurs reflexively (automatically) and is triggered by threat cues that operate preattentively or prior to awareness (Mathews & Macleod, 1986).

Table 8. Acquisition Model Summary Chart

1. Perception of "threat" to mortality
2. Increased level of sympathetic activation (SA)
3. Increased SA causes relative inhibition of left brain function (verbal, sequential, analytic, rational mode of information processing)
4. Increased SA permits relative regnancy of right brain function (visual, holistic, simultaneous mode of information processing) or hypnotic mode of information processing
5. Consequences:
   a. expansion of subjective time and doubling of stress hormone production and muscular bracing for each unit of clock time
   b. response and stimulus generalization
   c. relative amnesia for traumatic episode
6. If the person is also high on neuroticism or negative affectivity (NA) he is even more likely to learn and retain the trauma in memory
7. Memory circuits of high NA and high-hypnotic ability persons are more likely to learn and retain:
   a. aversive events
   b. unconscious muscular bracing sustained in periphery by overlearned single trial learning

In summary, the acquisition of chronic pain and anxiety responses may be based on chronic physiological mobilization and vigilance generated by unconscious memory circuits acquired during life-threatening, traumatic, and conditioned events. Chronic pain and unconscious physiological bracing are most likely to be acquired in hypnotic states by people high on catastrophizing and negative affectivity when they believe they are confronted by their own mortality. (See Table 8.)

Rationales for the Use of Psychological and Behavioral Procedures with Pain

There are several other general empirically established rationales for the use of psychological and behavioral procedures with acute and chronic pain problems. First, the most influential current theory of pain, the gate-control theory (Melzack & Wall, 1965), assigns a major role to descending inhibitory pathways from the brain through which psychological variables, such as attention, reinforcement, distraction, anxiety, placebo effects, depression, and hypnosis can profoundly influence the opening or closing of the gating mechanism in pain perception. The gate-control theory postulates a presynaptic mechanism modulating peripheral nociceptive input in the region of the dorsal horn of the spinal cord. All of the previously cited six psychological variables have been empirically shown to influence pain perception (Sternbach, 1968, 1974).

Second, it has been known for many years that though the pain threshold is fairly fixed and universal in man, the threshold of pain tolerance is profoundly influenced by a variety of cultural, personality, learning, and situational factors (Melzack, 1973). For example, pain expression seems to be determined by several factors. Pain expression is related to cultural learning and ethnic membership. For example, Zborowski (1969) showed that Old Americans and Irish Americans inhibit pain expression but that Italian and Jewish Americans encourage pain expression. Another major detriment of pain expression is individual personality. It has been found that the perception of pain is related to the degree of neuroticism (Bond, 1971, 1973) but that the expression of pain is related to the degree of extroversion (Lynn & Eysenck, 1961). Hence, neurotic introverts may suffer silently, but neurotic extroverts freely express their pain. It has been shown (Fordyce, 1976) that chronic pain behaviors are also controlled by reinforcing situational consequences. Pain behaviors can be reinforced by attention, monetary rewards, feedback, sympathy, and escape from unpleasant activities or situations. For example, Beecher (1959) found that the amount of pain medication requested and prescribed for tissue damage was more closely related not to the amount of tissue damage but to the situation where the damage occurred. A given injury in civilian life requires more morphine than the same injury in the combat zone. An injury in the combat zone may be perceived as a relief, because it assures that the person will be removed from the battlefield and perhaps his life will be saved. Beecher (1959) concluded that comparable amounts of tissue damage generate quantitatively variable requests for analgesics, depending on the situation in which the trauma occurred.

Third, the placebo response is another psychological factor that is very powerful but is poorly understood (Wickramasekera, 1977a, 1980, 1985). A review (Evans, 1974) of over 1,000 postsurgical pain patients has shown that a placebo, an inert substance, can under double blind conditions reduce by at least 50% postsurgical pain in, on the average, 36% of patients.

Fourth, it has been shown that attention and distraction can significantly modify the perception of pain caused by tissue damage (Melzack, 1973). An example is the football player who may seriously lacerate himself during a game but discovers the injury later in the locker room and only then perceives the pain.

Fifth, the reduction of depressive affect by drugs or psychotherapy can significantly increase pain tolerance (Sternbach, 1978). It appears that the depletion of central serotonin may account for increases in depression and chronic pain (Sternbach, Janowsky, Huey, & Segal, 1976). Anxiety can significantly amplify acute and chronic pain (Sternbach, 1974).

Sixth, there is now good evidence that people of high-hypnotic ability can significantly reduce experimentally induced pain (Hilgard & Hilgard, 1975) and there is less complete evidence that they can also reduce clinical pain (Gottfredson, 1973; Hilgard & Hilgard, 1975). Nearly 70% of people of high-hypnotic ability can reduce cold pressor pain significantly, whereas only 13% of people of low-hypnotic ability can do so. Hypnotic ability has been shown (Hilgard 1965) to be a measurable, stable, and partly genetically determined individual variable that has clear consequences for both the reduction and possibly also for the amplification of pain perception (Wickramasekera, 1979, 1981, 1983). It is likely that high-hypnotic-ability subjects have a lower pain tolerance or threshold level than people of low- or moderate-hypnotic ability if their cognitive ability to block pain is not mobilized (Wickramasekera, 1979, 1983).

Hypnosis for Pain

Hypnosis is a psychological method of pain reduction that can be remarkably effective with approximately 10% to 15% of the general population who have good hypnotic ability (e.g., Harvard scores between 9 and 12). Well controlled laboratory studies have found a correlation of .50 between hypnotic ability and the degree of acute pain reduction. Hypnosis is less likely to be effective with people of moderate- or low-hypnotic ability. This relationship between hypnotic ability and pain reduction is well established for acute experimental pain and is less securely established for clinical pain (Hilgard & Hilgard, 1975). This reduction of pain with hypnosis occurs with the sensory component of pain and not merely with the suffering (or reactive) component of pain. In fact, hypnosis is more reliably effective with pain of organic origin (e.g., surgery, cancer, obstetrics, dentistry) than pain of psychological origin (Hilgard & Hilgard, 1975). This appears to be true because the patient who has organic pain (surgical, etc.) is seldom or never motivated to retain it, whereas psychological pain is typically motivated or functional for the patient in some unclear or obscure way. Hypnotic pain-reduction techniques are equally applicable to many different types of clinical pain. For example, techniques like glove anesthesia, displacement of pain from one area to another, and escape from the pain through fantasy are useful with varied clinical pain conditions (dental, surgical, burns, labor and childbirth). Hypnosis appears not only to reduce the sensory component (analgesia) of pain, but can also reduce the reactive (suffering) component of pain if suggestions of mental and physical relaxation are given.

Hence, hypnosis can have analgesic and sedative effects. There is also some evidence that hypnosis may also have a placebo or nonspecific component for people who do not have hypnotic ability (Hilgard & Hilgard, 1975). In other words, labeling a procedure hypnosis may lead to some pain relief even for people who lack hypnotic ability. Modern hypnotic procedures are characterized by (a) greater patient participation in implementing the techniques (self-hypnosis), and (b) the hypnotist using more permissive and less authoritarian suggestions. There is also some evidence that the degree of pain relief from some other nonhypnotic methods (acupuncture, biofeedback, etc.) is related to hypnotic ability. For example some part of the efficacy of nonhypnotic methods like acupuncture (Katz, Kao, Spiegel, & Katz, 1974) and EMG biofeedback (Andreychuk & Skriver, 1975) seems related to hypnotic ability.

Biofeedback for Pain

Biofeedback can be defined as the use of instruments to provide a person with immediate and continuing informational feedback of typically unconscious changes in a biological response such as muscle tension, heart rate, blood pressure, or EEG responses. There are at least two rationales for the use of biofeedback with pain. First, certain types of pain (e.g., muscle tension headache, etc.) are based on sustained contraction of muscles on the scalp and/or neck (Wolff, 1963). EMG feedback has been used to reduce the muscle tension that partly accounts for the pain reports (Budzynski, Stoyva, & Adler, 1970; Cox, Freundlich, & Meyer, 1975; Wickramasekera, 1972, 1973). Second, high and sustained levels of muscle contraction may, if chronically maintained, limit mobility, and can potentiate the pain caused by tissue damage (Whatmore & Kohli, 1974). Stress and anxiety can induce reflex muscle spasm, vasomotor changes, and local ischemia, exacerbating pain syndromes that involve tendons and joints (Bonica, 1974). EMG biofeedback can be used to reduce the muscle spasm that is potentiating any pain of organic origin. Today the use of biofeedback to treat functional headache (muscular and vascular) is well established (Blanchard & Andrasik, 1982), but its application to other chronic pain problems is less secure (Turk, Meichenbaum, & Berman, 1979).

Biofeedback includes several techniques that use bioelectrical instrumentation to provide a patient with information about changes in biological responses of which the person is typically unaware. First, the biological response (e.g., EMG) to be controlled is identified and assessed to secure a baseline and moment-to-moment changes. This information is quantified and translated into information that is immediately fed back to the patient in a visual or auditory display. Biofeedback appears to recognize that the subjective sensation and subtle internal changes are associated with changes in specific biological responses.

Biofeedback has been used in the therapy of several types of pain, but the best established use is in the area of severe chronic muscular and vascular headache (see Figure 17). In a pioneering study, Budzynski and Stoyva (1969) were able to confirm Sainsbury and Gibson's (1954) observation of a correlation between tension in scalp and neck muscles and frontalis EMG activity. Wickramasekera (1972) was able independently to confirm Budzynski and Stoyva's (1969) findings that contingent EMG feedback alone will reduce the frequency and intensity of tension headache. These observations became the basis for a set of clinical procedures (training in reducing frontal EMG and home practice of relaxation) that have been shown reliably to reduce the intensity and frequency of muscle contraction headache during therapy and with long-term follow-up (Budzynski, Stoyva, & Adler, 1969; Budzynski, Stoyva, Adler, & Mullein, 1973; Cox *et al.*, 1975; Hutching & Reinking, 1976; Wickramasekera, 1973). Subsequent large-scale clinical applications and other replication studies have routinely confirmed the clinical efficacy (75%–80%) of the EMG biofeedback procedure for tension headache but it is still not clear what the active ingredients in the procedure are, and if the

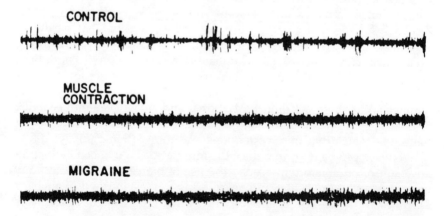

Figure 17. Frontalis EMG activity in headache patients and control subject; recordings obtained during a headache-free period (Bakal & Kaganov, 1977). Copyright 1977 by the American Association for the Study of Headache. Reprinted by permission.

procedure is always superior to simple progressive muscle relaxation therapy (Wolpe & Lazarus, 1966). There is evidence to suggest EMG biofeedback may be unnecessary for people of high-hypnotic ability to learn frontal EMG reduction (Qualls & Sheehan, 1981), and may, in fact, retard their rate of acquisition of the relaxation skill. But this group (high-hypnotic ability) is less than 10% of the general population. For people of high-hypnotic ability who have skeptical attitudes toward verbal-instructional procedures (hypnotic inductions, autogenic training, muscular exercises, etc.), EMG feedback may be at least initially the treatment of choice, because of the high credibility set and placebo effects generated by the medical-electronic instruments used in biofeedback (Wickramasekera, 1977a) that objectively validate self-efficacy.

The use of peripheral skin temperature feedback training and autogenic phrases was reported to be effective in reducing the frequency and intensity of migraine headache by Sargent, Green, and Walters (1972) and these results were confirmed by Wickramasekera (1973). Since then several other types of biofeedback investigations (Andreychuk & Skriver, 1975; Friar & Beatty, 1976; Medina, Diamond, & Franklin, 1976) have confirmed the efficacy of the temperature or pulse amplitude feedback procedures for the therapy of vascular headache. As with EMG biofeedback, the active ingredients and mechanisms have not been isolated nor has the size of the placebo component been identified, but repeated clinical trials have confirmed that the standard procedures are effective with a large percentage of patients (over 75%) with severe chronic vascular headache as determined by long-term (2 years) follow-up. It now appears that either EMG or temperature feedback will help vascular headache and the earlier claim of specificity (Wickramasekera, 1973) has not been supported.

It is less certain that biofeedback procedures alone will be effective with other non-headache-type pain syndromes (Coger & Werbach, 1975; Gentry & Bernal, 1977; Hendler, Derogatis, Avella & Long, 1977; Melzack & Perry, 1975; Newman, Seres, Yospe, & Garlington, 1978; Seres & Newman, 1976; Swanson, Swenson, Maruta, & McPhee, 1976; Wickramasekera, Truong, Bush, & Orv, 1976). But in combination with procedures like cognitive behavior modification, operant behavior modification, verbal relaxation instructions, psychotherapy, and hypnosis, biofeedback may significantly contribute to pain relief through cognitive mechanisms (objective validation of physiological self-control may generate increased self-esteem, perceived environmental mastery). These positive results, which are incompletely understood today, persist even on long-term (6 months) follow-up. The other types of pain syndromes treated with biofeedback include chronic rheumatoid arthritic pain,

(Wickramasekera *et al.*, 1976) chronic low back pain, peripheral nerve injury, cancer pain, phantom limb, stump pain, and posttraumatic pain (Melzack & Perry, 1975).

Several clinical rationales for the use of biofeedback as a primary or secondary procedure in the management of chronic pain have been proposed. Pain can have psychological and biological components. The psychological components of pain perception include anxiety, reinforcement, attention, depression, and suggestion (Hilgard & Hilgard, 1975; Melzack, 1973; Sternbach, 1978). Anxiety and fear can induce reflex muscle spasm, vasomotor changes, and local ischemia, all of which can amplify pain syndromes that involve muscles, tendons, and joints (Bonica, 1974). Suggestion and hypnosis can dramatically reduce pain perception (Hilgard & Hilgard, 1975) in superior hypnotic subjects. It seems that extended biofeedback training increases even temporarily the hypnotic ability (Wickramasekera, 1971) of people of low- or moderate-hypnotic ability (90% of the population), permitting them to use hypnotic mechanisms to reduce pain perception. There are logical and empirical grounds for believing (Edmonston, 1981) that extended clinical biofeedback training in combination with positive expectations can temporarily increase hypnotic ability (Wickramasekera, 1977b), making the benefits of hypnosis available to a large percentage of the population. Logically, the biofeedback training situation is similar to the sensory restriction situation and there is evidence that sensory restriction can temporarily increase suggestibility (Pena, 1963; Sanders & Reyher, 1969; Wickramasekera, 1969, 1970). In the biofeedback training situation the person sits for extended periods quietly limiting internal and external sensory input to a single auditory stimulus. Empirically, several studies have shown that EMG and EEG feedback can temporarily increase hypnotic ability (Engstrom, London, & Hart, 1970; London, Hart, & Lebovitz, 1968; Wickramasekera, 1971, 1973, 1977). This is not to imply that the informational feedback variable is unimportant in reducing pain perception but that it is inevitably confounded with increasing suggestibility in effective clinical biofeedback training. Effective clinical biofeedback training implicitly and explicitly positively manages the patient's expectancies before and during low-arousal training in ways that may even modestly increase the hypnotic ability of 90% of the population.

Biofeedback devices can be useful in helping the patient who is unaware of being physiologically activated. Objective credible evidence from an EMG or temperature monitor can motivate a patient to work at reducing an EMG signal or to attempt to warm his hands. The therapist may need to sample multiple physiological response systems (EMG, temperature, skin conductance, heart rate, etc.) to determine which patient response system is most reactive to psychosocial stressors and which functions as the patient's window of vulnerability. The window of vulnerability is that physiological system that is most reactive to stress, and is hence most likely to develop pathophysiology. On the other hand, the failure of a symptom to respond to low-arousal physiological feedback training from several response systems may indicate that the symptom is under the control of a more cognitive or social variable or variables and requires psychotherapy or behavior modification.

Behavior Modification for Pain

Behavior modification can be defined as the use of the principles of operant and respondent conditioning to alter either the perception of pain or pain behaviors. The general goals of behavior modification are to reduce the probability of pain behaviors by withdrawing any and all reinforcers for pain behavior and to increase the probability of health-promoting behaviors by reengaging, through selective reinforcement, the patient in life roles that compose the health-promoting behavior repertoire. The health-promoting behavior repertoire is composed of those normal behaviors (work, play, etc.) that make productive, coping, functional citizens. The basic assumption underlying the operant conditioning approach is that chronic pain behaviors (moaning, posturing, "down time") are controlled by factors (reinforcers) other than nociception (aversive sensations) alone. Respondent or Pavlovian conditioning can occur when the pain of tissue damage (UCR) has been paired or associated with neutral situations, sensations, or cognitions; so that these situations, sensations, or cognitions can operate like CS to elicit a conditioned pain response (Wickramasekera, 1977a, 1980, 1985). Imaginal or *in vivo* desensitization procedures (using relaxation or other counterconditioning stimuli) should reduce any respondently conditioned pain (CR) or anxiety responses (CR) to situations, sensations, movements, or cognitions (CS) that were previously paired with the pain of tissue damage (UCR). Anxiety, of course, can potentiate even minimal sensory pain by triggering muscle spasm and fearful affect. Also, the neutral aspect of stimuli (CS) like pills, injections, etc., reliably associated with the relief of pain through active ingredients (of morphine, aspirin, etc.) may, in highly conditionable subjects, reduce pain through placebo mechanisms (Wickramasekera, 1977a, 1980).

Cognitive behavior modification is an effort to self-regulate events (thoughts, anticipations, fantasies, images, etc.) occurring inside the "black box" or the head. This approach is based on the assumption that a patient's perceived pain response to an aversive stimulus (trauma) is very largely a function of the type of cognitive self-statements images, etc., he or she evokes before, during, and after aversive sensory stimulation. Laboratory studies have shown that the best predictor of patient response to an aversive stimulus or procedure is the patient's general cognitive attitude toward the event. Patients who catastrophize are very likely to experience high levels of pain. One study (Spanos, Radtke-Bodonik, Ferguson, & Jones, 1979) found that 85% of catastrophizers and only 39% of noncatastrophizers reported a decrease in pain tolerance during a cold pressor pain test. Catastrophizing consists of making self-statements like, "How I hate injections; I can't stand them; here we go again; that great big needle hurts awfully; I can't stand this suffering; I am going to go bananas." Confident use of cognitive strategies for coping with pain are the next best predictor of pain tolerance. There are several types of cognitive strategies that seek to alter the appraisal of the pain situation and/or to divert attention away from the pain. There are at least six common cognitive strategies that have been variously classified by Scott and Barber (1977) and Turk, Meichenbaum, and Genest (1983). (a) *Imaginative inattention* involves ignoring the painful stimulus by engaging in a vivid mental image incompatible with pain. For example, imagining attending a fun party or making love during aversive stimulation. (b) *Imaginative transformation* of pain involves interpreting the present sensations as something other than pain or minimizing those sensations as trivial or unreal. For example, imagining the pain-affected limb as numbed by Novocain or having mechanical limbs like the Six Million Dollar Man. (c) *Imaginative transformation of the context* involves changing the context of the painful situation. For example, "I am James Bond and have been shot in a limb while driving my car." (d) *Focusing attention on the physical features* of the environment. For example, getting absorbed in watching TV or counting the holes in the ceiling during pain induction. (e) *Mental distractions* involve focusing attention on various thoughts without producing vivid images. For example, doing mental arithmetic or singing battle songs during painful stimulation. (f) *Intellectualization* involves focusing attention on that part of the body that has been hurt, but doing so in an objective, detached, abstract way. For example, analyzing pain sensations in a detached, quantitative, scientific way and avoiding subjective involvement in the event.

There are several steps that are critical to implementing an effective behavioral pain therapy program. First, there is identifying and defusing patient resistance. This begins long before the initial patient contact and starts with educating referral sources to the nature of the procedures used, their rationales, limitations of the procedures, and data on their efficacy. It is also important to provide the referring sources with prompt feedback on the referral. It is important to be alert and aware of how the individual patient construes being in your waiting room, what the patient expects to find and hear, etc. The approach to the patient's intrapersonal private monologues during the initial visit can open or close the door to a therapeutic alliance. Second, it is critical immediately to help the patient start translating pain from a simple conventional acute tissue damage model to a three channel (verbal-behavioral-physiological) psychophysiological model in which different variables may control different channels. For example, the pain may reside mainly in the motor (behavioral) channel, and its increase or decrease may be simply a function of activity. Alternatively, the pain may, in rare instances, be exclusively in the verbal subjective or psychogenic channel that is mainly delusional in character but is associated with inhibition of motor activity. Of course, 95% of chronic pain is psychophysiological and involves complex interactions between cognitive anticipations, social and financial incentives and disincentives, residual tissue damage, and perhaps muscle spasm and peripheral vasoconstriction as a reaction to the tissue damage. The reactive muscle spasm, chronic mytonia, and peripheral vasoconstriction, plus the cognitive anxiety and uncertainty about the duration of the pain can further potentiate any sensory component of the pain. It is likely that the social and financial consequences of the tissue damage can reinforce the pain behaviors and the patient role can insulate the patient from the natural consequences of confronting his fears of returning to work and being unable to cope with any changes on the job. These are all complexities of chronic pain into which patients need to be led or educated.

Third, one must set realistic, limited goals for therapy. These goals have to be individualized, modest, and at least include some short-term goals. For example, reducing use of the narcotic pain medications and psychotropics, and increasing activities in relation to recreation or fun time. Another specific goal is to reduce down time (time spent sitting or lying down). These goals may include spending more time playing with grandchildren, eating out, going to church, losing weight, learning to swim, or walking for one hour in a mall. Acquisition of coping skills may include learning to use EMG feedback to reduce muscle spasm in the back or learning to warm one's hands to dilate peripheral blood vessels. For those who have hypnotic ability, the acquisition of self-hypnotic skills may be important in coping with pain. The skills could also include learning to identify topics, events, and persons who elicit a stress response in the patient and learning how to avoid, deal with, or desensitize one's reactions to these persons or events. This may also include learning to extinguish catastrophizing cognition and learning to replace them with coping cognitive self-statements and imagery. For example, learning to increase the frequency of self-statements like, "I can handle this present pain; I know it will reduce in intensity eventually; I can turn my attention to enjoyable memories until this passes."

Fourth, one should arrange conditions for the generalization and maintenance of progress. It is critical to ensure that coping skills and procedures learned in the clinic or consulting room transfer to the patient's natural habitat. An important part of this provision involves building short- and long-term follow-up of all patients into the initial role induction of the new patient. It also involves training the patient to practice learned skills in a natural habitat (at the "scene of the crime") and learning to recognize and mobilize resources in the patient's environment to support the acquired changes in coping with pain. During periods of acute exacerbation it is very easy for these patients to relapse into their previous maladaptive methods of dealing with stress and pain.

In summary, an individualized program of chronic pain management that includes a judicious blending of concepts and procedures from hypnosis, biofeedback, and behavior modification can significantly add to the efficacy of conventional medical methods of managing chronic pain. The integration of these concepts and procedures is still an art form for which no technical manual can be easily written, and that, like a complex surgical skill, can be learned only by the careful, direct observation of the clinical behaviors of skilled practitioners.

Clinical Guidelines for a Psychophysiological Approach to a Chronic Pain Patient

There are several common goals that all people who have chronic pain problems need to achieve in a graduated fashion.

1. A physical activity that is appropriate for the patient should be selected, one that can be performed regardless of weather (e.g., riding a stationary bicycle, walking in a mall, etc.) The activity needs to be very gradually increased in a quantitative, objective manner. Activity reduces the time available for pain ruminations, provides a sense of accomplishment, and combats introspective withdrawal and depression.

2. The patient needs to sign a contract to stop doctor shopping and to limit all pain and psychotropic medication refills to one physician who has completely investigated the patient's physical status and monitors his or her physical health. This should preferably be a neurosurgeon who has satisfied himself and the patient that nothing more can be done

for the patient in terms of surgery or drugs. This should be a neurosurgeon who has had several years of experience with chronic patients and one who has developed a lively sense of the limitations of surgery for chronic pain. It is crucial to defuse the patient's episodic tendency, when the pain temporarily increases, to seek new tests, new hospitalization, new medicines, and new surgeons.

3. The patient needs to be committed up front to a graduated decrease in the use of all prescription analgesic and psychotropic medications (with an exception of an antidepressant medication like Elavil). The patient should be warned in advance that this detoxification process will be painful, but that some modest relief lies on the other side of the detoxification process. The patient is told that acquisition and maintenance of the pain management skills that he or she will learn proceed best in an "unclouded" CNS. The patient is told that chronic usage of pain and psychotropic medications may in fact be hypoalgesic and interfere with normal sleep (Pilowsky, Crettenden, & Townly, 1985) and other physiological functions.

4. The patient is required to make a commitment up front to other health-promoting behaviors. These include at least one part-time or full-time money making activity. Gainful work ties us to life and reality, and can save self-esteem. Next, the patient may need to add at least one hobby or fun activity that is performed repeatedly several times per week. For example, photography, painting, sculpture, and wood carving. If the recreational activity is also money making the patient may be further along the road to rehabilitation. Finally, the patient needs to schedule at least one social activity (going to church, playing bridge with buddies, going fishing, etc.) that keeps him socially connected and involved in the life of other human beings. This may include volunteer work at a telephone switchboard, typing, and the like. "It's not what you have lost but what you have left that counts." The housewife who can't do her own chores can operate a telephone answering service to pay for a maid. The injured carpenter can become a locksmith. Fun activity that is creative or problem solving provides a reason for "getting out of bed" when one feels demoralized by constant pain. It combats the tendency to withdraw into a shell, become acutely aware of one's pain and lapse into invalidism.

Role Induction for Chronic Pain Patients

When I first meet a patient I ask why he or she is here and who made the referral. I inquire about the location, intensity, and duration of the pain or problem, and the conditions under which it improves or gets worse. I also inquire as to what therapies help and what do not help the problem. If the patient is currently in litigation, I suggest that the patient may want to wait until the patient receives the financial settlement before returning to me for evaluation. I point out that the patient should be practical because the injury sustained may deserve a nice settlement, and that if the patient should be accepted as a candidate for therapy and actually reduce the pain, he or she would risk losing a substantial financial settlement. The chances for a good financial settlement are better if the patient crawls into a courtroom rather than walks in. I request that before the patient makes a decision to continue with the other components (hypnosis test, psychophysiological stress profile test) of my evaluation, he or she discuss the legal-financial situation with an attorney. The patient should then have the attorney inform me in writing that it would be safe for the client to risk learning some methods of coping with the chronic pain problem. I also point out to the patient that chronic pain tends to "metastasize" and that if the patient does not aggressively and quickly work to arrest the spread of the pain, the pain eventually will take over the patient's life and reduce him or her to an invalid, a detached observer and no longer a participant in life. The patient is told that the sooner he or she makes the decision to learn to put the pain on a "back burner" and some fun activities regularly on a "front burner" in life, the prognosis for the condition will improve. I tell the patient that we cannot teach anyone to be rid of pain, but that one can learn to reduce the intensity of pain at first for only brief periods. Eventually these periods of reduced pain intensity will grow longer and the patient may actually have brief periods when the pain levels are quite low. I add that neither I nor anyone else can eliminate the pain forever. Learning to reduce the pain will be hard work and may lead to temporary increases of pain; that is, the pain may have to get worse before it gets better. The patient may have, at times, to take one step backward to take two steps forward. Only the patient can do this work and most of it will have to be done by the patient outside of the clinic (e.g., in the home). Also during the intake session, I tell the patient that the purpose of this intense evaluation is for me to evaluate the patient's candidacy for therapy; because our pain program has a good batting average, I am looking for a few good patients who want to work hard at coping better with their pain. The patient is told that our methods may not alter the sensory component of the pain but they can alter the reactive or suffering component. Muscular bracing and a sympathetic nervous system reactivity are natural consequences of pain that one can learn to alter, because they potentiate the sensory component of pain. The patient is told that one will be taught skills to replace the increasing pills the patient has been taking to reduce or abolish the pain. These skills take 80% of people 3 to 4 weeks to learn, or more precisely, to overlearn. The immediate results will be neither dramatic nor instantaneous but will be uneven, slow, and cumulative. I let the patient know that one will never be asked to do anything easy, and assure the patient that if there were an easy way out of the predicament, he or she would already have found it.

On the other side of some hard decisions and painful physical efforts there will be a quiet confidence in the skills the patient can use to manage the pain and to keep the pain from managing the patient. For example, the patient might be asked to pay progressively longer visits to a previous work environment from which he or she may have been absent for several months to a year. Fellow workers who have had to pick up the patient's slack may feel resentment toward the patient, thinking the patient is "gold bricking," etc. The patient may be anxious (phobic) or paranoid about returning to work even for a short visit. The patient's belief that fellow workers are angry and suspicious may mobilize anxiety and consequent reluctance even to return to that physical environment to check out the accuracy of the patient's beliefs of the coworkers' attitudes toward him or her. Yet it is important that the patient follow through on this assignment and monitor the pain levels before, during, and after such a visit and talk about his or her feelings about the experience.

In summary, in the first contact with the patient it is important for the patient to recognize that a candidacy for therapy is being evaluated. Membership in our pain program has to be earned and is not automatic. Second, the patient should understand that therapy involves learning to substitute pain management skills for pills. The process of skills acquisition is uneven but cumulative if the patient stays the course when the pain periodically gets worse, as it will. Next, and most importantly, the patient needs to get angry at the pain and perceive it as an ego-alien factor that limits the patient's functioning and that needs to be minimized and put in a small place in the patient's life. Finally, it is important that the patient is committed on a daily basis to practicing pain coping skills and gradually increasing physical activity.

Case Study of a Chronic Pain Patient

This 47-year-old, white, married male, father of three children (son 13, daughters, 21 and 23) presents with a back injury. Prior to the development of his present complaints, this patient had been a highly successful customs inspector who was so gifted at detecting the presence of illegal substances in luggage that he presented workshops on detection to peers all over the world. Prior to and during military service on the front line in Vietnam he had few or no somatic complaints and definitely no psychological or psychiatric complaints. He served in Vietnam as captain of a riverboat, retrieving bodies of dead American soldiers from the river. He was discharged with military honors and reported great contempt for soldiers who had psychological complaints (depression, anxiety, phobia, etc.). Soon after he returned to the United States he developed a variety of nonspecific physical complaints (e.g., pain, nausea, etc.) for which he was temporarily hospitalized. He returned to his previous job, where he had an accident leading to his present problems.

The patient currently reports pain in his low back with radiation into his left leg. The pain is constant and is increased by lying on his right side, sitting, or any increased activity. He takes up to 60 minutes to fall asleep, and he wakes up several times at night with pain. Also, at this time, his erections are unreliable and he frequently loses his erection soon after penetration. The patient is still interested in sexual activity. He appears depressed and anxious. He is the only provider in the family, and has not worked since the injury; he has many unpaid bills. The patient is a tall, 6-foot 8-inch, 240 lb. sturdy male whose manner was hostile and skeptical on initial contact with the present psychologist. He reported that he had tripped in a trailer and fallen backward 3 to 4 feet, landing on his hip. Within one hour after the fall, he had pain in his back, neck, shoulder unit, and left leg. He went to a general hospital where X rays were negative for fractures. He was treated with pain medications at home. A week later he was hospitalized for investigation of his back and neck pain; he again had a negative workup and was given pelvic traction three to four times a week without improvement of his pain. He was hospitalized on December 1982, and had a laminectomy at L5-6 disc. His pain improved for approximately 4 to 6 weeks but returned. He was hospitalized again in March 1983 and had a second laminectomy. His pain again improved for 3 to 6 weeks and returned. He had been evaluated with negative findings by neurosurgeons and orthopedic surgeons at two major medical centers. More surgery has been recommended but the patient is reluctant to proceed with further surgery. The patient has had numerous intensive trials of physical therapy, ice, and ultrasound to both hips, without relief of pain.

Following this patient's role induction (described in the previous section), the patient agreed to our assessment procedure and was accepted for treatment. The high-risk assessment revealed a patient who was positive on 4 of the 5 high-risk variables. His Harvard score was 12 (he was confirmed as an 11 on the Standard Form C), his neuroticism score was at the 87th percentile, his life change score was 1,178, his support systems were minimal and his satisfaction with them was low, and his coping skills were also very low. His level of muscle tension from frontalis was very high (EMG 22 UV p-p). This profile and its implications were presented to the patient. It was emphasized that his superior hypnotic ability implied that he could be inadvertently amplifying his pain, and possibly blocking from consciousness past events associated with the physiological mobilization (bracing) currently generating his levels of muscle tension. His neuroticism also increased the possibility that he would learn, retain, and be currently influenced by negative emotions that could also independently amplify his pain perception. This profile appeared to have a high face validity for the patient and significantly increased his rapport with the therapist. I further confirmed his high hypnotic ability by inducing, during the interview and with his permission, a partial temporary analgesia of his right hand. His attitude changed from one of hostility to one of interest and motivation. He came for weekly therapy sessions over a period of 5 months. Initially, my goal in therapy was to teach him to reduce muscular bracing in his upper and lower back and face. A combination of EMG biofeedback and hypnosis was utilized to reach these goals. Concurrently, he was required gradually to increase his physical activity, and began a strict regimen of walking. The patient learned self-hypnosis slowly but progressively and acquired some skill at reducing the intensity of his pain. Several times during episodes of acute exacerbation of his pain, he made plans to seek more medical consultations, tests, and surgery, but fortunately never followed through on those tentative plans. These episodes of pain escalation were associated with nightmares of Vietnam. As the horrors he had witnessed and participated in came to consciousness in his nightmares, the sustained muscular bracing in his body reduced and he had more and longer episodes of moderate or little pain.

He has become a wood carver and found this a lucrative source of part-time income and great creative pleasure. He has greatly increased his physical activity until he is walking 4 miles a day regardless of the weather. At the inception of therapy, I recorded a tape of self-hypnosis for him that he uses several times a day even to date. At this time, we have followed him for 3 years and he is committed to a 5-year follow-up.

Summary and Conclusion

A recent review of the behavioral treatment of chronic pain (Linton, 1986) reached several important conclusions. (a) The methodology of the studies in the behavioral treatment of chronic pain has improved in number and controls to the point that valid conclusions can be drawn from the studies. For example, multiple and broad outcome measures and control conditions characterize the majority of the studies. (b) Operant programs are clearly effective in decreasing medication consumption and in increasing activity levels. (c) Relaxation-based techniques (progressive muscular relaxation, biofeedback, etc.) and cognitive coping techniques are clearly effective in reducing pain intensity ratings. (d) Therapeutic effects continue into follow-up but patients' compliance with assigned techniques is reduced. (e) Behavioral treatment techniques seldom produce 100% improvement. These conclusions fit our clinical observations but fail to stress a crucial clinical procedure. This procedure is the initial patient interview, or what I call the role induction. The role induction can very significantly determine the degree of patient engagement with the therapy program, and its eventual clinical outcome.

References

Andreychuck, T., & Skriver, C. Hypnosis and biofeedback in the treatment of migraine headache. *International Journal of Experimental and Clinical Hypnosis*, 1975, 23(3), 172–183.

Aronoff, G. M. [Editorial]. *Clinical Journal of Pain*, 1985, 1, 1–3.

Barton, J., Haight, R., Marsland, D., & Temple, T. Low back pain in the primary care setting. *Journal of Family Practice*, 1976, 3, 363–366.

Beecher, H. K. *Measurement of subjective responses: Quantitative effects of drugs.* New York: Oxford University Press, 1959.

Blanchard, E. B., & Andrasik, F. Psychological assessment and treatment of headache: Recent developments and emerging issues. *Journal of Consulting and Clinical Psychology*, 1982, 50, 859–879.

Blackwell, B. Biofeedback in a comprehensive behavioral medicine program. *Biofeedback and Self-Regulation*, 1981, 6, 445–472.

Bond, M. R. The relation of pain to the Eysenck Personality Inventory, Cornell Medical Index and Witley Index of Hypochondriasis. *British Journal of Psychiatry*, 1971, 119, 671–678.

Bond, M. R. Personality studies in patients with pain secondary to organic disease. *Journal of Psychosomatic Research*, 1973, 17, 257–263.

Bonica, J. J. (Ed.). *International symposium on pain. Advances in neurology* (Vol. 4). New York: Raven Press, 1974.

Bonica, J. J. Pain research and therapy: Past and current status and future needs. In L. K. Y. Ng & J. J. Bonica (Eds.), *Pain, discomfort and humanitarian care.* New York: Elsevier, 1980.

Bowers, K. S., & Meichenbaum, D. *Unconscious revisited.* New York: Wiley Interscience, 1984.

Brena, S. F. The mystery of pain: Is pain a sensation? *Management of patients with chronic pain.* Jamaica, New York: Spectrum Publications, 1983.

Budzynski, T. H., & Stoyva, J. M. An instrument for producing deep muscle relaxation by means of analog information feedback. *Journal of Applied Behavior Analysis*, 1969, 2, 231–237.

Budzynski, T. H., Stoyva, J. M., & Adler, C. Feedback-induced muscle relaxation. In T. Barber, L. Di Cara, J. Kamiya, N. Miller, D. Shapiro, & J. M. Stoyva, (Eds.), *Biofeedback and self-control*. Chicago: Aldine-Atherton, 1970.

Budzynski, T. H., Stoyva, J. M., Adler, C. S., & Mullaney, D. J. EMG biofeedback and tension headache: A controlled outcome study. *Seminars in Psychiatry*, 1973, 5, 397–410.

Chapman, C. R., Casey, K. L., Dubner, R., Foley, K. M., Gracely, R. H., & Reading, A. E. Pain measurement: An overview. *Pain*, 1985, 22, 1–31.

Coger, R., & Werback, M. Attention, anxiety, and the effects of learned enhancement of EEG in chronic pain: A pilot study in biofeedback. In B. L. Crue, Jr. (Ed.), *Pain: Research and treatment*. New York: Academic Press, 1975.

Costa, P. T., & McCrae, R. R. Hypochondriasis, neuroticism and aging: When are somatic complaints unfounded? *American Psychologist*, 1985, 40, 19–28.

Cox, D. J., Freundlich, A., & Meyer, R. G. Differential effectiveness of electromyograph feedback, verbal relaxation instructions, and medication placebo with tension headaches. *Journal of Consulting Clinical Psychologists*, 1975, 43, 892–898.

Crue, B. L. Multidisciplinary pain treatment programs: Current status. *Clinical Journal of Pain*, 1985, 1, 31–38.

Edmonston, W. E. *Hypnosis and relaxation*. New York: Wiley, 1981.

Edwards, P. W., Zeichner, A., Kuczmierzyk, A. R., & Boczkowski, J. Familial pain models: The relationship between family history of pain and current pain experience. *Pain*, 1985, 21, 379–384.

Engstrom, D. R., London, P., & Hart, J. I. EEG alpha feedback training and hypnotic susceptibility. *A.P.A. Proceedings*, 1970, 5, 837–838.

Evans, F. J. The power of a sugar pill. *Psychology Today*, April 1974, pp. 55–59.

Eysenck, H. J. Psychophysiology and personality. In A. Galse & J. A. Edward (Eds.), *Physiological correlates of human behavior*. London: Academic Press, 1983.

Flor, H., & Turk, D. C. Etiological theories and treatments for chronic low back pain: I. Somatic models and interventions. *Pain*, 1984, 19(2), 105–121.

Fordyce, W. E. *Behavioral methods for chronic pain and illness*. St. Louis: C. V. Mosby, 1976.

Forster, P. M., & Govier, E. Discrimination without awareness? *Quarterly Journal of Experimental Psychology*, 1978, 30, 282–295.

Friar, L. R., & Beatty, J. Migraine: Management by trained control of vasoconstriction. *Journal of Consulting Clinical Psychologists*, 1976, 44, 46–53.

Gentry, W. P., & Bernal, G. A. Chronic pain. In R. B. Williams & W. D. Gentry (Eds.), *Behavioral approaches to medical treatment*. Cambridge, MA: Ballinger, 1977.

Gottfredson, D. K. Hypnosis as an anesthetic in dentistry. Doctoral dissertation, Department of Psychology, Brigham Young University. *Dissertation Abstracts International*, 1973, 33, 7–13: 3303.

Hendler, N., Derogatis, L., Avella, J., & Long, D. EMG biofeedback in patient with chronic pain. *Diseases of the Nervous System*, 1977, 38, 505–574.

Hilgard, E. R. *Hypnotic susceptibility*. New York: Harcourt & Brace, 1965.

Hilgard, E. R., & Hilgard, J. R. *Hypnosis in the relief of pain*. Los Altos, CA: Kaufmann, 1975.

Hult, L. Cervical, dorsal, and lumbar spinal syndromes: A field investigation of a non-selected material of 1200 workers in different occupations with special reference to disc degeneration and so-called muscular rheumatism. *Acta Orthopedica Scandinavia*, 1954, 17, (Suppl.) 1–102.

Hutching, D. F., & Reinking, R. H. Tension headaches: What form of therapy is most effective. *Journal of Biofeedback and Self-control*, 1976, 1, 183–190.

Jaynes, J. *The origin of consciousness in the breakdown of the bicameral mind.* Boston: Houghton Mifflin, 1977.

Johnson, A. D. *The problem claim: An approach to early identification.* Department of Labor and Industries, State of Washington (mimeo), 1978.

Karron, J., DeGoode, D. E., & Tait, R. A comparison of low back pain patients in the United States and New Zealand: Psychosocial and economic factors affecting severity of disability. *Pain,* 1985, *21,* 77–89.

Katz, R. L., Kao, C. Y., Spiegel, H., & Katz, G. J. Pain, acupuncture, hypnosis. In J. J. Bonica (Ed.), *Advances in Neurology* (Vol. 4). New York: Raven Press, 1974.

Kerr, F. W. L. The structural basis of pain: Circuitry and pathways. In K. Y. L. Ng & J. J. Bonica (Eds.), *Pain, discomfort, and humanitarian care.* New York: Elsevier, 1980.

Kihlstrom, J. F. Hypnosis. In M. R. Rosenzweig & L. W. Porter, (Eds.), *Annual Review of Psychology, 36,* 1985, 385–418.

Kihlstrom, J. F. The cognitive unconscious. *Science,* 1987, *237,* 1445–1452.

Kimble, G. A. *Hilgard and Marquis' conditioning and learning* (2nd ed.). New York: Appleton-Century-Crofts, 1961.

Levine, J. Pain and analgesia: The outlook for a more rational treatment. *Annals of Internal Medicine,* 1984, *100,* 269–276.

Lewicki, P. *Nonconscious social information processing.* New York: Academic Press, 1986.

Linton, S. J. Behavioral remediation of chronic pain: A status report. *Pain,* 1986, *24,* 125–141.

Loeser, J. D. Neurosurgical control of chronic pain. *Archives of Surgery,* 1977, *12,* 880–883.

Loeser, J. D. Nonpharmacologic approaches to pain relief. In L. K. Y. Ng & J. J. Bonica (Eds.), *Pain, discomfort, and humanitarian care.* New York: Elsevier, 1980.

London, P., Hart, J., & Lebovits, M. EEG alpha rhythms and hypnotic susceptibility. *Nature,* 1968, *219,* 71–72.

Lynn, R., & Eysenck, H. J. Tolerance for pain, extraversion and neuroticism. *Perceptual and Motor Skills,* 1961, *12,* 161–167.

Mathews, A., MacLeod, C. Discrimination of threat cues without awareness in anxiety states. *Journal of Abnormal Psychology.* 1986, *95*(2), 131–8.

Medina, J. L., Diamond, S., & Franklin, M. A. Biofeedback therapy for migraine. *Headache,* 1976, *16,* 115–119.

Melzack, R. *The puzzle of pain.* New York: Basic Books, 1973.

Melzack, R., & Dennis, S. G. Neurophysiological foundations of pain. In R. A. Sternbach (Ed.), *The psychology of pain.* New York: Raven, 1978.

Melzack, R., & Perry, C. Self-regulation of pain: Use of alpha feedback and hypnotic training for control of chronic pain. *Experimental Neurology,* 1975, *46,* 452–469.

Melzack, R., & Wall, P. D. Pain mechanisms: A new theory. *Science,* 1965, *150,* 971–979.

Newman, R. I., Seres, J. L., Yospe, L. P., & Garlington, B. Multidisciplinary treatment of chronic pain: Long-term follow-up of low back pain patients. *Pain,* 1978, *4,* 283–292.

Ng, L. K. Y., & Bonica, J. J. *Pain, discomfort and humanitarian care.* New York: Elsevier, 1980.

Pagni, C. A., & Maspes, P. E. A critical appraisal of pain surgery and suggestions for improving treatment. *Recent advances on pain pathophysiology and clinical aspects,* Springfield, IL: Charles C Thomas, 1974.

Payne, B., & Norfleet, M. A. Chronic pain and the family: A review. *Pain,* 1986, *26,* 1–22.

Pena, F. *Perceptual isolation and hypnotic susceptibility.* Unpublished doctoral dissertation, Washington State University. Pullman, Washington, 1963.

Pilowsky, I., Crettenden, I., & Townly, M. Sleep disturbance in pain clinic patients. *Pain,* 1985, *23,* 27–33.

Qualls, P. J., & Sheehan, P. W. Electromyograph biofeedback as a relaxation technique: A critical appraisal and reassessment. *Psychological Bulletin*, 1981, *90*, 21–42.

Robinson, D. Psychobiology and the unconscious. In K. S. Bowers & D. Meichenbaum (Eds.), *Unconscious revisited*. New York: Wiley-Interscience, 1984.

Sainsbury, P., & Gibson, J. G. Symptoms of anxiety and tension and the accompanying physiological changes in the muscular system. *Journal of Neurology, Neurosurgery, and Psychiatry*, 1954, *17*, 216–224.

Sanders, R. S., & Reyher, J. Sensory deprivation and the enhancement of hypnotic susceptibility. *Journal of Abnormal Psychology*, 1969, *74*, 375–378.

Sargent, J. D., Green, E. E., & Walters, E. D. Autogenic feedback training in a pilot study of migraine and tension headaches. Unpublished manuscript, 1972.

Schmorl, G., & Junghanns, H. *Die gesunde und kranke Wirbelseule im* Roentgenbild. Leipzig: Thieme, 1932.

Scott, D. S., & Barber, T. X. Cognitive control of pain: Effects of multiple cognitive strategies. *Psychological Record*, 1977, *27*, 373–383.

Seres, J. L., & Newman, R. I. Results of treatment of chronic low back pain at the Portland Pain Center. *Journal of Neurosurgery*, 1976, *45*, 32–36.

Shevrin, H., & Dickman, S. The psychological unconscious: A necessary assumption for all psychological theory? *American Psychologist*, 1980, *35*, 421–434.

Skinner, B. F. *Science and human behavior*. New York: Macmillan, 1953.

Spanos, N. P., Radtke-Bodonik, L., Ferguson, J. D., & Jones, B. The effects of hypnotic susceptibility, suggestions for analgesia, and the utilization of cognitive strategies on the reduction of pain. *Journal of Abnormal Psychology*, 1979, *88*, 282–292.

St. Jean, R., & McLeod, C. Hypnosis, absorption and time perception. *Journal of Abnormal Psychology*, 1983, *92*, 81–86.

Sternbach, R. A. *Pain: A psychophysiological analysis*. New York: Academic Press, 1968.

Sternbach, R. A. *Pain patients: Traits and treatment*. New York: Academic Press, 1974.

Sternbach, R. A. Treatment of the chronic pain patient. *Journal of Human Stress*, 1978, *4*, 11–15.

Sternbach, R. A., Janowsky, D. S., Huey, L. Y., & Segal, D. S. Effects of altering brain serotonin activity on human chronic pain. In J. J. Bonica & D. Albe-Fessard (Eds.), *Advances in pain research and therapy* (Vol. 1). New York: Raven Press, 1976.

Swanson, D. W., Swenson, W. M., Marita, T., & McPhee, M. C. Program for managing chronic pain: Program description and characteristics of patients. *Mayo Clinic Proceedings*, 1976, *51*, 401–408.

Sweet, W. H. Animal models of chronic pain. *Pain*, 1981, *10*, 275–295.

Turk, D. C., Meichenbaum, D. H., & Berman, W. H. Applications of biofeedback for the regulation of pain: A critical review, *Psychological Bulletin*, 1979, *86*(6), 1322–1338.

Turk, D. C., Meichenbaum, D., & Genest, M. *Pain and behavioral medicine—A cognitive-behavioral perspective*, New York: Guilford Press, 1983.

Turner, J. A., Calsyn, D. A., Fordyce, W. E., & Ready, L. B. Drug utilization patterns in chronic pain patients. *Pain*, 1982, *12*, 357–363.

Watson, D., & Clark, L. A. Negative affectivity: The disposition to experience aversive emotional states. *Psychological Bulletin*, 1984, *96*, 465–490.

Watson, D., & Tellegen, A. Toward a consensual structure of mood. *Psychological Bulletin*, 1985, *98*, 219–235.

Whatmore, G. B., & Kohli, D. R. *The physiopathology and treatment of functional disorders*. New York: Grune & Stratton, 1974.

White, J. C., & Sweet, W. H. *Pain and the neurosurgeon: A forty-year experience*. Springfield: Charles C Thomas, 1969.

Wickramasekera, I. The effects of sensory restriction on hypnotic susceptibility. *International Journal of Clinical and Experimental Hypnosis*, 1969, *17*, 217–224.

Wickramasekera, I. The effects of sensory restriction on susceptibility to hypnosis: A hypothesis and more preliminary data. *Journal of Abnormal Psychology*, 1970, *76*, 69–75.

Wickramasekera, I. Effects of EMG feedback training on susceptibility to hypnosis: preliminary observations. *Proceedings of the 79th Annual Convention of the American Psychological Association*, 1971, *6*, 785–787.

Wickramasekera, I. EMG feedback training and tension headache: Preliminary observations. *American Journal of Clinical Hypnosis*, 1972, *15*(2), 83–85.

Wickramasekera, I. The application of verbal instructions and EMG feedback training to the management of tension headache: Preliminary observations. *Headache*, 1973, *13*(2), 74–76.

Wickramasekera, I. The placebo effect and biofeedback for headache pain. *Proceedings of the San Diego Biomedical Symposium*. New York: Academic Press, 1977. (a)

Wickramasekera, I. On attempts to modify hypnotic susceptibility: Some psychophysiological procedures and promising directions. *Annals of the New York Academy of Sciences*, 1977, *796*, 143–153. (b)

Wickramasekera, I. *A model of the patient at high risk for chronic stress related disorders.* Paper read at Annual Convention of the Biofeedback Society of America. San Diego, California, March, 1979.

Wickramasekera, I. A conditioned response model of the placebo effect: Predictions from the model. *Biofeedback and Self-Regulation*, 1980, *5*, 5–18.

Wickramasekera, I. Clinical research in a behavioral medicine private practice. *Behavioral Assessment*, 1981, *3*, 265–271.

Wickramasekera, I. A model of people at high risk to develop chronic stress related symptoms. In F. J. McGuigan, W. E. Sime, and J. M. Wallace (Eds.) *Stress and Tension Control*. New York: Plenum, 1983.

Wickramasekera, I. A conditioned response model of the placebo effect: Predictions and postdictions from the model. In L. White, B. Tursky, & G. Schwartz, (eds.), *Placebo: Clinical phenomena and new insights*. New York: Guilford Press, 1985.

Wickramasekera, I., Truong, X. T., Busch, M., & Orr, C. The management of rheumatoid arthritic pain: Preliminary observations. In I. Wickramasekera (Ed.), *Biofeedback, behavior therapy and hypnosis*. Chicago: Nelson-Hall, 1976.

Wiesel, S., Feffer, H., & Tsournas, N. *The incidence of positive CAT scans in an asymptomatic group of patients.* Volo Award Paper read at Annual Meeting of the International Society for the Study of Lumbar Spine, Montreal, Canada, 1984.

Wilson, S. C., & Barber, T. X. The fantasy-prone personality: Implications for understanding imagery, hypnosis and parapsychological phenomena. In A. A. Sheikh (Ed.), *Imagery: Current theory, research, and application*. New York: Wiley, 1982.

Wolff, H. F. *Headache and other head pain* (2nd ed.). New York: Oxford University Press, 1963.

Wolpe, J., & Lazarus, A. A. *Behavior therapy techniques*. New York: Pergamon Press, 1966.

Zborowski, M. *People in pain*. San Francisco: Jossey-Bass, 1969.

9

HIGH-RISK PROFILE
Assessment, Patient Feedback, and Therapy Planning

Assessment Questions and Assumptions

There are five types of questions the therapist should ask about each patient profile. First, for this patient, what is the most distressing chronic symptom or symptoms (e.g., back pain on walking, headache, angina) and what is the frequency (times per day or hour), intensity (patient's subjective rating, absent 0–5 severe), duration (length of symptomatic episode), the antecedents (psychological mood and situational) and the consequences (onset or offset of aversive events, attention, sympathy, etc.) of this distressing symptom or symptoms. Investigating these questions involves finding out why an acute problem became chronic in this case. Second, what factor or factors does the patient believe have caused or is presently maintaining the distressing symptom or symptoms. Third, what conceptual or procedural links can be made between the patient's beliefs about the etiology or present condition of the disorder and the five components of the high-risk profile. Fourth, what elevations or deficits discovered through the patient's performance on the high-risk profile (Wickramasekera, 1979) can account for parts or all of the patients presenting problems. In other words, what predisposes, triggers, and buffers are operating in this case at this point in time. Fifth, what maladaptive, unattended, or unconscious and overlearned beliefs and behavioral responses block this patient's assimilation of major life changes (e.g., rape, physical impairment, death, loss of job, loss of lover, loss of child, etc.) in intimate relationships (commitment, sex, affection, confiding) and work (commitment, production, challenge, control) relationships. In intimate relationships it is crucial to be able to feel committed; and to be sexually, affectionally, and verbally uninhibited with at least one person. In the work situation too, it is important to feel committed to what one is doing and to feel some degree of control over the products of one's work and to be challenged by them. Impairments of adaptation in areas of work and love are destructive to normality. Unconscious (unattended) and overlearned belief filters or schemata the patient holds may block the assimilation of and adaptation to a traumatic incident or major life change. For example, the premature death or betrayal of a loved one may be incongruent with one's unconscious, unattended, or over-learned belief in a just world. This unconscious cognitive incongruence may obstruct the assimilation and adaptation to this irreversible life change. Repeated episodes of unstable angina or a myocardial infarction in a young adult may not fit the overlearned belief "I am intact and invulnerable." A discrepancy between unattended and overlearned un-conscious beliefs and everyday empirical experiences can generate feel-ings of incoherence, disorientation, and hopelessness. A serious breach of personal or professional standards may be incongruent with the deep unattended belief "I do not do bad things." This guilt may torture the person. A series of incomprehensible personal and/or professional losses or failures may be incongruent with the unconscious belief that "my world has meaning and I am in control of my life." Deep uncon-scious or overlearned beliefs like I am "unworthy" or "incompetent" can be threatened by life events like the prospect of promotion, mar-riage, or love. These threats to unattended and overlearned or uncon-scious deep schemata can unwittingly trigger intrusive ruminative epi-sodes, attack, or escape behaviors that block or impede functional adaptation to major life changes that have, in fact, occurred. For exam-ple, symptoms like chronic anxiety, depression, dissociative acting-out episodes, guilt, insomnia, rheumatoid arthritis, torticollis, chronic pain, or an ulcer can occur in response to the loss of a loved one or a major personal or professional failure.

There are now converging bodies of empirically and experimentally established literatures (selective attention, subliminal perception, etc.) documenting the hypothesis that large amounts of behaviorally influen-tial complex cognitive activities can occur outside of consciousness (Bowers & Meichenbaum, 1984; Dixon, 1981; Kihlstrom, 1987; Shevrin & Dickman, 1980). The clinician who ignores the patient's and his own unconscious cognitive events is likely to be clinically ineffective and to risk symptomatic relapses.

These overlearned but unattended (Bowers, 1984) unconscious be-liefs may be accessed and altered by several promising techniques, de-pending partly on the hypnotic ability of the patient. In patients of high-hypnotic ability, hypnotic suggestions that dreams will occur in the coming days and weeks that are relevant to underlying beliefs and problems is often adequate. Such patients should also be told to keep a dream diary by their bed. The high-hypnotic-ability patient can also be instructed to have a hypnotic dream about unconscious beliefs in the consulting room. For patients of low- or moderate-hypnotic ability, low-arousal (physiological relaxation) training and diachotic listening is often effective in accessing unconscious beliefs. The patient in low-arousal training should be told to report all spontaneously occurring images, impressions, and sensations during low arousal, however irrelevant or silly they may seem. The diachotic listening procedure can be used to deliver suggestions to night dream at home or have relevant images during low-arousal induction in the consulting room. Suggestions delivered after 1½ to 3 hours in a sensory restriction chamber can also facilitate accessing unconscious beliefs in low- or moderate-hypnotic ability patients. The following is an illustration of how low-arousal induction (EMG feedback training) can be used to access unconscious overlearned beliefs. A female patient of low-hypnotic ability who presented with severe headaches (see case described on page 218) was also excessively perfectionistic and believed in her own sense of indispensability on her job. One day while coming out of low arousal in my laboratory she reported the following unexpected clear and very vivid image. She saw "a little girl with blond hair and freckles and a pasted on smile who always wanted to please her family and relatives." The patient immediately recognized the little girl as her early self that was even today very influential in her job-related activities. The patient's recognition and ownership of this image led immediately to profound, broad, and rapid behavioral, physiological (drop in mean baseline EMG) changes and medication reduction. The frequency and intensity of her headaches also dropped dramatically. Previously, several weeks of EMG feedback and home relaxation practice had led to only small reductions in headache activity and no changes in medication. But clearly the previous low-arousal training (EMG feedback) appears to have facilitated the probability of accessing this cogently diagnostic image of an unconscious or dissociated self. Having this hypnagogic image was as useful to this patient's problem solving as was Kekule's hypnagogic image of hexagonal benzene structure to chemistry. The psychophysiological therapist should arrange conditions (low-arousal training and use of patient self-report questionnaire of images, sensory restriction chamber, dream diary, diachotic listening procedure, etc.) to increase the probability of accessing unconscious overlearned beliefs that are obstacles to the assimilation and adaptation to present life events.

Discussion of Assessment Questions

Question 1. What is the most distressing symptom from the patient's viewpoint? This need not be the most critical patient problem from the therapist's viewpoint. For example, for the patient it may be tachycardia episodes, headache pain, or an ulcer, but from the therapist's expert viewpoint it may be premature ejaculation, marital stress, parents who infantalize the patient, or a lack of self-assertion on the job or in bed, or at home. It is important (a) to keep the focus initially on the patient's definition of the problem; (b) to investigate the conditions under which the distressing symptom can be turned on and off; and (c) to reproduce in the consulting room, if only for a few minutes or seconds, the symptom or a similar symptom, by replicating the suspected pathological conditions. Successful manipulation (on–off) of the presenting symptom or a related symptom for a few seconds in the consulting room early in therapy (even in the initial interview) can capture the patient's attention, imagination, and provide even an illusory sense of control over the symptom. The labeling of the symptom, the calling it out, sending it back, and the identification of the conditions of recall and dismissal appear to domesticate what to the patient has appeared to be a demoralizing, overwhelming, and unruly problem. It is good to know it can be ruled by someone.

For example, if the patient complains of anxiety, pain, or some motor dysfunction, he can be asked what can be done here and now for only a few minutes to call forth the symptom (increase its frequency or intensity) before it is allowed to return to a resting baseline. Or the patient may be told to try and have a few extra headaches or anxiety episodes so that we can secure a conservative base rate or a good baseline before we alter the symptom in therapy. These symptomatic episodes are to be carefully tracked and recorded on graph paper. The analogy of the mechanic needing to see the car malfunction in the mechanic's garage before it can be fixed is sometimes useful. If the patient has superior hypnotic ability, as revealed by the hypnotic tests on the High-Risk battery, one can be confident that one is dealing with an imaginative, empathic, creative person who can, in response to hypnotic suggestions (without prior training) experience an anesthesia or catalepsy over parts of the body. An anesthesia or levitation can be induced over an area of the body (e.g., hand) unrelated (always) to the symptom (head pain) to show the patient how the therapy can work. This patient can also be confidently told that he or she has a rich interior life that may include ESP experiences that others may not even suspect. The accuracy of this observation may prove startling and capture the patient's attention and imagination.

If the patient's presenting symptom is anxiety, the subjective units of disturbances scale is explained (SUDS scale). Perfect tranquility is anchored as 0 and 50 is anchored as intolerable or massive fear or panic that requires getting out of the situation. The patient is asked for two SUDS levels, first "right now" or at this moment in time; and second, what the SUDS level was when the patient or therapist entered the consulting room. The patient can be asked what the SUDS level would be if the patient were asked to stand up and recite a poem or read from a book on the therapist's shelf or be told to go over to the receptionist's desk and congratulate her or criticize her on her telephone manner. The patient can next be asked to do one or more of the tasks just mentioned and to monitor and record on paper his or her SUDS level in action. If the SUDS level increases, the patient is asked carefully to note any changes in location and quality of physical sensations (e.g., loud and rapid pulse, can't get breath, dry throat, blank mind, feet feel restless, feelings of numbness in hands, or legs, butterflies in stomach, tightness in chest, neck, jaws, or upper back) and deliberately to focus on these sensations and to intensify them. As often occurs with ANS symptoms, attempts deliberately to evoke them simply weakens and extinguishes them, concurrently reducing the patient's fear of them. In this way even in the initial clinical interview the patient who feels overwhelmed by the symptom can be encouraged to view the symptoms as unwelcome outsiders and to take a detached, objective, analytical, curious, and scientific view of them. As if they were even briefly somehow "outside" of him and responsive to some internal or external control in intensity, duration, and frequency. Often such demonstrations capture the patient's imagination, impart even briefly a sense of being on top of rather than under the problem, and even provide an illusory sense of control of the symptoms. In any event, these opening maneuvers convey cogently but nonverbally to the patient that the therapist is not frightened by the symptoms and has in fact a strong academic interest in the patient's private distress.

In the initial clinical interview the patient can be told to keep a stress diary in which one records the frequency, duration, and intensity of daily hassles, level of physical exercise, and incidents of negative emotional arousal. Such records kept for 5 or 7 days prior to, for example, a migraine headache, can encourage curiosity about mind–body relationships and nourish psychological introspection. Figures 18, 19, and 20, from a recent study (Levor, Cohen, Naliboff, McArthur, & Heuser, 1986), illustrate the above suggestions.

The initial interview is always terminated by telling the patient that we are evaluating his or her application for candidacy for therapy at the Behavioral Medicine Clinic and Stress Disorders Laboratory. One is a

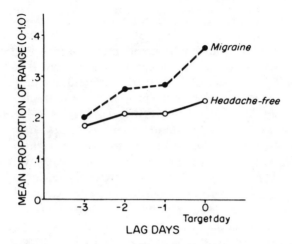

Figure 18. Mean levels of feelings (emotional arousal) for migraine and headache-free target days over 3 days of lag. Reprinted from Levor *et al.*, 1986.

candidate first, and may be accepted as a patient later. Patienthood is reserved for a few good people who demonstrate during the assessment process a commitment to recovery. Since our time and energy are limited, we devote ourselves only to those few people who are likely to profit from our interventions. In order to determine if the candidate has the type of profile that may qualify him or her for patienthood and that

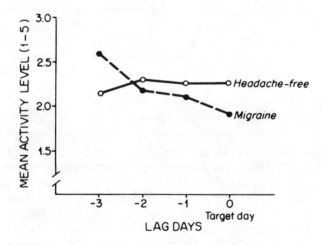

Figure 19. Mean levels of physical activity for migraine and headache-free target days over 3 days of lag. Reprinted from Levor *et al.*, 1986.

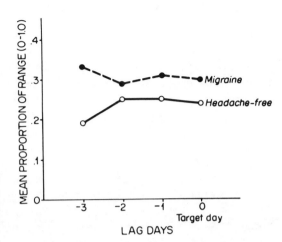

Figure 20. Mean levels of stressful events for migraine and headache-free target days over 3 days of lag. Reprinted from Levor *et al.*, 1986.

may account for the symptoms, we need to begin by conducting several tests. First, there is a paper-and-pencil self-report battery that measures certain aspects of high- and low-hypnotic ability, catastrophizing, neuroticism, major life change, minor hassles, support system, and coping skills. The rationale for the self-report package is that it reduces the cost of accurately and systematically collecting information about important aspects of a patient's personal functions and social-physical situation. It is important to be explicit about the rationales for each test with the patient. Second, the patient is told that he or she will take a safe, standardized, objective test of hypnotic ability called the Harvard Test, administered by a videotape. This test will tell us how much hypnotic ability the patient has. This information can be used for several purposes: to select treatments that are more likely rapidly to benefit the patient and to provide information on what the patient's private world is like in terms of empathy, perception, imagery, memory and mood, and how this patient stylistically prefers to process information. Third, the patient will take a psychophysiological stress profile and a waking and sleep behavioral EEG. The stress profile will provide information on the patient's most reactive biological organ system or window of vulnerability. The behavioral EEG will tell us about this patient's ability to fall asleep, lateralize information processing, and the incidence of certain nonspecific physical symptom and subcortical EEG rhythms (Struve *et al.*, 1986). The patient is warned that the diagnostic tests can be boring and time-consuming and that the patient should choose now to go forward with the tests or to leave the clinic altogether. Many small explicit moments of choice or decision are arranged during the candidacy investigation. When this is done kindly but firmly and always with clear rationales, the patient's commitment to therapy tightens. Hence a role-induction technique that looks initially like an obstacle course for picking out only "the strong and the brave" for therapy becomes, in fact, a motivational procedure that mobilizes and challenges even the docile and ordinary person to produce at an extraordinary level to secure entry into an apparently exclusive and elite club. This impression was initially supported by clinical observation and now by two consecutive empirical studies of the drop-out rate at our clinic. Our drop-out rate has in fact dropped from Study 1 to Study 2 (see Figure 14, p. 154) because the role-induction technique (Chapters 6 and 7) has been tightened and used more systematically by all staff members and doctoral students at our clinic. Few, if any, patients are turned off or away by the role induction when it is used confidently, firmly, and warmly. In fact, it has the paradoxical effect of mobilizing the patient up front to a tightening conscious commitment of time and energy to hard therapeutic work.

If this patient's chronic symptoms started as an acute episode, it becomes important to know why this particular patient has tarried in the sick role (Parson, 1951). The role of sickness can be attractive because it absolves one of responsibility for one's symptoms, and because it exempts one from normal chores and obligations. Lingering in such a role may result from patient features (for example, some high hypnotizables readily accept an infantile patient role and people high on neuroticism typically have lower pain tolerance thresholds, etc.), features of the disease (chronic intermittent or episodic nature of the disease onset, e.g., vascular or muscular headaches, or rheumatoid arthritis), features of the situation (motivation to escape from crummy job or marriage), or the financial incentive (e.g., sick pay, compensation, etc.) that sometimes accompanies disability.

Question 2. It is important to discover what the patient believes triggered the symptom and what factors are maintaining it. Often patients who present physical complaints without identifiable pathophysiology believe that they are suffering from an undetected and undiagnosed physical illness (e.g., tumor), or from exposure to a serious unidentified environmental pollutant or an interpersonal or role-related stressor. It is important for the therapist to reach for and to state explicitly what was only dimly and implicitly focused in the patient's mind. The patient may think the therapist is reading his mind. It will not hurt the therapist to be seen as a competent mind reader or to be seen as expecting some competence and hard work from the patient. These early nonverbal maneuvers implicitly make a silent alliance with the healthy side of the patient. This healthy side has often in the past taken a wait-and-see attitude. This cannot continue. The patient needs to be confronted with his or her beliefs and their implications. If the patient really still believes he or she is suffering from an undiagnosed physical illness, the patient needs to spend more time and money on more pilgrimages to more temples of healing (Mayo Clinic, Duke Medical Center, Scripps Medical Center) and be exposed to more hazardous diagnostic tests and more exploratory surgical procedures before becoming a legitimate candidate for a psychophysiological investigation of the complaint. The patient should come back to us only after having exhausted more medical centers, more cash, and having contracted more iatrogenic disease. Until then the patient may not be treatable.

Question 3. What links can be made between the patient's ideas about the causes and the timing or onset of the disorder on the one hand, and on the other hand what family factors, social interactions, and personal psychological factors (in terms of distress, perception, empathy, catastrophizing, unattended beliefs, imagination, etc.) as reported by the patient can be linked to risk factors on the patient's high-risk profile. It is critical credibly to link the patient's private phenomenology of the disorder with objective risk factors for illness. For example, the patient who is high on hypnotic ability can be shown how an exquisite sensitivity to one's own and others' feelings, and low tolerance for pain outside the hypnotic situation can potentiate psychosocial or other traumas at home or work. Examples from the patient's empathic experiences at movies, concerts, etc., can be elicited to demonstrate this link. The patient who ruminates on stressors may be shown the elevations on negative affectivity or neuroticism, the physiological stress profile marked by short latency, and large or sustained physiological responses that delay in returning to prestress baselines. The patient is reminded of his or her difficulty in shutting off aversive cognitive tapes (unpleasant memories or apprehensions) once they are started. The ruminator nearly always demonstrates a hypervigilant or red-alert status marked by delayed returns to prestress baseline levels. High life change scores, low coping-skill scores, and deficits in the use or availability of support systems can be easily related to patient theories of feeling overwhelmed and demoralized 6 months or one year ago, before the current symptoms started.

Question 4. What elevations and/or deficits in predisposing, triggering, and buffering factors does this patient demonstrate? The patient is

Factors That Will Attenuate
Relationship Between Stress And Symptoms

1. High Social Support
2. High Satisfaction With Social Support
3. High Coping Skills

Density Of

1) Major Life Changes --------> Mental or Physical Symptoms

or

2) Minor Hassles (Micro-stressors)

Factors That Will Potentiate
Relationship Between Stress And Symptoms

1. High or Low Hypnotic Ability
2. High Catastrophizing
3. High Neuroticism

Figure 21. The factors that moderate the relationship between stress and symptoms.

shown the profile and the five risk factors are presented as underlying risk factors but not necessarily causes of the symptoms. (See Figure 21.)

It should be pointed out that as the patient accumulates positive findings on one or more of the risk factors, the probability of mental or physical distress increases. Feedback can be prefaced with a statement like, let me now share with you the good news and the bad news. Feedback on the high-risk profile should always start with that risk factor that has the highest face validity for the patient and appears to be most clearly and directly relevant to the patient's distress. For example, if headaches are the presenting problem and particularly if the patient is low on either hypnotic ability or neuroticism, you will look for evidence of elevated baseline EMG, cold hands, or some other physiological indication of sustained red-alert or chronic fight or flight response. Persons low on hypnotic ability and/or neuroticism respond poorly to psychological interpretations of their physical symptoms or to the implication that they may participate (a self-criticism) in producing an illness. For most patients who are high on hypnotic ability psychological explanations will be acceptable, particularly soon after taking the Harvard Test. Their personal experience of their own response to test suggestions (e.g., amnesia, experience of loss of voluntary control of their own muscular responses, hallucinations, etc.) will reduce any lingering skepticism about the effects that psychological variables (cognitions, etc.) can have on physical symptoms and health. One should always end the feedback with a specification of what changes in the high-risk profile are expected at the end of therapy and with a discussion of the risk factor that is likely to have the least face validity for the patient but that can arouse curiosity. For example, the patient can be told that at the end of active therapy, the patient's hypnotic ability, support system, and coping-skill scores should be higher and the neuroticism, catastrophizing, and hassles scores should be lower. The patient should be told that the focus of therapy is first to put out the fire but that in terms of preventing relapse it is very important to find the matches. The patient is also asked if he or she would like to learn about those unattended and overlearned deep unconscious programs that have predisposed the patient to transduce psychosocial conflicts into somatic symptoms.

Eventually the clinical significance of elevations or deficits on all patient positive risk factors should be explained. For example, to the patient high on hypnotic ability it can be said, "You can be supersensitive to or markedly reduce internal and external sensory events to an extraordinary degree, when and if you choose to do so, for brief or extended periods of time." The patient low on hypnotic ability can be told, "You are not particularly aware of or likely to talk much about your inner feelings (anger, fears, sadness, etc.) and reactions. You tend to prefer objective, quantitative ways of looking at the world and you tend to be skeptical of fuzzy concepts, but once convinced of anything you tend to stubbornly hold to your beliefs."

The fourth set of questions the therapist should ask pertains to the common underlying psychophysiological mechanisms, the common triggers, and the common buffers of human mental and physical dysfunction and disease. It is at this level of analysis that psychosocial information becomes transduced by the brain into biological events. But there are nearly always in individual cases some unique psychological and physiological factors missed by the high-risk profile and related to previous overlearning, diet, environmental, and genetic differences that also need to be considered in diagnosis and therapy. These unique factors should be identified and assessed during the clinical interview, feedback, and therapy sessions because these factors can set the boundary conditions for growth and change. The primary common predisposing psychophysiological mechanisms of dysfunction and disease are (a) high- or low-hypnotic ability, (b) excessive sympathetic reactivity predisposing to neuroticism or negative affectivity (Watson & Clark, 1984; Watson & Tellegen, 1985), and (c) catastrophizing (Ellis, 1962). The first factor is mainly a central nervous system factor, the second an autonomic nervous system factor, and the third an interactional factor. High- or low-hypnotic ability *per se* does not necessarily guarantee mental or physical illness, in fact there is some evidence that measured hypnotic ability is negatively correlated with serious psychopathology (Spiegel, Detrick, & Frischolz, 1982). But when people who are located at either extreme of hypnotic ability, who lack coping skills, and who lose satisfaction with their support systems, are exposed to a high density of major life changes and/or minor hassles, they are more likely than people of moderate-hypnotic ability to develop mental or physical disorders, particularly if they are elevated on catastrophizing and neuroticism. In many, but not all ways, people at both extremes of hypnotic ability are more alike than those in the middle range of ability. This is a curious paradox that has to be observed clinically to be appreciated. For example, low-hypnotic ability may in fact be an active inhibition of the abilities abundantly present in the highs.

High-Hypnotic Ability

The high-hypnotic-ability patient can generate very rich fantasy almost to the point of hallucinatory intensity and inadvertently alter perceptions, memory, and mood in maladaptive ways. Acute alterations in these functions can become chronic through learning and reinforcement mechanisms. This capacity for fantasy, if focused maladaptively, can temporarily be either immobilizing or disruptive of ongoing everyday employment (e.g., public speaking phobia) and intimacy (e.g., premature ejaculation or secondary impotence) functions. This capacity to anticipate and remember pain and fear at excessive magnification levels can disrupt smooth motor and behavioral operations by clouding consciousness or generating physiological hyperarousal that may lead to stable neurochemical changes. These high-hypnotic-ability patients can anticipate and be exquisitely hypersensitive to physical or psychological traumas, such as pain or fear. They hurt earlier, deeper, more broadly, and if they are high on neuroticism (NA), for longer periods than other people. Once the high-hypnotic-ability person's fears or suspicions are mobilized, they tend to spiral outward, picking up increasingly remote associations that are only topographically similar, but are fed back along a final common pathway into the vortex of initial suspicion as irrefutable evidence of the initial fear or suspicion. They can learn bad health habits (e.g., substance abuse, interpersonal dependency, etc.) or superstitious contingencies too quickly, and if high on neuroticism (NA), remember them for too long a time. They can block from memory significant lessons or events that they may need to remember (e.g., life- or self-esteem-threatening traumas), to process, and to integrate into consciousness to protect themselves from future pain or to adapt to a new environment or situation. They can keep important secrets from themselves. In the case of the patient who is high on hypnotic ability, it may be useful to make sense out of the symptomatic distress by telling him the story of Alexander's horse, which is described on page 70. The patient needs to be alerted to the need to keep his "shadow" behind him, so that he is empowered by his talents and not crippled by them. In other words, the patient needs to learn to redirect creative energy and talents into art, science, recreation, work, or love. A simple, direct, sincere, and compassionate conversation (with or without a hypnotic induction) can be used as suggestions to enable the patient to access unconscious information. It is impossible to deal effectively with the patient of high-hypnotic ability without subscribing to a model of the psychological unconscious (Bowers, 1984; Shevrin & Dickman, 1980). Secrets like the following unconscious parental injunctions or nonverbal statements can potently influence behaviors: "You should never try to do anything you might fail at. You cannot do better than your brother, mother, or sister. You do not deserve to be happy. This is a just world and you should be treated justly." Such unconscious overlearned and unattended beliefs can potently regulate adult choices and the amount and duration of personal energy expenditures in areas of love, work, and play. Simple, direct, or indirect suggestions or rhetorical questions can be used with or without a hypnotic induction to help these patients identify unconscious thoughts and feelings that are associated with their symptoms. Suggestions can also be used to enable these high-hypnotic-ability patients to dream on preselected topics that may be pertinent to their conflict. These patients are often able to have profound experiences of abreaction in response to waking techniques in the consulting room like role playing or talking or writing to an absent but hallucinated significant other (dead or absent parent, boss, or spouse) with whom they have unfinished business. In the context of systematic desensitization, with each escape from cognitively rehearsing phobic material into relaxation the patient can be told to go deeper. This repeated confronting and escaping from the phobic material into relaxation can become a very potent and reliable deepening technique for some patients. High-hypnotic-ability patients also need carefully to recognize their prospensity to make broad generalizations and they need training in processing information with skeptical-critical discrimination and analytic-sequential style, a style that forces them to specify each step in their thinking and forces them critically to evaluate the evidence for each step.

Academic courses in logic and computer science are often useful to force these high-hypnotic-ability patients to recognize the implicit assumptions they make in their conceptual processes. These patients may need to practice careful problem definition, to specify the components in the remediation process, and to use a graduated approach to problem solving. A practical way of examining some of the covert or implicit assumptions underlying their behavior is to ask them to read for self-diagnosis, and to bring in for discussion, the book *I Can If I Want To* (Lazarus & Fay, 1975). Therapeutic suggestions given to people of high-hypnotic ability can be very effective if simply delivered in a conversational style that is marked by a sincere, compassionate manner. High-hypnotic-ability patients should be told of their powerful ability to block from awareness significant facts or to amplify internal or external sensory events. This ability can be inadvertently abused to produce anxiety, somatic, or phobic symptoms in themselves. These patients respond well to ego-strengthening suggestions. ("Your nerves will grow stronger and steadier each time you practice this exercise." "You may be surprised to notice how much faster you can recover from stressful stimulation since you started relaxation exercises." "You may notice that you are not as easily distressed, disappointed, angered or hurt as you used to be and that you bounce back from irritation faster.") The patient of high-hypnotic ability needs to practice critical, skeptical, and analytic thinking in everyday life. Courses in science and engineering foster critical-analytical types of information processing that reduce the tendency to generalize too soon from isolated instances to general classes of phenomena that may be topographically similar but are functionally different (e.g., things that look and sound alike may be very different in function and structure).

People who do not know their history, according to the philosopher, are doomed to repeat it. Patients of high-hypnotic ability should be confronted up front during the feedback session with their superior capacity for anticipation and fantasy, for the voluntary control of memory, of perception, of states of consciousness, and of mood. It should be pointed out that these assets can also be focused in ways and on things that can create problems for the patient or disrupt normal everyday functions. These potential dysfunctions of memory, mood, or perception need to be related to specific distressing aspects of the problem and/or symptoms the patient presents. For example, a patient with a Harvard score of 12, exposed to severe mental trauma (deaths and dismemberment of enemies and buddies) in Vietnam denied any mental distress (e.g., anxiety, guilt, depression) or character weakness (tears or fears) at the time in Vietnam, saying that he put these traumatic incidents out of his mind to do his job and to provide leadership to his men. But soon after he returned to the United States he developed multiple severe physical complaints of pain, motor function, and peculiar sensations for which he was treated with physical therapy, major narcotics, minor psychotropics, and eventually multiple exploratory surgeries. He eventually reached me, 14 years later, dependent on narcotics, psychotropics, and iatrogenically diseased. Therapy for him first consisted of confronting him with his superior hypnotic ability through suggestions temporarily to alter his perception (e.g., visual hallucinations), memory, and mood in the consulting room. Because he was not psychologically minded these subjectively compelling hypnotic experiences surprised him. The next step was to teach him how to mobilize this ability voluntarily for self-regulation of pain and mood. Hypnosis was also used to ventilate his burden of anger, guilt, and fear about Vietnam and to finish his unfinished business with hallucinated dead comrades.

A doctoral level aeronautical engineer with a Harvard score of 11 had recently experienced multiple personal hassles and several major life changes (moving, divorce, several rapid promotions to more hazardous and responsible jobs, etc.) in response to which he developed several chronic, phobic, and psychophysiological job-related complaints (phobias, headaches, respiratory and cardiovascular distress). These major life changes (e.g., promotions) had reduced his support systems and released a cascade of minor job-related hassles (hiring, firing, supervising, etc.). Therapy for him also consisted of recognizing and refocusing his hypnotic ability on self-regulation of perception and mood and systematic desensitization of his phobias.

A housewife with a Harvard score of 12 who made an average of two emergency room visits per month, presented with intermittent abdominal pain with swelling and chronic low back pain, secondary to a minor auto accident. The patient was dependent on numerous narcotics, minor psychotropics, and was polysurgically addicted (14 exploratory surgeries on stomach and abdomen) and seeking more surgeries. Unassimilated psychic experience, incorrectly interpreted previously as hallucinations (Stevenson, 1983) reliably triggered the pain, abdominal swelling, and emergency room visits. Accepting, exploring, and reframing these psychic events (out-of-the-body experiences) as mind–body integrative experiences and not psychosis was correlated with rapid remission of pain, discontinuing analgesics and emergency room visits, and remission of abdominal swelling for 8 years at follow-up. Previously, pain, emergency room visits, and abdominal swelling had occurred at least twice per month for 15 or more years, typically after a very vivid out-of-the-body experience. A 16-year-old female exposed to high-density serious life changes (parental divorce, loss of mother, loss of brother, relocation across country, new friends, changed school) was in a life-threatening automobile accident from which she escaped with only minor bruises, scratches, and shock. But within days she developed severe chronic neck, head, and shoulder pain that was resistant to all conventional medical therapy (analgesic drugs, hot and cold packs, traction, physical therapy, etc.) for over one-and-a-half years in the absence of any identifiable pathophysiology. Therapy focused on mobilizing her superior hypnotic ability to reduce muscle spasm, and to process and integrate the major unassimilated life changes. She needed to confront and repair her reduced self-esteem related to the recent loss of major support systems. She also needed to abreact the recent threat to her mortality during the accident and the associated, overlearned, but unattended mytonia elicited by the shock of the accident.

The patient's subjective personal experiences of hypnosis (sensations of floating, tingling, sinking, amnesia, etc.) during the Harvard Test, his response to test suggestions, and his experience of "involuntariness" will provide subjective confirmation of the therapist's statement of the unusual abilities the patient has to alter perception, mood, and memory. These subjective experiences should be recalled, recorded, and discussed because these sensations can be suggested to speed up and deepen future inductions. Further armed with the knowledge of the patient's high Harvard score the therapist can confidently "state" that the patient has had several unusual experiences or naturally occurring altered states of consciousness (ASC) that he previously has never or seldom shared. These unique compelling "secret" experiences that most people of high-hypnotic ability have had can then be elicited and may be tied to aspects of their present symptoms and Harvard score. The therapist's ability to post-dict the patients past "secret experiences" will impress the patient and boost the therapist's credibility or social reinforcer (Gewirtz & Baer, 1958) value to the patient.

Low-Hypnotic Ability

People of low-hypnotic ability are at risk because they are hyposensitive to their own feelings and have a profound capacity to deny or ignore emotional or even physical distress. Emotional imagery (Lang, 1979) has been shown to be a good predictor of positive psychotherapy outcome. It appears that people of low-hypnotic ability generate emotional imagery at very low frequency in everyday life. Biofeedback techniques are particularly helpful to such people because the machines amplify their dim awareness of emotional changes and physical sensations in objective and quantifiable ways. In the sense that the machine puts a low-hypnotic-ability person's "insides on the outside" (a meter, tone, TV screen, graph, etc.). This accurate, moment-to-moment, fedback, and amplified awareness of bodily sensations compensates for their hyposensitivity to internal events. The biofeedback loop amplifies the hookup between the cortical and subcortical (peripheral ANS events) centers. This enhanced awareness of internal emotional events can be developed further with assigned reading from books like *Why I Am Afraid to Tell You Who I Am* (Powell, 1969). Books like this can provide informational (rational) motivation for self-exploration and the verbal practice of vulnerability and risk taking that is crucial for successful psychotherapy. After each low-arousal trial (relaxation practice), which should start briefly (2 minutes) but gradually grow longer (15 minutes), the patient should be systematically questioned about spontaneous physical sensations, spontaneous feelings, and spontaneous images and intrusive thoughts that occurred during the relaxation episode. This can be systematically explored with the subjective-response inquiry (see Appendix G). The purpose of this exercise is to train the patient to focus and become curious about spontaneously occurring internal sensations, imagery, and emotional events. It also helps to develop a tolerance for fading "generalized reality orientation" (Shor, 1979). Low hypnotizables have a particularly inflexible grip on practical pedestrian reality and are reluctant to fantasize and daydream. These procedures will, in fact, at least temporarily increase their hypnotic ability and indirect or direct suggestions given to them during or immediately upon exiting the low-arousal state will have an enhanced probability of acceptance (Wickramasekera, 1977). In other words, they will be most receptive to new information or cognitive reframing intervention immediately upon exiting the relaxed state. Low hypnotizables profit from keeping temperature diaries or stress diaries to help them recognize the contingency between psychosocial stress (emotions like fear, anger, sadness, and rejection) and physiological changes or symptom onset (e.g., headaches, angina). Sensory restriction procedures (Suedfeld, 1980; Wickramasekera, 1977) can also be used to enhance the low-hypnotic-ability persons' awareness of emotional and physical changes.

The patient with low-hypnotic ability is nearly always locked into the critical, analytic-skeptical mode of information processing. Their basic asset and liability is their perceptual rigidity. Such patients are impressed only by objective quantitative, empirical data, graphs, curves, and hardware. St. Thomas is the prototype of the low hypnotizable who needed empirically to verify Christ's risen identity by placing his own fingers in the wounds and scars of the crucifixion. But once he was convinced, his faith, tradition tells us, carried him beyond the outermost edges of the Roman Empire across the world to India. St. Peter, a prototype of the high-hypnotic-ability person, acquired his faith on one trial learning, the fishing incident on the lake, but lost it as quickly when confronted by fear ("and the cock crowed twice"). Lows will dismiss psychological events (fear, anger, despair) unless they can be shown, not told, that they have biological consequences (e.g., headaches, chronic pain, and ulcers). They are like the pathologist who said, "I believe in nothing that I am told, and only half of what I can see." These people's beliefs are very resistant to change but once altered are very stable. Attempts to modify their beliefs require objective and quantitative packaging. For example, they may need to be shown how performance pressure (e.g., a mental arithmetic task) can constrict the blood vessels in their hands (drop hand temperature), or how anger can speed their heart rate or increase their blood pressure. They are skeptics who are persuaded only, but easily, by hardware or quantitative empirical packaging, particularly if the demonstration can be replicated. These patients need to develop an early warning system (attention to what they are subjectively feeling) that increases their awareness of the contingency between psychological states and physiological changes. Otherwise they transduce psychological responses (e.g., fear) into physiological responses (pain). Initially their learning to recognize, label, and discriminate subjective feelings may need to involve instruments that put their insides on the outside (on meters, digital printouts, etc.) where they can see or hear them. Biofeedback devices provide them with credible evidence of mind–body interaction. These patients need to practice risk taking in the sense of emotional vulnerability (sharing their positive and negative feelings) with significant others with concurrent physiological tracking to help them recognize the magnitude of cognitive emotional effects on physiology. They also need to practice cognitive and perceptual flexibility, or "acting as if." Role playing the behavior of another person can help them become more perceptually flexible and empathic. Scientific props like computer screens, graphs, physiographs, etc., can provide the cognitive incentives to mobilize these people's beliefs into behavioral role playing.

High Catastrophizing (Panicking) Cognitions

High catastrophizing (Ellis, 1962) is probably a learned response that is moderately correlated with neuroticism. It is probably learned through modeling (Bandura, 1969) from significant others (mother, father, or grandmother). These patients tend to make mountains out of molehills. It is important to show the patient the hypothalamic-pituitary-adrenal-axis and how catastrophizing cognitions can put and keep the sympathetic branch of the ANS on red-alert, increasing muscle tension, heart rate, blood pressure, peripheral vasoconstriction, etc. The

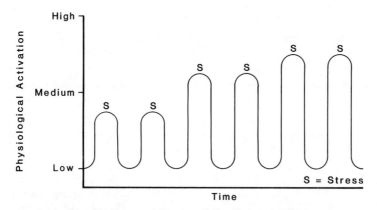

Figure 22a. Hypothetical normal pattern: no delay in return to baseline.

Netter (1962) plates can be helpful in this illustration. Habitual catastrophizing unnecessarily and intermittently activates the fight or flight
response, probably gradually elevating baseline muscle tension, and
perhaps in some people, cardiovascular responses like hypertension.
(See Figures 22a, 22b.)

Catastrophizing patients need to learn to substitute coping verbalizations for catastrophizing verbalizations. These people often scru-
tinize trivial and transitory events and appraise and cognitively react to
them almost reflexively as if they were intolerable and permanent life-
threatening predicaments marked by phobic, anxiety, or pain behaviors.
In many instances these events may be internal or external cues of which

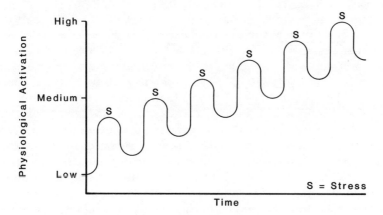

Figure 22b. Hypothetical abnormal pattern: acute stress becomes chronic pattern of bracing
caused by delay in return to baseline. Elevated baseline pattern above.

they are unaware (Mathews & MacLeod, 1986). These patients' perceptions of the present appear in those situations in which they are vulnerable (e.g., their health, their self-esteem) to be reliably locked into the anticipation of future escalating pain and tragedy. A patient who is elevated on this variable should first be helped to identify the specific self-statements the patient makes in specific stressful situations (e.g., "Nothing good ever happens to me. I am incompetent. Why is this happening to me?. I can't stand this. This is impossible to endure. I know I will fail. I know I have a brain tumor or cancer. This pain will increase each minute. This is horrible."). Keeping a diary of stressful events, making self-ratings of the intensity of these events (mild, moderate, severe), and attempting to identify the self-statements and internal or external cues that are associated with the catastrophizing response provides the patient with an opportunity for a more objective, analytic view of his or her own overlearned and unattended but counterproductive reactions to recurrent real life events. The most unique feature of the catastrophizer is the reliable propensity to retrieve from the future the worst possible outcomes or consequences. This self-fulfilling prophecy phenomenon is most potently and purely demonstrated in catastrophizing. Particularly in the instance of pain tolerance during medical or dental procedures. The self-monitoring exercise (e.g., keeping a diary) *per se* will produce a short-term decline in these catastrophizing self-statements and even some reduction in the intensity of the patient's clinical symptoms. But these results will be short-lived unless the patient replaces his reduced catastrophizing self-statements with a different preattentive bias occurring before awareness and a more proactive positive response set. The modification of this preattentive bias occurring outside of awareness may require special tools, such as dichotic listening or subliminal stimulation (Dixon, 1981; Forster & Govier, 1978; Shevrin & Dickman, 1980). The use of two tape recorders and the dichotic procedure can be quite effective in modifying the preconscious appraisals. One tape contains random numbers to be repeated concurrent with the subliminal listening to a therapeutic message on the other tape. The patient who habitually catastrophizes needs not only to reduce the frequency of negative self-statements but to increase the frequency of self-statements of calm acceptance. He needs to deeply accept the fact that in his life and everybody else's lives there is a daily inevitable quota of unwanted happenings. For example rejection, failure, disappointment, and injury are inevitable events in human life and relationships. Our only choice is (a) to choose how we will respond to these unwanted events and (b) to recognize which of these events can be avoided in the future and at what price.

First, the patient needs to recognize that reacting automatically with the negative self-statements only amplifies misery and reduces efficiency in coping with the stressful event. "There is no percentage in it." Second, the patient needs to find a quiet time and place to sort out which recurrent adverse events are inevitable and which are not. He needs deeply and fully to accept and calmly even forgive his maker (God) for those miseries that cannot be changed, and these are many. The clay pot needs to forgive the potter for imperfections in the potter's skills and the limitations of the materials the potter used. Those miseries that can be changed should be approached calmly and planfully, not by criticizing, punishing, or condemning the people or events involved as unfair, inferior, incompetent, or unlikeable but by encountering these people or events with calm, sincerity, compassion, and acceptance that models both kindness to self and others. It is important to recognize that many evils are never eradicated but are simply displaced by missionary zeal and that other evils are simply creative energies in need of positive redirection.

It is important for the patient to recognize that catastrophizing is a learned behavior, usually from observing the reactions of significant others or parents. It can be unlearned and replaced with an attitude of stoicism, often without loss of significant personal achievement and accomplishment.

Neuroticism (Negative Affectivity) and Excessive Sympathetic Reactivity

Patients elevated on the Neuroticism factor need to be told and shown (physiological data on strip charts, etc.) that they have inherited or overlearned a tendency early in life to overreact to threat. Their perceptions of the present and future are excessively filtered through memories of past anxiety or pain. They are locked into their past by limiting memories of pain and hurt. Nevertheless, they need to risk themselves in the present because in the final analysis, life is lived forward and understood backward. Their self-limiting beliefs and anticipations can imprison them in their past. High neuroticism is most effectively reduced, probably only temporarily, by a combination of cognitive and psychophysiological exercises. The patient can profit from identifying his irrational (Ellis, 1962) beliefs (I should not fail; The world should be just and fair, etc.) and actively attempting to challenge these beliefs cognitively and behaviorally. Reading and daily using a book like *I Can If I Want To* by Lazarus and Faye (1975) can facilitate identifying, challenging, and altering irrational beliefs. Just as the latter process is necessary for the high catastrophizer, it is equally necessary for the patient elevated on neuroticism. There is a need to calmly recognize and to deeply, philosophically accept the fact that in everybody's life there will every day be a quota of unwanted happenings (e.g., rejection, failure, or disappointment). It is also important to recognize that often evil or misery is not eradicated but rather it is only displaced (all solutions inevitably produce new problems) and that every distress that we feel (phobia, jealousy, rejection, sadness, anxiety attack, etc.) passes with time. We can grow stronger by facing horrors, if we can look at them as opportunities or challenges to surmount our current limitations. Also, daily practice of low-arousal procedures (biofeedback, muscular relaxation, autogenic training, self-hypnosis, etc.) will reduce chronic subjective distress and/or negative affectivity even when there are no symptomatic changes (Blanchard *et al.*, 1986; Sovak, Kunzel, Sternbach, & Delassio, 1981). For the management of particularly distressing specific situations or beliefs, specific procedures like desensitization, response prevention, and flooding can be quite helpful. These patients need to learn psychophysiological stress-reduction skills (low arousal or relaxation induction) now, and use them periodically for the rest of their lives. Elevations on neuroticism or negative affectivity identify people who react too strongly and for too long to threats or unwanted happenings. Psychologically, they tend to be selectively hyperattentive to past aversive memories. They tend to ruminate on their past faults, failures, and hurts. These people need actively to work at altering their negative memory patterns and aversive cognitive rehearsals. Usually distraction (McCaul & Malott, 1984) in work or play is the most effective short-run technique to disrupt their trains of aversive thoughts (e.g., guilt, shame, fear, pain, sadness). Psychophysiologic conditioning procedures like relaxation training, biofeedback, systematic desensitization, flooding, and so forth, and/or drugs are an essential and necessary component in the therapy of patients who are elevated on this variable. After the elevations are reduced by psychophysiological stress-management skills or drugs, there is a need periodically (twice per week) to monitor and use the procedure because baseline reactivity appears to return slowly to pretherapy levels unless actively opposed by the regular practice of psychophysiological skills. For these patients long-term (5-year) follow-ups at periodic intervals (3 months) are critical to prevent episodic symptomatic relapses from becoming chronic histories.

Initially this variable should be presented to the patient as a learned or inherited physiological response tendency (Collins, Cohen, Naliboff, & Schandler, 1982; Flor, Turk, & Birbaumer, 1985; Krantz & Manuck, 1984; Philips, 1977). It can be illustrated by either high and sustained or variable and slow recovery of frontalis muscle tension, skin conductance, heart rate, systolic and diastolic blood pressure, or low peripheral skin temperature. The patient should be told that he has the kind of autonomic nervous system (sympathetic) that responds too quickly with the fight or flight (red-alert) response and delays in returning to normal alert even after the stressor has passed. When something negative happens, the patient is reminded, the patient very often has difficulty blocking the aversive event from his mind. The patient tends to ruminate on negative memories. This delay in returning to the prestress baseline is what makes the patient dysfunctional. The patient goes on red-alert too easily and stays up there too long, even after the threat of danger has passed. This feature can be credibly demonstrated by showing the patient the physiological response latency, magnitude, and/or delay in returning to baseline (prestimulation level of response of his most reactive organ system or "window of vulnerability") after stressful stimulation. The patient is told that therapy for this component requires checking and ensuring through regular practice (of psychophysiological stress management skill) that this window of vulnerability remains closed, particularly when entering stressful situations. Often there is a marked discrepancy between paper-and-pencil measures of this variable (neuroticism scores) and the data from the psychophysiological profile. There are some patients who look visibly calm and relaxed on the surface, and even on a self-report measure like the Eysenck Neuroticism Scale are like a "swan on a lake." But the psychophysiological profile reveals that they are kicking or agitated like hell "underneath" or inside.

Showing the patient the actual raw data (e.g., like a strip chart recording) from the psychophysiological stress profile can be very effective in confirming the patient's belief in the validity of the elevation on this factor. Also, demonstrating the discrepancy between the patient's blind SUDs rating and the actual fontalis EMG measure can be like starting a catheter directly into the patient's mind (belief system). The procedure potently bypasses the defenses of skepticism and denial. With high-hypnotic-ability patients it has to be used cautiously because it may, in fact, intensify their symptoms.

A patient with an elevated N score is very likely to have a variety of physical complaints in the absence of documented pathophysiology. This may be important to know if one is running an HMO. The patient is told that certain psychophysiological skills (e.g., muscle relaxation training, autogenic training, self-hypnosis, biofeedback) can temporarily reduce the baseline level of arousal and/or the tendency to delay in recovering from stressful events, but that preventative maintenance of the skill is essential, because the patient may have a natural biological tendency to elevated baselines in various vulnerable organ systems. Hence, regularly scheduled monitoring of baselines (in the patient's specific window or windows of vulnerability (e.g., EMG, blood pressure) and preventative doses of physiological skill practice is necessary on at least a biweekly basis for at least 5 years. This is essential to prevent acute episodes from becoming a chronic relapse. Hence, at the very start of therapy (during assessment and feedback), or during "the honeymoon," the patient is introduced to the requirement of long-term 5-year follow-up on at least a monthly basis. Later, a once-in-3-to-6 months follow-up can prevent relapses and protect his own financial investment in the initial cost of therapy. Keeping several patients in this holding pattern for at least 5 years is not only good for science (to verify efficacy of therapy techniques and spontaneous remission rates with long-term follow-up) but it also makes good business sense (protects patients' initial investment in therapy, provides a means of filling in gaps in the therapist's schedule because of cancellations or during dry episodes). Patients in the holding pattern can descend periodically for reexamination of their stress management skills and monitoring of their physiological baselines. What is good for science in the long run may turn out also to be good for business.

Major Life Changes

Retrospective and prospective studies have shown a modest correlation (rarely over .30) between increasing life change and the onset of sudden cardiac death, myocardial infarctions, accidents, athletic injuries, leukemia, diabetes, tuberculosis, and several minor medical complaints (Depue & Monroe, 1986; Rabkin & Struening, 1976). This indicates that major life changes *per se* account for seldom more than 9% of the variance in symptomatology. It is stated that when the Life Change Units (LCU) exceed 300, the probability of illness within 3 to 6 months of accumulating this (LCU) approximates 80% (Petrich & Holmes, 1977). It appears that the features of life change that are most crucial for illness onset are (a) undesirability, (b) magnitude, (c) time clustering, and (d) uncontrollability (Thoits, 1983). (See Figure 23.)

The patient who is positive for major life change should be shown the profile and LCU score. Patients intuitively recognize that increasing life change may demand increases in the amount and rate of psychological and physiological energy required to adapt to change. Patients easily recognize that negative changes particularly (death, divorce, financial loss, getting fired from a job, etc.) are likely to trigger stress reactions. Patients who have a high life change score (over 500) should be encouraged to talk about their feelings about these changes and how they impacted everyday life and function at the time. This exercise will frequently trigger several "insights" into their present situation and how much in control or out of control of their life they feel today and how much control they felt in the past. The patient should be encouraged to place their life changes in a broader philosophical perspective of psychological growth (Maslow, 1954) and/or religious faith. For example, many such interpretations are illustrated by the book, *When Bad Things Happen To Good People* (Kushner, 1981). Many of these major life changes, if anticipated, can be planned and prepared for psychologically and materially (e.g., insurance, saving, new coping skills, and systematic desensitization and education). Hence, these physical or psychological traumas or changes can be negotiated with a sense of control that can significantly reduce the physical and psychological pain of their impact (Thompson, 1981). Also it may be important for some people to psychologically process (talk about) and to assimilate these changes to provide enough time to permit the dust to settle and to know that this pain or hurt also will pass. Or to reframe the change in the manner of Anna Eleanor Roosevelt when she said, "You gain strength, courage and confidence by every experience in which you really stop to look fear in the face. You are able to say to yourself, 'I lived through this horror. I can

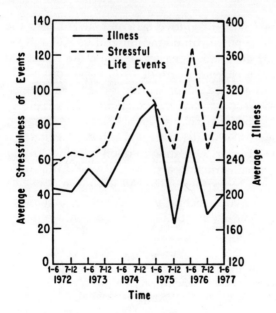

Figure 23. Stressful life events and illnesses over time. Reprinted from Kobasa *et al.*, 1982.

take the next thing that comes along. . . .' You must do the thing you think you cannot do" (Roosevelt, 1960). In those cases where the patient is in a position to control the number of his life changes (e.g., accepting a new job, having a child, returning to school when the nest empties, moving), it may be wise to spread the changes over a wider period of time (2 years rather than 6 months) by graduating the rate of change. Generally it is important for the patient to be able to see change as an opportunity or challenge to grow rather than as a burden to be endured like a victim. Obstructions need to be seen not as obstacles but as stepping stones. In the final analysis a religious faith that is subjectively credible but that need not be subject to any determination of objective truth can be the best buffer of major life stress. Sir Walter Raleigh, when confronted with death, wrote:

> Even such is Time, which takes in trust
> Our youth, and joys, and all we have;
> And pays us but with age and dust,
> Which in the dark and silent grave,
> When we have wandered all our ways,
> Shuts up the story of our days:
> And from which earth and grave and dust
> The Lord shall raise me up, I trust.
>
> —Sir Walter Raleigh
> Found in his Bible after his execution

A religious faith (cognitive schema) that makes the "slings and arrows of outrageous fortune" meaningful or redemptive makes *assimilation* of major life changes easier. When a life disaster (birth of a deformed child or accidental death of a young person) makes it difficult to sustain faith in a just God or world, a cognitive schema that regards "God" as imperfect or as having only limited power in the universe and regarding ourselves as picking up his slack, by doing his unfinished work with our own hands, feet, and minds, facilitates the process of assimilating a disaster. Our unique nobility comes from our voluntary participation in constructing a more just world than the one we were born into. It can be further enhanced if we see ourselves as forgiving Him ("God") for constructing us of imperfect materials but giving us tasks that surmount our abilities. The eleventh-century Persian poet Omar Khayyám says,

> Oh Thou, who man of baser Earth didst make.
> And ev'n with Paradise devise the Snake:
> For all the Sin wherewith the face of Man
> Is blacken'd—*Man's* Forgiveness give—and take.

Subjectively credible articles of faith that are stated in the form of paradoxes are particularly resistant to disconfirmation by empirical experience. For example, statements like, "Unless you lose your life you shall not find it." "You have to take one step back to take two steps forward." "You have to let go to hold on." These types of universal cognitive schema framed as paradoxes can facilitate the assimilation of aversive life changes that if left psychophysiologically undigested can generate physical and mental symptoms. For subjects of high-hypnotic ability, packaging the schema in attractive visual, auditory, and/or tactile kinesthetic images alone is often enough to ensure psychophysiological assimilation. For people of low- or moderate-hypnotic ability, low-arousal training (Wickramasekera, 1971, 1973, 1977) and cognitive rehearsal of the trauma in the low-arousal state can facilitate psychophysiological assimilation. After the previously cited type of desensitization, the low- or moderate-hypnotic-ability patient is more likely to discuss the incident in counseling with emotional involvement and insight about its present consequences.

Hassles

Hassles have been defined as irritating, frustrating, distressing demands and troubled relationships that plague us day in and day out (Lazarus, DeLongis, Folkman, & Given, 1985). Examples of hassles are traffic jams, delays, not getting enough sleep, disagreements, unpleasant surprises, and losing a wallet. These are seen as microstressors that are more malignant because unlike major life change events they occur much more frequently (Depue & Monroe, 1986). In a sense they are the chronic small events that occur daily, weekly, and monthly. "It is not the mountain in front of you but the grain of sand in your shoe" that can make you dysfunctional. It is likely that some major life changes trigger a cascade of chronic minor role related strains, for example, the birth of a child who is sickly initiates multiple visits to the doctor, marital conflicts, medical expenses, and sleepless nights. The death of a spouse may force a widow to assume total responsibility for the housework, child care, laundry, cooking, and so forth, in addition to a full-time job.

In fact, hassles and other chronic microstressors appear to be more strongly related to the onset of mental and physical disorders than major life change (Kessler, Price, & Wortman, 1985). The effect of microstressors appears to be predictive even after the effects of major life changes on health has been statistically removed (DeLongis, Coyne, Dakof, Folkman, & Lazarus, 1982, Lazarus et al., 1985, Zarski, 1984). Major life changes may trigger a ripple effect, causing multiple chronic minor hassles that persist long after the major life change is over. On methodological grounds, Dohrenwend and Shrout (1985) claimed that the reason hassles correlate so well with symptoms is because of the confounding of psychological symptoms (hassles) with other mental symptoms. Nothing correlates with symptoms like other symptoms. Patients who show elevations on the number or intensity of hassles need to be helped to sort out if these hassles are related to specific roles (e.g., work, father, husband, wife) or if they are unrelated events (auto repairs, traffic jams) that are distressing. Because of the frequency and duration of these microstressors no single simple sweeping solution can be found. Often any single solution produces a new set of microstressors. A divorce may be a solution to minor chronic marital conflicts, but it can create a new set of financial, social, household, child-care problems. It appears that a cultivated attitude of intellectual curiosity but general emotional detachment is the best strategy to deal with the microstressors. The Q.R. technique developed by Charles Stroebel (1982) appears to be the best current single technique with which to handle these microstressors.

Support Systems

Social support, either through direct protective effects or by buffering the negative consequences of major life changes or minor hassles, reduces the probability of physical or psychological symptoms. The evidence for this hypothesis ranges from animal laboratory studies to large-scale epidemiologic studies of mental and physical disease (Depue & Monroe, 1986). But the mechanisms of the protective or buffering effect are unknown and the methodology of measurement of effects has defects (DuPue & Monroe, 1986). Important practical dimensions of social support include (a) living arrangements (alone or with others), (b) frequency of social contact, (c) participation or use of social support, and (d) satisfaction.

Social support in a practical sense refers to functions performed for a distressed person by significant others such as family members, friends, co-workers, relatives, or neighbors. These functions include (a) instrumental aid (e.g., a ride to work, use of an auto, a loan), (b) socioemotional aid (e.g., statements or demonstrations of caring, validation of self-worth or beliefs, respect, empathy, ventilation or nonjudgmental listening, and group belonging), and (c) informational aid (shared opinions or facts relevant to current stressors, etc.) (Thoits, 1986).

The data from Nuckolls, Cassell, and Kaplan (1972) (see Figure 24) clearly demonstrate the relationship between life change before and during pregnancy, support systems (TAPPS), and physical complications in pregnancy. When the amount of life change is high before and during pregnancy but support systems are high the rate of complica-

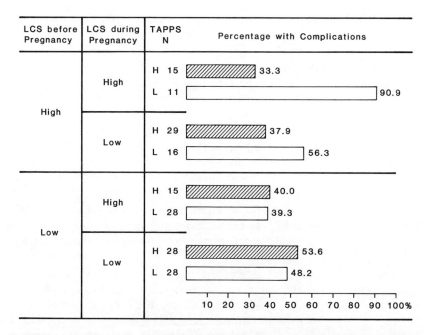

LCS before Pregnancy	LCS during Pregnancy	TAPPS N	Percentage with Complications
High	High	H 15	33.3
		L 11	90.9
	Low	H 29	37.9
		L 16	56.3
Low	High	H 15	40.0
		L 28	39.3
	Low	H 28	53.6
		L 28	48.2

Figure 24. Comparison of percentage of patients with complications by high and low TAPPS (Support System) scores, life change scores controlled. High—boxes with diagonal lines; low—clear boxes. Definition of complications: (1) blood pressure elevation during pregnancy or during both labor and postpartum period—(a) systolic blood pressure of over 139mm, or (b) systolic elevation of over 30mm, or (c) diastolic blood pressure of over 89mm; (2) proteinuria in combination with any of these blood pressure elevations; (3) preeclampsia; (4) hyperemesis; (5) premature membrane rupture in the absence of cephalo-pelvic disproportion; (6) prolonged labor in the absence of cephalo-pelvic disproportion; (7) apgar rating of infant of less than 7; (8) birthweight of less than 2500 grams; (9) spontaneous abortion, stillbirth or neonatal death within first 3 days. From "Psychological Assists, Life Crisis, and the Prognosis of Pregnancy" by K. B. Nuckolls, J. Casell, & B. H. Kaplan, *American Journal of Epidemiology*, 1972, *95*, 431–441. Reprinted by permission.

tions is only 33.3%. But when the level of support systems (TAPPS) is low for the same data the rate of complications is 90%.

If a patient's high-risk profile shows that the patient is deficient in either number of social support persons or his degree of perceived satisfaction with available support persons, specific vulnerabilities have been identified for which fairly specific remedies are available. First, the vulnerability identified is very likely to have high face validity or to match dimly or clearly the patient's perception of his or her own phenomenological view of his or her life situation. It takes little abstract or inferential reasoning for patients to make this self-diagnosis. "You have many friends but you are very much alone" (if there are many support persons but if levels of satisfaction with them is low), or if the profile indicates few or no support persons ("You are very much alone, and I wonder why this is true").

If there are no support persons this may result generally from inter-personal inhibitions on the part of the patient (guilt, shame, fear of rejection, social discomfort, etc.) or from an actual lack of social and assertive skills and information. In rare instances the loneliness is chosen and is a positive philosophical asset (e.g., for a monk). Assertive skills include the (a) ability to say no; (b) the ability to ask for favors or to make requests; (c) the ability to express positive (loving, gentle) and negative feelings (irritation, frustration); and (d) the ability to initiate, continue, and terminate general conversations (Lazarus, 1976). These social skills have to be taught and practiced verbally and nonverbally (Serber, 1976) if they are likely to be used in the patient's natural habitat. Role playing with video feedback is an excellent tool to expand the social repertoire.

Specific interpersonal inhibitions may be caused by specific cog-nitive-emotional beliefs that can be remediated by specific cognitive and behavioral exercises described very concisely and accurately by Lazarus and Fay (1975). This excellent little paperback book should be prescribed for patients with common maladaptive belief systems. The patient should be asked to read the book for self-diagnosis of irrational beliefs and next should be assigned behavioral activities to challenge these beliefs. There may be deficits in specific kinds of self-exploratory and self-disclosure skills the patient may need to learn and practice under therapist supervision and with therapist support. More specifically, the patient may need to practice vulnerability or social risk taking, first in the safety of the therapeutic relationship and later in his own school, work, or home environments. Powell's excellent book (1969) can prompt, motivate, and help guide this critical process even outside the consulting room. Strong and chronic negative emotions (strong auto-nomic arousal), like guilt, shame, performance pressure, and fear of failure or rejection may be blocking or disrupting the initiation and practice of socially important behaviors (e.g., public speaking anxiety, erectile dysfunction, premature or retarded ejaculation, lack of orgasm, vulnerable expressions, apologies, tender loving expressions), verbal behaviors, expressions of anger, and the like. These emotional inhibi-tions once identified by patient and therapist working as co-investiga-tors can be remediated by specific behavioral techniques like systematic desensitization, flooding, assertive training, EMG biofeedback, role playing, sex therapy, or hypnotherapy (Wickramasekera, 1976).

Powerful social support can be delivered by a psychotherapist who has high credibility in the patient's eyes for the patient's specific problems. A good psychotherapist is essentially a flexible support system. Social support can also be delivered credibly by a person or persons who are socially similar, seem relatively more expert than the patient, or who are calmly confronting or have confronted similar stressors. The aid from therapist or lay person can either directly alter threatening aspects of the situation (e.g., provide relevant and accurate information, a skill, a loan, a place to sleep and eat, or facilitate self-diagnosis) or buffer the impact of the stressor through emotional support (ventilation, abreaction, etc.).

Coping Skills

As Freud remarked, there are two areas of life, work and love, in which successful coping is critical to good mental and physical health. A third area, aging gracefully, is particularly significant for a society composed of a growing number of old people. The phenomena of widening and increasing loss is an inevitable consequence of simply growing old. To live long enough is to lose everything—profession, status, possessions, property, friends, family, strength, health, taste, teeth, and sight.

Coping can be defined as cognitive and behavioral responses made to master, tolerate, or reduce demands that strain or exceed a person's resources (Kessler et al., 1985). Some investigators state that there is cross-situational consistency (Pearlin & Schooler, 1978; Stone & Neale, 1985) in how people cope but others (Folkman & Lazarus, 1984) have disputed this. Some investigators state that people are aware and can report accurately on how they cope whereas others have questioned this (Kessler et al., 1985). It appears that coping works through three mechanisms: (a) altering the problem directly, (b) changing one's way of looking at the problem, and, (c) reducing the emotional distress provoked by the problem. It appears that the more varied an individual's coping repertoire the more protected that person is from future distress and that certain coping techniques may, in fact, be symptoms of illness or disorder (e.g., food or alcohol abuse) or associated with greater role stress (Menaghan, 1983). There is also evidence that unsuccessful coping can result in more negative consequences ("initiate a malignant spiral") than for those who do not even try to cope (Kessler et al., 1985).

Many of our concepts and procedures in the domain of coping are based on the investigation of weaklings or pathological role models. The illustrious American novelist, William Faulkner, on the occasion of his acceptance of the Nobel Prize in Literature (1949) stated: "I believe that man will not merely endure: he will prevail." It is unfortunate that our psychological models of coping are based on the observation of people whose functioning was marginal or impaired.

A positive coping skill approach should be based on the recognition that people can not only merely endure stressful events, but can transcend them, if they learn and overlearn (mastery) certain cognitive-emotional attitudes (cognitive and perceptual flexibility, compassion, stoicism, etc.) and low-arousal (relaxation) or high-arousal (ritual or cultural dancing) psychophysiological skills.

Kobassa, Maddi, and Kahn (1982) have identified three measurable psychological dispositions that compose a trait called hardiness that seems to be cross-situationally stable. The Kobassa *et al.* (1982) model more nearly approximates a model of transcendent coping skill. The subcomponents in hardiness include (a) commitment, (b) control, and (c) challenge. *Commitment* means a tendency to actively involve oneself in (rather than detach from) whatever one is doing or encountering. This may mean that if anything is worth doing it is worth doing to the best of one's ability. Or perhaps that it is better to be a lusty sinner than a sickly saint or paradoxically that it is better to do evil than to do nothing. "Committed persons have a generalized sense of purpose that enables them to identify with and find meaningful the events, things, and persons in their environment" (Kobasa *et al.*, 1982, p. 169). Commitment is particularly important in the areas of love and work.

"*Control* disposition is expressed as a tendency to feel and act as if one is influential (rather than helpless) in the face of the varied contingencies of life" (p. 169). This implies a perception of oneself as having a definite influence through the exercise of imagination, knowledge, skill, and choice.

"The *challenge* disposition is expressed as the belief that change rather than stability is normal in life and that the anticipation of changes are interesting incentives to growth rather than threats to security. Challenge mitigates the stressfulness of events on the perceptual side by coloring events as stimulating rather than threatening" (p. 170).

It is very likely that commitment, control, and challenge are most efficiently taught through role models or assigned readings or observations in literature and poetry. Hardiness can also be taught through the inspirational viewing of plays and films or the investigation of historical figures who illustrate courage and commitment in little and great things in the face of adversity. These assignments then need psychotherapeutic processing in terms of the patient's own values, ideals, methods, fears, inhibitions, and capacity for perceptual flexibility and risk taking. We currently measure baseline coping skills with the Learned Resourcefulness Scale (LRS) (Rosenbaum, 1980). Coping skills are defined as "a compendium of skills by which an individual controls the interfering effects that certain internal events (such as emotion, pain, or undesired thoughts) have on the smooth execution of a desired behavior" (Rosenbaum, 1985, p. 300).   The components the scale assesses are (a) the use of cognitions and self-instructions to cope with emotional and physiological response, (b) the application of problem-solving strategies (e.g., planning, problem definition, evaluating alternatives, and anticipation of consequences), (c) the ability to delay gratification, and (d) a general belief in one's ability to self-regulate internal events. The 36 items on the LRS depict specific behavior in specific interactions. But the instructions are described in general ways to make them applicable to a wide range of individuals. Hence, the therapist can determine in which of the four general areas of learned resourcefulness this particular patient's coping deficits exist. Discussion of a patient's profile and a remediation plan can be outlined and field tested.

Therapy Planning

Some temporary remission of clinical symptoms begins when the patient is given an appointment and assumes patienthood. This happens because significant others start to treat the patient differently (better) when he or she assumes the patient role. The patient may be regarded as not responsible for the symptoms, which reduces the general pressure on the patient and one may temporarily start to feel better in spite of one's symptoms. The patient may be exempted from normal tasks, chores, and obligations because he or she is "sick." Significant others do not want bad reports of their behavior carried to the therapist so they may temporarily start to treat the patient more kindly because he is "sick." This honeymoon continues during the diagnostic, assessment, and feedback phases. The patient may begin to feel better, is less demoralized, and even enthusiastic and ready to commit to therapy.

During this honeymoon phase it is critical to predict how painful and at times how discouraging and long therapeutic work will seem to be. This is the time to predict that episodic symptomatic relapses and regressions are inevitable milestones on the road to recovery. So that when the inevitable relapses occur the patient can recognize them as passing milestones on the road to recovery rather than looking at them as evidence of therapeutic failure. It is crucial during this honeymoon phase to structure the patient's attitude in regard to future disappointments and relapse as the natural byproducts of genuine therapeutic movement. Because psychophysiological therapy is a complex learning process of skill acquisition, it is useful to illustrate the course of therapy by showing the patient a graph of the normal individual human learning curve. (See Figure 25.)

It is important to point out the phenomenon of trial-and-error learn-

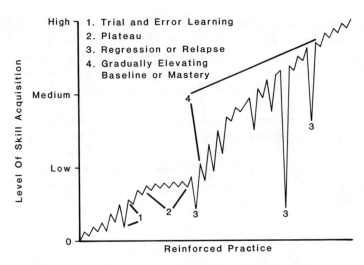

Figure 25. Changes in level of skill with reinforced practice.

ing, plateaus, of relapses and regression, and of a gradual but cumulative elevation in the baseline of mastery that occurs when complex skills have become overlearned and are emitted almost automatically under the right social and environmental conditions (SDs). The general goals of therapy are to reduce the patient's risk for illness by altering the patient's position on as many of the five risk factors on which he or she is positive. The following case studies will illustrate the approach.

Case Study of a Low-Hypnotic-Ability Patient

Figure 26 (p. 219) is the profile of a 41-year-old white married female, living in a small midwestern town, who presents with a 16-year history of severe chronic bilateral headaches that in the last 2 years have become intolerable, continuous, and varying only in intensity. She has no prodrome but she has severe nausea and vomiting when the intensity increases. There is a positive family history but the headache appears to be a mixed muscular-vascular chronic headache. The patient has seen multiple physicians for her head pain, including several neurologists, ear, nose, and throat specialists, and internists. The referring neurologist reports that she has been tried on a variety of medications over the last 16 years, none of which have resulted in adequate control of her headaches. She has also been hospitalized several times for the control and investigation of her head pain, but neurological tests, including CAT scans, are negative. For the same period, the patient has

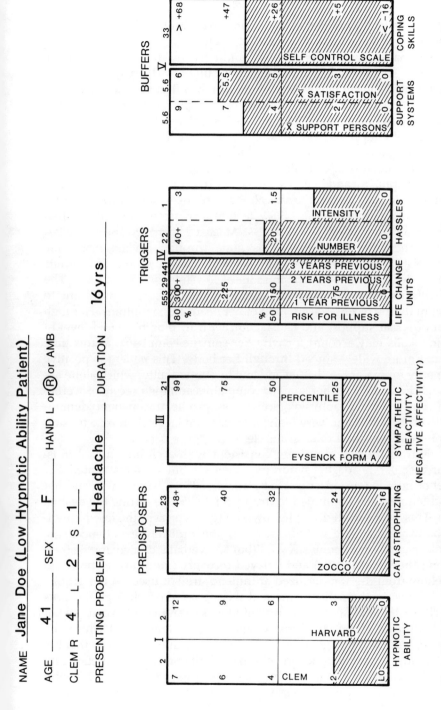

Figure 26. Patient profile for high-risk model (Wickramasekera 1979) Jane Doe (low-hypnotic-ability patient). I = Bakan (1969), Harvard Group Scale; II = Zocco (1984); III = Eysenck (1968), Sympathetic Reactivity Profile, (Wickram, 1976); IV = Holmes (1981); V = Sarason et al. (1583), Rosenbaum (1980).

also had several episodes of abdominal pain and multiple abdominal surgeries (oopherectomy, hysterectomy, etc.).

The patient was quite skeptical and even negativistic in the initial interview. Her level of hypnotic ability is quite low (Harvard 2) and this is confirmed by the fact that the bulk of her reflective eye movements (See Appendix C for CLEM Test) are to the right. This type of patient is very likely to transduce psychosocial stress into somatic symptoms and tends to be critical and skeptical in her approach to new information. Her long history of therapeutic failure appears to have further eroded her faith in doctors and reinforced her skepticism. Her very low scores on catastrophizing and negative affectivity (neuroticism) suggests that at least consciously she is quite stoical, is not prone to self-criticism, and is not psychologically minded. Such factors increase the probability that she will somatize psychosocial stress. At least 3 years ago and in the last year particularly, the patient has gone through several major life changes as indicated by very high major life change scores. She admits to a moderate level of microstressors of low intensity in her life. The high life change score and low-hypnotic-ability score is sufficient to account for the recent exacerbation of her headache symptoms. Her high level of social support and satisfaction with it, plus her good level of coping skills may account for why her somatic complaints at this time are not more widely spread through her body. This patient is positive primarily for major life change and low hypnotic ability, which alone are enough to account for her somatic complaints and their recent exacerbation. On the psychophysiological stress profile this patient demonstrated cold hands and very high and sustained levels of muscle tension monitored from the frontalis muscle. (See Figure 27.)

Both of these findings are consistent with a chronic mixed muscular-vascular headache syndrome. This patient underestimated her level of muscle tension or stress by almost 50% of what it was and her hand temperature continued to drop (78°F to 75.2°F) during the evaluation. This hyposensitivity to her own body is typical of the low-hypnotic-ability person. It also indicates that she probably experienced the whole evaluation as quite stressful (but she verbally denied any distress during the stress profile) and delayed recovery (no return to prestress baseline) from the standardized arithmetic stressor used on the profile.

Because of the patient's marked skepticism of psychological factors the clearest point of entry into her mind was to show and explain to her her high level of objective physiological muscle tension (of which she was unaware and that genuinely surprised her) and to point out that her cold hands, probably indicating chronic peripheral vasoconstriction and a chronic red-alert status of which she was unaware. These EMG and temperature data were impressive and credible to the patient. Her high

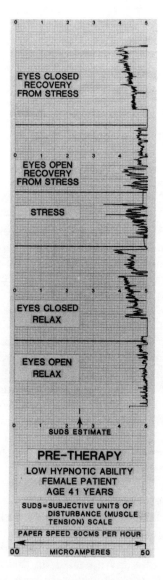

Figure 27. Pretherapy low-hypnotic ability (female patient, age 41 years).

score on major life change was used to help her to recognize that she had, in fact, been going through multiple psychosocial adjustments that could be stressful (e.g., new job as a minister in a church in which she was the only unordained female minister). Even this patient was able to recognize that these major life changes (moving, new jobs, etc.) were stressful. Her low-hypnotic ability was framed as a skepticism that was probably partly an outcome of all her previous therapeutic disappointments, and I told her that this skepticism would eventually make any new biofeedback learning slower and more difficult for her. She was told that unfortunately her burden of skepticism would render her unable to approach new learning like a child with innocence and faith. It was her fate to make this therapy harder and slower for herself. This framing was challenging for the patient and she asked to be taught self-hypnosis and biofeedback immediately so that she might prove me wrong by learning faster than other patients and with an open mind. I told her I would reluctantly accept her as a patient but that she should be prepared for a long and slow psychophysiological skill-learning process. The patient was taught the 1-2-3 self-hypnosis exercise and told to practice 10 times per day every 2 hours for 3 minutes to bring down her baseline muscle tension. During the demonstration and teaching of the 1-2-3, she was monitored on the frontal EMG and shown how the self-hypnosis did in fact drop her frontal EMG from 30 UVp-p to 11.5 UVp-p, and increased her hand temperature from 71°F to 72.9°F. The patient was also asked to keep on her person at all times a stress diary in which she was to record (at the scene of the "crime") all irritations, frustrations, disappointments, and hurts that occurred during her day and to place a rating of mild, moderate, or severe next to each. She was also made a muscle relaxation tape and told to practice for 30 minutes twice per day. She was told to record all her headache activity during waking hours for frequency and intensity. It was predicted that after several sessions of therapy the first changes she would notice would not be in her duration of headache pain but in the intensity of her headache pain. After the patient had acquired some skill at physiological relaxation and was frequently reporting subjective sensations of tingling, heaviness, and numbness during relaxation, she was helped to recognize the contingency between changes in her level of headache activity and changes in the intensity of psychosocial stressors recorded in her stress diary. When her stress diary showed that most of her symptoms and changes in skin temperature were job related she began to admit that she was very much afraid of making any mistakes on this job (God's work as a minister to others) and that she felt very indispensable and vulnerable on the job. She stated that as the only woman she felt a need to be perfect or a superwoman. I pointed out that even Superman had a need to become a vulnerable bumbling Clark Kent. The strain of constant perfection was too heavy a burden for any single person to carry constantly. As she began to talk with tears about her psychological states of fear, doubt, uncertainty, and vulnerability, her headache pain started to fade. This change in perception of her work would not only alter her physiological response to stress but would also alter her perception and manner of coping with other psychosocial stressors. Discussion, ventilation, confiding, and assertion could be alternatives to somatization. As this patient started to recognize the contingency between her headache pain and her psychosocial stressors (perfectionism, indispensability, invulnerability), her physical complaints generally reduced and she started to talk about her fears, doubts, and her guilt related to work and home. She is now coming out of the somatic closet and presenting her distress psychologically rather than somatically. Her headaches have improved over 80% and she is becoming a psychotherapy candidate. During her last self-hypnosis EMG biofeedback session in my office she reported an unsuggested, unexpected, and spontaneous visual image of "a little girl with blond hair and freckles and a pasted on smile who always wanted to please her family and relatives." The patient stated that she recognized the little girl as a part of herself that was still very much in control of her today and needed to let go of the adult she was now. She accused me in anger of using age regression suggestions to produce the image of the little girl. I tacitly accepted the accusation. She found this unsolicited image fascinating and felt it summarized the causes of her headaches. She now recognizes the need still to practice self-relaxation daily but is now essentially a psychotherapy candidate. Posttesting shows an increase (5) in her Harvard score.

Case Study of a High-Hypnotic-Ability Patient

Figure 28 (p. 224) is the profile of a 41-year-old white single male, a resident of northern California, with a Bachelor of Science degree in electrical engineering presenting unilateral (left) neck pain that at times radiates into his left shoulder. The patient has a long and stable employment history that is currently threatened by his chronic pain. The pain is constant and varies only in intensity. The patient has been evaluated and unsuccessfully treated by 10 different medical specialists, ranging from orthopedists and neurosurgeons to internists and psychiatrists using drugs, TNS, physical therapy, traction, etc. The patient believes that the cause of his pain is physical damage to a tendon or ligament that physical inspection under surgery will reveal. This patient was actively searching for a surgical solution when he was referred to me. He came to the initial interview with me only out of courtesy to his referring internist who urged him to consult me before surgical exploration.

Evaluation on the high-risk profile revealed a normal male who is very high in hypnotic ability (Harvard score 12). This high level of hypnotic response surprised the patient himself and was inconsistent with

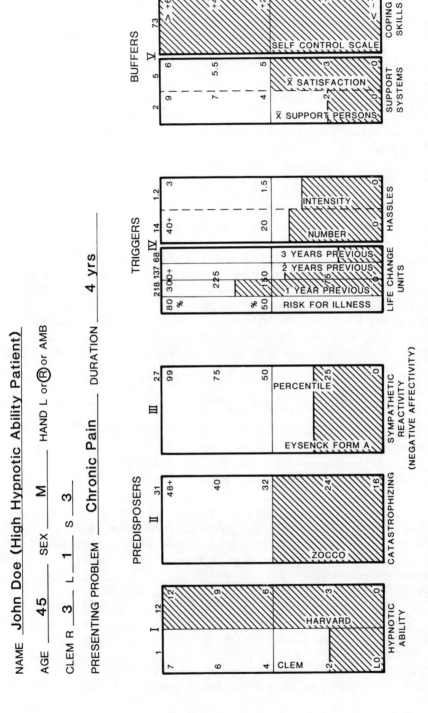

Figure 28. Patient profile for high risk model (Wickramasekera 1979) John Doe (High-hypnotic-ability patient). I = Bakan (1969), Harvard Group Scale; II = Zocco (1984); III = Eysenck (1968), Sympathetic Reactivity Profile, (Wickram, 1976); IV = Holmes (1981), Kanner *et al.* (1981); V = Sarason *et al.* (1983), Rosenbaum (1980).

his self-image. The patient's level of frontal EMG was only moderately high (10.2–8.8 UV.p-p) during the first 80% of strip chart recording and dropped sharply (4.3 UVp-p) during the last few minutes of the recording when he was asked to close his eyes and relax. But the patient's verbal report very significantly underestimates his actual levels of muscle tension in his head and neck. (See Figure 29.)

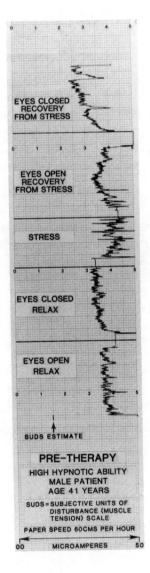

Figure 29. Pretherapy high-hypnotic ability (male patient, age 41 years).

This ability dramatically to drop frontal EMG without prior training is often consistent with high-hypnotic ability (Wickramasekera, 1977). The patient's skin conductance was also moderately high (7.0–7.5 μohms) and was quite reactive (8.9–6.7 μohms) to psychosocial performance stress (mental arithmetic), suggesting that he is in fact internally more acutely agitatable than the calm collected exterior he presents visually. His low verbally reported neuroticism score confirms his observed tendency on the frontal EMG to underestimate his level of physiological activation.

The onset of his chronic pain is related to a "pop" in his neck that he heard in the early hours of the morning 4 years ago while getting ready to leave on a long auto trip with his second wife and his first wife's parents. Four hours into the trip the pain in his neck got so bad that he had to seek medical attention. Parenthetically, the patient added that his first wife had been murdered at work 2 years previously by an unknown assailant, when she was 4 months pregnant with their first child. He also reported some guilt about not taking her prior complaints about prowlers at work more seriously and not viewing her dead body when he got to the scene of the crime. He reports that he was devastated by his first wife's sudden death and his double loss. He reported that "a vast black cavern opened up before him on her death and that he fell into this cavern." He stated that he remarried too soon after her death and that the second marriage did not work out because his second wife could no longer endure living in "the home and shadow of his first wife." Since the divorce from his second wife, he has lived alone and is trying to put the memories and pain of his first wife's sudden death and their very deep love out of his mind. He has been in conventional psychotherapy for over one year and feels that he has processed most of the sadness of his sudden loss, but his neck pain has grown steadily worse and is spreading into his left shoulder.

Since the patient was committed to a somatic explanation of his pain, his moderately elevated frontal EMG was used as the likely point of entry into his belief system. Further, the marked discrepancy between his actual EMG level and his large underestimation of his muscle tension was further used to reinforce how unaware he was of muscle tension in his head and neck. It was suggested that this muscle tension could be a primary factor in his neck and shoulder pain, because contracted muscles become painful. The patient was told that some event originating in his cerebral cortex was probably responsible for sending signals to keep the muscles in his neck and shoulder contracted and painful. He was told that a permanent cure for his pain would include two components. First, reducing the local muscle contractions in his neck and shoulder and, second, attenuating the contraction signal coming from the brain (cerebral cortex).

Because he had good hypnotic ability he was taught the 1-2-3 self-hypnosis procedure and he reported a modest reduction in his pain level during practice. He was asked to practice it at least 10 times per day every day for at least one month. During the demonstration of the procedure in the office the patient was monitored by EMG and skin conductance. His attention was drawn to the very large objective drop in EMG and skin conductance that was associated with the 3-minute 1-2-3, self-hypnosis procedure. It was made explicit that the practice of the self-hypnosis technique was associated with biological changes (EMG and skin conductance) in his body. This rapid (one session) physiological response to self-hypnosis was also consistent with his high Harvard score (12). The patient was also shown his baseline EMG and skin conductance levels at the first therapy session and told that if he practiced the 3-minute self-hypnosis exercise 10 times each day both baselines (EMG plus skin conductance) would be lower on baseline measurement in his therapy session next week. Our standard practice of first measuring baseline physiological levels at the start of each therapy session provides us with an objective method of verifying patient compliance with self-hypnosis homework.

The patient returned to the second therapy session one week later reporting that for the first time in 4 years he had actually had brief periods (5 to 10 minutes) when he was totally pain free in spite of reducing his use of pain medication during the week. The first part of the session was spent having the patient look at the Netter plates (Netter, 1962) of the brain and CNS, particularly those showing the pathways from the cortex to the sternocleidomastoid and trapezius muscles. The patient was told that he may have inadvertently learned to send an electrical signal from his motor cortex to his neck muscles, activating muscular contractions and "a reverbating electrical circuit" that is now dysfunctional and needs to be turned off at the central (brain) and local (neck and shoulder) centers. The patient was hypnotized and asked to imagine the color, the shape, the activity, and the components in this pain circuit from his cortex to his neck and shoulder. He was then told to imagine himself adjusting the components, the shapes, and the colors in the circuit to reduce the activity of the circuit. Later, he reported adjusting down a large visualized gain switch, which episodically rotated itself up under psychosocial stress. He was told to imagine himself reducing the activity of this circuit each time he practiced self-hypnosis. Finally, he was asked how the events of his first wife's death might have predisposed him to acquiring this pain circuit. He had no answer and was therefore told that he would have one or more dreams in the coming weeks in which parts of the answer would be presented in his dreams. Next week, the patient reported several dreams in which his first wife appeared. He reported that those dreams had made him aware of the fact that she is still very much with him even though she has been dead several years. The next week, he reported the first incident of visual contact and visitation with her since her death, which was either a hallucination or a genuine ESP incident. She came to him in "a golden light and spoke directly to his mind" about her love for him, but she left abruptly when he asked her when he would meet her again and the sex of their unborn child. He was troubled by the incident and the recognition that he still had unfinished business with her. Meanwhile he continued to report shorter episodes of pain and less intense pain even though he was not using any pain medication. In subsequent sessions, he spent half the session using the EMG and conductance signals on a computer screen to verify with delayed feedback his growing proficiency in rapidly and reliably dropping his EMG and skin conductance signals. He reported feeling proud of his ability to manipulate his EMG, skin conductance, and pain levels. With patients of high-hypnotic ability the primary use of biofeedback devices is objectively to verify and validate their natural skill at physiological self-regulation. Direct and continuous physiological feedback is frequently very disruptive of the acquisition of physiological self-regulation skills in such patients. A part of these sessions were devoted to finishing in role-played fantasy his business with his dead wife and talking about his present complicated love relationships with two women. The patient's experiences in hypnosis have convinced him of the reality of his unconscious mind. He decided to seek advice from his "unconscious mind" about which relationship he should dissolve and which he should pursue. In one hypnotic session in my laboratory, the patient reported hearing my voice telling him which woman to "let go of." I did not challenge the testimony of his ears but I asked him if he was sure I had spoken. He started the next session by telling me that he was confident that the voice he heard came from out of his own unconscious mind and that he knew that I had not spoken. I assured him that it never was my voice he heard and that I was glad that his unconscious mind had spoken to him and that it deserved respectful attention. He thanked me for this insight and mailed me a letter between sessions telling me that for the rest of his life he would be grateful to me for teaching him to care and attend to his unconscious mind.

   At termination of psychophysiological therapy, the patient had been pain free for 2 months and was off all pain medications for 5 months. He is currently in long-term follow-up and I will be seeing him once per month for the next 5 years to ensure that any relapses are defused before they turn into more serious chronic problems.

References

Bandura, A. *Principles of behavior modification*. New York: Holt, Rinehart & Winston, 1969.

Blanchard, E. B., Andrasik, F., Applebaum, K. A., Evans, D. D., Myers, P., & Barron, K. S. Three studies of the Psychologic changes in chronic headache patients associated with biofeedback and relaxation therapies. *Psychosomatic Medicine*, 1986, *48*, 73–83.

Bowers, K. S. On being unconsciously influenced and informed. In K. S. Bowers & D. Meichenbaum (Eds.), *The unconscious reconsidered*. New York: Wiley, 1984.

Bowers, K. S., & Meichenbaum, D. (Eds.), *The unconscious reconsidered*. New York: Wiley, 1984.

Collins, G. A., Cohen, M. M., Naliboff, B. D., & Schandler, S. L. Comparative analysis of paraspinal and frontalis EMG, heart rate, and skin conductance in chronic low back pain patients and normals to various postures and stress. *Scandinavian Journal of Rehabilitation Medicine*, 1982, *14*, 39–46.

DeLongis, A., Coyne, J. C., Dakof, G., Folkman, S., & Lazarus, R. S. Relationship of daily hassles, uplifts, and major life events to health status. *Health Psychology*, 1982, *1*, 119–136.

DePue, R. A., & Monroe, S. M. Conceptualization and measurement of human disorder in life stress research: The problem of chronic disturbance. *Psychological Bulletin*, 1986, *99*, 36–51.

Dixon, N. F. *Preconscious processing*. England: Wiley, 1981.

Dohrenwend, B. P., & Shrout, P. E. "Hassles" in the conceptualization and measurement of life stress variables. *American Psychologist*, 1985, *40*, 780–785.

Ellis, A. *Reason and emotion in psychotherapy*. New York: Lyle Stuart, 1962.

Faulkner, W. Nobel Prize acceptance speech. In H. Frenz (Ed.), *Nobel lectures: Literature, 1901–1967*. New York: Elsevier/North Holland, 1969.

Flor, H., Turk, D. C., & Birbaumer, N. Assessment of stress-related psychophysiological reactions in chronic back pain patients. *Journal of Consulting and Clinical Psychology*, 1985, *53*, 354–364.

Folkman, S., & Lazarus, R. S. If it changes it must be a process: A study of emotion and coping during three stages of a college examination. *Journal of Personality and Social Psychology*, 1984, *48*, 150–170.

Forster, P. M., & Govier, E. Discrimination without awareness? *Quarterly Journal of Experimental Psychology*, 1978, *30*, 282–295.

Kessler, R. C., Price, R. H., & Wortman, C. B. Social factors in psychopathology: Stress, social support and coping processes. *Annual Review of Psychology*, 1985, *36*, 531–572.

Kihlstrom, J. F. The cognitive unconscious. *Science*, 1987, *237*, 1445–1452.

Kobasa, S. C., Maddi, S. R., & Kahn, S. Hardiness and health. *Journal of Personality and Social Psychology*, 1982, *42*, 168–177.

Krantz, D. S., & Manuck, S. B. Acute psychophysiologic reactivity and risk of cardiovascular disease: A review and methodologic critique. *Psychological Bulletin*, 1984, *96* (3), 435–464.

Kushner, H. S. *When bad things happen to good people*. New York: Schocken Books, 1981.

Lang, P. J. A bio-informational theory of emotional imagery. *Psychophysiology*, 1979, *16*, 495–512.

Lazarus, A. A. On assertive behavior: A brief note. In I. Wickramasekera (Ed.), *Biofeedback, behavior therapy, and hypnosis.* Chicago: Nelson-Hall, 1976.

Lazarus, A. A., & Fay, A. *I can if I want to.* New York: William Morrow, 1975.

Lazarus, R. S., DeLongis, A., Folkman, S., & Given, R. Stress and adaptational outcomes: The problem of confounded measures. *American Psychologist*, 1985, *40*, 770–779.

Levor, R. M., Cohen, M. J., Naliboff, B. D., McArthur, D. & Heuser, G. Psychosocial precursors and correlates of migraine headache. *Journal of Consulting and Clinical Psychology*, 1986, *54*, 347–353.

Maslow, A. H. *Motivation and personality.* New York: Harper, 1954.

Mathews, A., & MacLeod, C. Discrimination of threat cues without awareness in anxiety states. *Journal of Abnormal Psychology*, 1986, *95*, 131–138.

McCaul, K., & Malott, J. M. Distractions and coping with pain. *Psychological Bulletin*, 1984, *95*, 516–533.

Menaghen, E. G. Individual coping efforts: Moderators of the relationship between life stress and mental health outcomes. In H. B. Kaplan (Ed.), *Psychosocial stress: Trends in theory and research.* New York: Academic Press, 1983.

Netter, F. *The CIBA collection of medical illustrations: Vol. I. Nervous system.* New York: CIBA, 1962.

Nisbett, R. E., & Wilson, T. D. Telling more than we can know: Verbal reports on mental processes. *Psychological Review*, 1977, *84*, 231–259.

Nuckolls, K. B., Cassell, J., & Kaplan, B. H. Psychological assets, life crisis, and the prognosis of pregnancy. *American Journal of Epidemiology*, 1972, *95*, 431–441.

Parson, T. *The social system.* New York: Free Press, 1951.

Pearlin, L. I., & Schooler, C. The structure of coping. *Journal of Health and Social Behavior*, 1978, *19*, 2–21.

Petrich, J., & Holmes, T. H. Life change and onset of illness. *Medical Clinics of North America*, 1977, *61*, 825–839.

Philips, C. A psychological analysis of tension headache. In S. Rachman (Ed.), *Contributions to medical psychology.* Oxford, England: Pergamon Press, 1977.

Powell, J. *Why am I afraid to tell you who I am?* Chicago: Argus Communications, 1969.

Rabkin, J. G., & Struening, E. L. Life events, stress, and illness. *Science*, 1976, *194*, 1013–1020.

Roosevelt, A. *You learn by living.* New York: Harper, 1960.

Rosenbaum, M. A schedule for assessing self-control behaviors: Preliminary findings. *Behavior Therapy*, 1980, *11*, 109–121.

Rosenbaum, M., & Ben-Atri, K. Learned helplessness and learned resourcefulness: Effects of noncontingent success and failure on individuals differing in self-control skills. *Journal of Personality and Social Psychology*, 1985, *48*, 1, 198–215.

Serber, M. Teaching the nonverbal components of assertive training. In I. Wickramasekera (Ed.), *Biofeedback, behavior therapy, and hypnosis.* Chicago: Nelson-Hall, 1976.

Shevrin, H., & Dickman, S. The psychological unconscious: A necessary assumption for all psychological theory? *American Psychologist*, 1980, *35*, 421–434.

Shor, R. The fundamental problem in hypnosis research as viewed from historic perspectives. In E. Fromm & R. E. Shor (Eds.), *Hypnosis: Developments in research and new perspectives.* New York: Aldine, 1979.

Sovak, N., Kunzel, M., Sternbach, R. A., & Dalessio, D. J. Mechanism of the biofeedback therapy of migraine: Volitional manipulation of the psychophysiological background. *Headache*, 1981, *21*, 89–92.

Spiegel, D., Detrick, D., & Frischolz, E. Hypnotizability and psychopathology. *American Journal of Psychiatry*, 1982, *139*, 431–437.

Stevenson, I. Do we need a new word to supplement "hallucination"? *American Journal of Psychiatry*, 1983, *140*, 1609–1611.

Stone, A. A., & Neale, J. M. New measure of daily coping: Development and preliminary results. *Journal of Personality and Social Psychology*, 1985, *46*, 892–906.

Stroebel, C. F. *The quieting reflex.* New York: Putnam, 1982.

Struve, F., Wickramasekera, I., Giannetti, R., Johnson, C., Atkins, E., Hubbard, M., & Muten, E. *Electroencephalographic and psycholophysiological differentiation of behavioral medicine patients: An empirical investigation.* Paper presented at the 33rd Annual Scientific Meeting of the Academy of Psychosomatic Medicine, New York, November 1986.

Suedfeld, P. *Restricted environmental stimulation: Research and clinical applications.* New York: Wiley, 1980.

Thoits, P. A. Dimensions of life events that influence psychological distress: An evaluation and synthesis of the literature. In H. B. Kaplan (Ed.), *Psychosocial stress: Trends in theory and research.* New York: Academic Press, 1983.

Thoits, P. A. Social support as coping assistance. *Journal of Consulting and Clinical Psychology*, 1986, *54*, 416–423.

Thompson, S. Will it hurt less if I can control it? A complex answer to a simple question. *Psychological Bulletin*, 1981, *1*, 89–101.

Watson, D., & Clark, L. A. Negative affectivity: The disposition to experience aversive emotional states. *Psychosocial Bulletin*, 1984, *96*, 465–490.

Watson, D., & Tellegen, A. Toward a consensual structure of mood. *Psychological Bulletin*, 1985, *98*, 219–235.

Wickramasekera, I. Effects of EMG feedback training on susceptibility to hypnosis: Preliminary observations. *Proceedings of the 79th Annual Convention of the American Psychological Association*, 1971, *6*, 785–787. (Summary)

Wickramasekera, I. The effects of EMG feedback on hypnotic susceptibility: More preliminary data. *Journal of Abnormal Psychology*, 1973, *82*, 74–77.

Wickramasekera, I. (Ed.). *Biofeedback, behavior therapy, and hypnosis.* Chicago: Nelson-Hall, 1976.

Wickramasekera, I. On attempts to modify hypnotic susceptibility: Some psychophysiological procedures and promising directions. *Annals of the New York Academy of Sciences*, 1977, *296*, 143–153.

Wickramasekera, I. *A model of the patient at high risk for chronic stress related disorders: Do beliefs have biological consequences?* Paper presented at the Annual Convention of the Biofeedback Society of America, San Diego, March, 1979.

Zarski, J. J. Hassles and health: A replication. *Health Psychology*, 1984, *33*, 243–251.

10

SELF-HYPNOSIS AND THE COMMON COMPONENTS OF OTHER STRESS-REDUCTION TECHNIQUES
A Theory

> I believe the idea of a "right" to health should be
> replaced by that of a moral obligation to preserve
> one's own health. The individual then has the
> "right" to expect help with information, accessible
> service of good quality, and minimum financial
> barriers. Meanwhile the people have been led to
> believe that national health insurance, more
> doctors, and greater use of high-cost, hospital-
> based technologies will improve health.
> Unfortunately, none of them will.
> —John H. Knowles, M.D.
> Science, 1977

Medical high technology and superior medical skills cannot substitute for individual responsibility for health care today. One of the primary causes of chronic disease today is our psychological and psychophysiological reactions to psychosocial stress and our maladaptive (smoking, obesity, drug abuse) ways of coping with psychosocial stress. These psychological

A part of this paper was first read as an invited presentation to the American Association for the Advancement of Tension Control, Chicago 1977, and a summary of it without reference to self-hypnosis was printed in the proceedings of the American Association for the Advancement of Tension Control. This paper was also read at the American Psychological Association Convention in Toronto, 1978, at the annual convention of the Illinois Psychological Association in 1978, and at the annual convention of the American Association for the Advancement of Science, Houston, Texas, 1979.

and psychophysiological reactions are consequences of fixed perceptions of threat and fixed perceptions of the ways of coping with threat. Hence, giving patients tools and the responsibility to use these tools to alter their own perception of threat is a major step toward restoring individual responsibility for health care. Self-hypnosis may be a useful prototype of such a tool to alter fixed perceptions of threat arousal and resolution.

Fromm (1972) predicted that self-hypnosis would attract increasing scientific investigations in the future. Self-hypnosis (Weitzenhoffer, 1957) appears to be a prototype of several other stress-reduction techniques currently marketed to control psychological stress (Lazarus, 1966). The five best known methods are (a) Transcendental Meditation (TM) (Wallace & Benson, 1972), (b) autogenic training (Schultz & Luthe, 1959), (c) relaxation (Jacobson, 1970), (d) systematic desensitization (Bandura, 1969; Wolpe, 1973), and (e) frontal EMG biofeedback (Budzynski, Stovya, Adler, & Mullaney, 1973).

Where data is available, careful study demonstrates that there are some individual differences in clinical response to these five psychological stress-reduction methods (Woolfolk & Lehrer, 1984). The effective components, if any, in these superficially disparate procedures are still unclear. The mechanism or mechanisms of change in behavioral and physiological symptoms, when the five techniques are used, have contradictory explanations.

On initial inspection, these stress-reduction techniques are procedurally like self-hypnosis with respect to the following features. They are (a) self-initiated, (b) self-regulated, and (c) the learning of the techniques follows a graduated, educational model. In addition, these techniques share with self-hypnosis the use of four other common procedural variables: (d) sensory restriction, (e) relaxation practice, (f) credibility enhancing packaging, and (g) structuring of therapeutic expectations. I hypothesize that these seven procedural commonalities will enhance the probability that the trainee will have access to at least one or more of three useful therapeutic mechanisms (enhanced hypnotizability, "allocentric mode of perception," [Schachtel, 1959], and enhanced cognitive control of physiological functions), that can reduce psychophysiological and behavioral symptoms. These three therapeutic mechanisms, when used consistently with psychophysiological disorders, promise to provide an effective, cheap, and safe method of resolving psychological stress through the alteration of perception, without the use of drugs and surgery. I believe that the investigation of the parameters of self-hypnosis will further clarify the mechanisms and parameters of change in the five previously cited and apparently disparate stress-reduction techniques.

Psychological Stress

Psychological stress (Appley & Trumbull, 1967; Lazarus, 1966) has been implicated in the exacerbation or etiology of several psycho-physiological disorders, including headaches, peptic ulcers, essential hypertension, ulcerative colitis, and bronchial asthma (Weiner, 1977; Wolff, 1963). Analyses of psychological stress emphasize the critical role of cognition (e.g., appraisal and labeling) in the sequence of events that comprise psychological stress (Arnold, 1969; Mandler, 1975). They suggest that it is unlikely that physiological arousal alone, without aversive cognitive labeling (perception of danger or threat) of the arousal and situation is a sufficient condition for the acquisition and maintenance of chronic stress-related disorders, such as chronic pain, anxiety, peptic ulcers, and insomnia.

The stressors that impinge on these patients seldom involve tissue damage, but they do involve a perception of danger or threat to the well-being of the person. Frequently, the stressors are problems in living that present in vague, ambiguous forms that gradually, over many years, elicit cumulative physiological arousal and/or ambivalent feelings in these patients. These psychosocial stressors may include an unhappy marriage, a problem child, a hypercritical boss, an unrealistic perfor-mance standard, a major loss or death, rejection, or loneliness. These complex psychosocial challenges in living cannot be adequately remedi-ated by primitive, fight or flight methods of coping or alternatively, by the exclusive and habitual use of modern drugs and surgery to reduce the psychophysiological arousal these challenges provoke. Their resolu-tion requires at least a fresh perception of the challenge, and creative approaches to coping with it.

Self-Hypnosis and the Alteration of the Perception of Stressors

There is growing conviction that a self-help or self-responsibility approach will be one of the essential components in the management of our current health problems (Knowles, 1977). Self-hypnosis is taking responsibility to manage one's cognitive, behavioral, and physiological responses within genetic and environmental constraints. Autosugges-tion or self-hypnosis, by definition, is giving hypnotic suggestions to one's self to self-induce an altered state of consciousness characterized by alterations in perception, mood, and memory. One of the best docu-mented consequences of altering consciousness is the alteration of com-mon perceptions (Ludwig, 1969; Tart, 1969). Weitzenhoffer (1957) claimed that theoretically self-hypnosis and heterohypnosis should have the same parameters and he states that Hull (1933) had presented some evidence supporting this position. Recent empirical studies (Johnson, 1979; Ruch, 1975) appear to support Weitzenhoffer's position. But Fromm (1972) pointed out the lack of direct research evidence that heterohypnosis and self-hypnosis are "similar experiential phenomena" and she and her associates (Fromm, Bopxer, Brown, Hurt, & Oberlander, 1981) have found important similarities and differences between self-hypnosis and heterohypnosis. Fromm (1972) predicted a "great upsurge of scientific interest" in self-hypnosis in the future. This prediction may be valid because of the growing need for a cheap, effective, and reliable method of coping with psychosocial stress-related illnesses. Self-hypnosis may be a skill that can provide an alternative to the widely used pills and surgery currently used to treat chronic-stress-related illness.

There are a variety of passive solitary (meditation, biofeedback, autogenic training) and active (religious dances, running, chanting, etc.) techniques of inducing altered states of consciousness (Ludwig, 1969) that appear to involve at least elements of self-hypnosis. But, conventionally, the label *self-hypnosis* is attached to a procedure practiced quietly, inwardly, and in a relatively immobile state. This analysis will assume some continuity between heterohypnosis and self-hypnosis (Fromm *et al.*, 1980; Johnson, 1979; Ruch, 1975). Self-hypnosis is a psychophysiological technique that can be used to self-induce an altered state of consciousness characterized by enhanced hypnotizability or primary suggestibility and increased cognitive control of physiological functions (Herzfeld & Taub, 1977; Sarbin & Slagle, 1972; Zimbardo, Maslach, & Marshall, 1972). But there is probably a third characteristic of this altered state, imaginative involvement (Hilgard, 1970) and increased creativity (Dave, 1979; Johnson, 1981), which is even more important, but difficult to document (Bowers, 1978; Raikov, 1976). The importance of enhanced creativity lies in the simple fact that most psychological stress (and its destructive biological consequences) is initiated and maintained not by tissue damage, but by the perceived threat (Mason, 1971) to the well-being of the person. Fixed perceptions of threat, anticipations of damage, and the rigid meanings we assign to inevitable psychosocial events (death, uncertainty, rejection, failure) may trigger impulsive maladaptive behaviors (e.g., substance abuse, violence), premature resignation in the face of adversity (e.g., illness behavior and depression), or chronic vigilance and physiological hyperarousal (e.g., primary hypertension, pain). Catastrophizing cognitive (Beck, 1976; Ellis, 1962) habits can enhance the perception of threat, promote behavioral avoidance, and chronic physiological arousal. Aversive cognitive labels can lock into perception as stressors common and inevitable psychosocial events (failure, death, delays, uncertainty, rejection, etc.). When perceived rigidly as stressors, rather than opportunities for growth, these events are often maladaptively coped with by chronic and excessive physiological arousal (which can trigger somatic symptoms like peptic ulcers or muscular or vascular pain syndromes), negative cognitive ruminations (causing anxiety and/or depression), neurotic avoidance (phobias, obsessions-compulsions), or acting-out behaviors (reckless driving causing automobile accidents, substance abuse). Beliefs about stressors can have biological and behavioral consequences (Wickramasekera, Paskewitz, & Taube, 1979). Self-hypnosis may provide a cheap, effective, and reliable technique to alter perceptions and beliefs about stressors and their resolution.

Common Procedural Components

In spite of many differences between these five stress-reduction techniques at a theoretical, historical, cultural, and philosophical level, they appear to have some similarities.

The most obvious way in which these five techniques are alike is first with respect to their similarity to self-hypnosis. As in self-hypnosis, patients or trainees are introduced to these methods by a therapist, guru, or trainer who uses a (1) graduated educational model.

As in self-hypnosis, there is an emphasis on (2) self-initiation or active patient participation, and on (3) self-regulation of the process or on the responsibility of the patient for the success of the process. Teaching the technique involves a graduated approach to skill acquisition, homework assignments, emphasis on repeated practice at home or work, guidelines for dealing with problems, and periodic review or supervision with a trainer. Clearly all these techniques appear to use a graduated educational model that makes trainees active participants in their own rehabilitation.

All five stress-reduction techniques encourage or require the trainee to (4) restrict sensory stimulation during the exercises. For example, subjects are asked to close their eyes, lie or sit still, and/or to concentrate attention on a repetitive stimulus (e.g., biofeedback) or phrase (e.g., meditation).

These techniques all encourage the patient to relax his muscles, let go, and to (5) reduce the patient's level of physiological arousal. This is done by reducing motor activity, repeating verbal suggestions of relaxation and warmth, tensing and relaxing muscles, alternating between focusing on phobic and relaxing images, or trying to reduce the frequency of a tone or light that is correlated with a reduction in arousal in a physiological function.

All these techniques explicitly or implicitly engage the patient's belief system with (6) credibility manipulations and cognitive motivations. The technique's credibility may be boosted by its association with high-credibility belief systems like science, medicine, the human potential movement (Barber, 1976) or even the mysterious and the esoteric that already have high credibility for at least some patients. Credibility appears to be at least a function of selective confirmed experiences and reinforced events (Wickramasekera, 1976). The variety of belief systems (science, medicine, human potential, and mystery) that rationalize these stress-reduction techniques permits an accommodation somewhere on the belief spectrum of the bulk of idiosyncratic needs and beliefs, that varied people under stress bring to professional and lay healers. We are introduced as children to exaggerated images of the power and mystery of hypnosis, medicine, and science by the mass media (movies, TV, popular books, newspapers). Cognitive motivation for participation in hypnosis or self-hypnosis may be latent in some people long before the patient enters the waiting room. Recently, efforts (Barber, 1969; Hilgard, 1965) have been made with some success to package hypnosis in the methodology of science, to legitimize it by association with medical education (Hilgard, 1965), and even to marry it to the human potential movement (Barber, 1976).

TM training, for example, is introduced with a display of charts and graphs and a lecture on the alleged scientific validation of TM at the Harvard Medical School and other temples of scientific-academic respectability. Progressive relaxation (Jacobson, 1970) stresses its roots in the muscle physiology laboratory and EMG measurement. Desensitization (Wolpe, 1973) is introduced to a patient in clinical practice with reference to its roots in the conditioning laboratory and its presumed origins in experimental-scientific psychology (Buchwald & Young, 1969). Clinical biofeedback uses impressive scientific-medical instruments and, in fact, appears to have such high scientific face validity that it requires no explicit presentation of credentials. Autogenic training is always preceded by a serious ritualistic medical measurement of vital functions (pulse, blood pressure, etc.), which can implicitly create the impression that grave and healing events are at hand. The graphing and counting rituals of science and medicine can function as discriminative stimuli for reducing confusion and anxiety and generally operate as safety signals indicating the impending offset of pain and fear (Wickramasekera, 1977a, 1980). The labels and trappings of science and medicine are the most potent placebo stimuli in Western industrialized society (Wickramasekera, 1977a, 1980). The scientific and medical packaging of these five procedures may increase their credibility and attractiveness for many people in distress. All of these five techniques appear to the lay person to have something concrete for mind and body, and hence, they may have more face validity (Anastasi, 1961) than conventional psychotherapy or counseling. But not everything that has high face validity is necessarily empirically true or effective. In spite of Christopher Columbus and his empirical investigations, the hypothesis that the earth is flat continues to enjoy high face validity for some primitive people.

The complex and broad belief systems that accompany these five techniques provide the kind of durable (resistant to disconfirmation by specific negative instances) and cross-situationally consistent cognitive motivation to mobilize hope (Frank, 1965). Medical interventions have shown that the most effective treatment program (primary prevention) is that which requires the least personal effort (Saward & Sorensen, 1978). For example, interventions like the public health management of water, sewage, and fluoridation, neither request nor require patient participation. Psychological, unlike medical interventions (injections, surgery, pills), require much personal effort and time, and also intrude on the patient's priorities and life-style. Strong cognitive motivation is crucial to psychological techniques. A personally relevant, complex, comprehensive and cross-situational, consistent belief system that is fairly resistant to disconfirmation by specific negative instances is essential to motivate compliance in the face of slow skill acquisition, uncertainty, distraction, and episodic clinical relapse. Science and medicine, today, generate more faith than the old gods. The dogmas of older and more complex religions once provided this cognitive motivational component for adaptive behavior. They motivated behavior by stating their primary tenants in paradoxes that insulated the tenants from logical analysis and also immunized them from disconfirmation by negative instances encountered in everyday empirical experience. Today in the Western world, the marketability or motivational value of a belief is in direct proportion to the extent to which it is packaged in the wrappings of science and medicine. The new stress-reduction techniques, as I have pointed out, are packaged for high credibility in the trappings of science and medicine.

In addition, all these techniques explicitly or implicitly (7) structure positive therapeutic expectations. All the stress-reduction techniques claim clinical efficacy and their claims are supported by some empirical data, clinical anecdotes, testimonials, and plausible clinical rationales (Woolfolk & Lehrer, 1984).

There is good consensus in the psychotherapy and the medical literatures that positive therapeutic expectations (in patient and therapist) can powerfully influence clinical outcome with biological and psychological disorders (Beecher, 1959; Goldstein, 1962; Frank, 1965; Shapiro, 1971). These effects may have several mechanisms (Wickramasekera, 1976, 1980). But the most systematically and objectively investigated mechanisms are related to the placebo effect in drug and surgical studies. The medical literature shows that the effects of an active drug can be attenuated, potentiated, or reversed by expectational manipulations (Shapiro, 1971). Beecher (1959) and Evans (1974) reviewed, in all, 36 double blind studies and found that a placebo reduced organic pain by half of its original intensity in 36% of patients. There are currently at least three explanatory models of the placebo effect. The suggestion hypothesis (Barber, 1963; Shapiro, 1971), the anxiety reduction hypothesis (Evans, 1974; Orne, 1974), and recently I have proposed (Wickramasekera, 1977a, 1980) a conditioned response hypothesis of the placebo effect. All three models regard positive patient expectations as a critical component in generating positive clinical outcome.

Common Therapeutic Mechanisms

It is hypothesized that patient use of these seven common procedural components will be associated with enhanced hypnotizability or primary suggestibility (Eysenck & Furneaux, 1945), accessing the allocentric mode of perception, and enhanced cognitive control of physiological functions. It is further hypothesized that these three elements are sufficient conditions for positive clinical outcome with functional stress-related disorders.

Enhanced Hypnotizability

There is growing evidence for a relationship between the degree of the subject's hypnotizability and probability of a positive clinical outcome (Barabasz, Baer, Sheehan, & Barabasz, 1986; Bowers & Kelly, 1979; Perry, Gelfand, & Marcovitch, 1979; Wickramasekera et al., 1979) with several clinical symptoms. Based on evidence to be presented later, there is reason to believe that the repeated use of these five stress-reduction techniques will either temporarily or permanently increase the practitioner's baseline hypnotizability or primary suggestibility. This enhanced hypnotizability can be used to potentiate instructions within therapy to attend to and to absorb for use in problem-solving factual information that might be ignored or considered irrelevant in the everyday waking state.

> In order to effect a cure a condition of "expectant faith" was induced in sick persons. . . . We have learned to use the word "suggestion" for this phenomenon, and Mobius has taught us that the unreliability which we deplore in so many of our therapeutic measures may be traced back actually to the disturbing influence of this very powerful factor . . . it is disadvantageous, however, to leave entirely in the hands of the patient what the mental factor in your treatment of him shall be. In this way it is uncontrollable; it can neither be measured nor intensified. Is it not then a justifiable endeavor on the part of a physician to seek to control this factor, to use it with a purpose, and to direct and strengthen it? This and nothing else is what scientific psychotherapy proposes. (Freud, 1959, pp. 250–251)

For example, Spiegel's (1976) self-hypnotic procedure for smoking control draws the patient's attention to important but ignored information. For example, he says, "You cannot live without your body. . . . This [to stop smoking] is your way of acknowledging the fragile, precious nature of your body" (Spiegel, 1976). The enhanced hypnotizability state may increase the probability of behavioral compliance with homework assignments. Homework requires numerous and extended blocks of time that could intrude on life-styles. The practice of new skills (e.g., relaxation, pacing, etc.) and insights (e.g., recognize that "I am catastrophizing") in the home or work setting can improve clinical outcome. Doing anything in the natural environment that distracts from or is incompatible with vigilance, muscular bracing, and catastrophizing (Ellis, 1962) can be therapeutic. The increased state of suggestibility can be used to instruct the patient selectively to perceive evidence of progress and to inhibit attention to counter evidence. This programming of attention may be particularly important in the early stages, when new therapeutic behaviors are weak and unreliable. Verbal instructions (Bandura, 1969), delivered in an enhanced suggestible state, can be used to create a cognitive set favorable to the acquisition or extinction of operant, respondent, and vicarious conditioning mechanisms (Wickramasekera, 1976). In a small minority of subjects, verbal instruction given in this potentiated suggestible state may lead directly and immediately to behavioral and visceral changes.

Allocentric Mode of Perception

During self-hypnosis and practice of the other five stress-reduction techniques, there is an increased probability of an alteration in the mode of perception of everyday events and problems (Bowers, 1978; Dave,

1979; Johnson, 1981). The creative aspects of an altered state of consciousness have been psychologically described by Kris (1951), Schachtel (1959), and others. Perception is altered in a way that increases the probability that events and problems in living (Szasz, 1960) will be looked at freshly. Schachtel (1959) called this the "allocentric mode of perception" and described it as follows:

> This openness means that the sensibilities of the person, his mind, and his senses, are more freely receptive, less tied to fixed anticipations and sets, and that the object is approached in different ways, from different angles, and not with any fixed purpose to use it for the satisfaction of a particular need, or the testing of a particular expectation or possibility. (p. 245)

The ability to look freshly at a stressor as an opportunity can have profound behavioral and biological consequences for attending to neglected aspects of the stressor and generating new coping techniques to resolve the challenge (Wickramasekera et al., 1979). Cognitive vigilance, physiological hyperarousal, muscular bracing (Whatmore & Kohli, 1974), and behavioral avoidance can cease. The patient may shift down from red-alert to a quiet task-oriented approach characterized by curiosity about the stressor in the larger environment, the mobilization of new coping resources (skills and information), and a commitment to risk taking with new coping strategies in the pursuit of short-term goals graduated in difficulty level.

The allocentric mode of perception that can occur in self-hypnosis and hypnosis increases the probability of creatively approaching old problems in living (Bowers, 1978; Dave, 1979; Johnson, 1981), finding meaning in what seemed meaningless, looking freshly at everyday events, and noticing alternatives where none seemed to exist before. These subtle attitudinal and perceptual changes can have far-reaching positive behavioral and biological consequences in terms of reduced sympathetic activation, which can feed back to reinforce the perceptual changes in the subject, increasing a sense of self-efficacy (Bandura, 1977). The patient may become more willing to take risks, acquire new skills, and persist in coping behaviors in the face of uncertainty or delayed reinforcement. The absence of an adaptive set of perceptions and beliefs can be at least as crippling to self-mobilization as the absence of an arm or leg (Wickramasekera, 1977b; Wickramasekera et al., 1979).

Cognitive Control of Physiology

Repeated practice of self-hypnosis or the other five stress-reduction techniques can lead to growing potency and reliability in the cognitive control of physiological functions. The increased cognitive control of physiological functions (Paul, 1966, 1969; Roberts, Kewman, & Mac-Donald, 1972; Schultze & Luthe, 1959; Surwit, 1978; Wallace & Benson, 1972; Zimbardo, Maslach, & Marshall, 1972) a patient often experiences with self-hypnosis or the other five techniques can add considerably to the patient's self-esteem. The patient's ability to control the frequency or intensity of a specific biological symptom like headaches, skin disorders, and asthma (DePiano & Salzberg, 1979) can boost self-efficacy. "An efficacy expectation is the conviction that one can successfully execute the behavior required to produce an outcome" (Bandura, 1977). Self-efficacy is postulated by Bandura (1977) to be the primary determinant of the intensity and duration of coping behaviors, assuming the patient has the relevant skills and incentives. The availability of these coping behaviors determines if stress change is associated with progress or regression. This enhanced sense of self-efficacy can be a specific antidote for the sense of fatalism and pessimism that predictive longitudinal studies have found to characterize patients prone to stress disorders (Hinkle, 1961; Valliant, 1978).

Sensory Restriction and Enhanced Hypnotizability

It appears that sensory restriction procedures are generally associated with an increase in human suggestibility and potentiated expectations (Adams, 1964; Azima, Vispo, & Cramer-Azima, 1961; Hebb, 1966; Lilly, 1956; Lindsley, 1957; Suedfeld, 1969; Zukerman & Cohen, 1964). These reports have been critically and exhaustively reviewed in at least two authoritative texts (Rasmussen, 1973; Zubek, 1969) and will not be elaborated on further.

Reviews (Adams, 1964; Suedfeld, 1969, 1980) support the thesis that in a clinical situation, some subjects show a positive therapeutic response to even a single session of mild to moderate sensory restriction. But these studies do not illuminate the mechanism of change in clinical status. I hypothesize that the mechanism of clinical response is enhanced primary suggestibility or hypnotizability (Eysenck & Furneaux, 1945). I also hypothesize that the systematic and frequent practice of the therapeutic regimens of self-hypnosis, autogenic training, progressive muscular relaxation, Transcendental Meditation, EMG or temperature biofeedback, and symbolic systematic desensitization increase the probability of numerous brief consecutive periods of sensory restriction which, in turn, increases the person's baseline hypnotizability either temporarily or permanently. All of the above stress-reduction techniques require the trainee to restrict sensory stimuli during the exercises. For example, subjects are asked to close their eyes, ignore auditory stimuli, lie or sit still, and concentrate on a repetitive stimulus (tone or light) or phrase. Sensory restriction periods may have cumulative suggestive effects through the mechanisms of potentiated primary suggestibility or hypnotizability.

The studies to be cited later, however, constitute the first controlled, direct, and explicit empirical demonstrations that sensory restriction procedures reliably and at least temporarily increase primary suggestibility (Eysenck & Furneaux, 1945) or hypnotizability. Previous studies of sensory restriction focused mainly on secondary suggestibility or persuasibility and did not incorporate pre-post measures of known reliability and validity. Increased personal sensitivity to complex expectational manipulations is most potently indexed by changes in primary suggestibility (Eysenck & Furneaux, 1945).

Several controlled and independently replicated studies demonstrate that sensory restriction procedures increase primary suggestibility or hypnotizability at least temporarily (Barabasz, 1982; Cobb & Shor, 1964; Leva, 1974; Pena, 1963; Sanders & Rehyer, 1969; Wickramasekera, 1969, 1970). Studies have found large increases in hypnotizability in fully plateaued Ss following sensory restriction. The subjects ($N>151$) in these studies ranged from college students to prisoners. Sensory restriction was induced with comparable procedures and the pre-post measurement of susceptibility was done with Stanford Scales, which are measures of hypnotic ability of established reliability and validity. Sensory restriction conditions were established by stressing the need for silence and immobility as subjects reclined on a small, comfortable bed. Subjects wore padded earphones, heard white noise, wore opaque goggles and loose-fitting, heavy cotton gloves that reached their wrists. The duration of sensory restriction varied in the studies cited (1 hour to 6 hours), but the similar results provided independent confirmation of the hypothesis. For example, I was unaware of Pena's (1963) pioneering work until I attempted to publish my results,[1] and I was unaware of Sanders and Rehyer's (1969) study until its publication. There is, however, only one study (Levitt, Brady, Ottinger, & Hinesley, 1962) that used three "resistant" student nurses that fails to confirm the previously cited hypothesis. The remarkable degree of similarity among the majority of the investigators with respect to procedures and conclusions based on a total of over 151 subjects, and who were unaware of each others' work, lends some support to the hypothesis that sensory restriction may en-

---

[1]Pena's work was brought to my attention by Prof. E. R. Hilgard (personal communication, 1969).

hance hypnotizability, at least temporarily. For clinical purposes, a temporary and small, but reliable change may be quite sufficient to increase perceptual and behavioral changes in patients. These temporarily altered perceptual and behavioral changes can have natural consequences (e.g., primary or secondary reinforcements that stabilize these changes through other behavioral and psychological mechanisms; i.e., operant, respondent, and vicarious conditioning mechanisms) This increased hypnotizability induced through numerous brief periods of sensory restriction (the inevitable procedural consequence of repeated practice of any of the five stress-reduction techniques), can make people more responsive to any explicit therapeutic expectations (instructions) and/or the implicit therapeutic demand characteristics (Orne, 1962) that are built into all clinical situations. In all clinical situations, there is a tacit assumption shared by patients and staff that compliance with clinical procedures means that recovery from illness is at hand. The sensory restriction component built into all of these stress-reduction procedures may potentiate for patients the credibility of the therapeutic milieu, and the belief systems on which these clinical stress-reduction interventions are based. Unfortunately, there are, to date, no pre-post studies showing that the systematic and long-term practice of self-hypnosis, autogenic training, symbolic desensitization and Transcendental Meditation[2] enhances hypnotizability. Experimental tests of this hypothesis are simple and particularly testable with pre-post measures of hypnotizability (e.g., Stanford Form A and B) in patients before and after for example systematic desensitization. I have predicted (Wickramasekera, 1976) that such studies will find at least modest to large increases in hypnotizability in people who consistently practice these stress-reduction techniques. I will now review studies that have shown that the practice of progressive muscular relaxation and frontal EMG feedback is also reliably associated with at least temporary but modest increases in hypnotizability.

Muscle Relaxation and Enhanced Hypnotizability

Self-hypnosis, Transcendental Meditation, autogenic training, progressive muscular relaxation, systematic desensitization, and frontal EMG biofeedback all encourage or require the patient to relax his or her

---

[2]In 1971, I proposed to the Illinois Department of Mental Health a study to investigate the effects of Transcendental Meditation with standardized pre-post measures of hypnotizability. But the study was never completed beyond the pilot stage for several reasons, including the inadequately curious attitude of the local TM groups.

muscles, let go, and to reduce his or her level of physiological arousal. This low-physiological-arousal component built into all of the five stress-reduction techniques probably inhibits the efficiency with which the left or dominant hemisphere processes information and increases the opportunities for the involvement of the nondominant right hemisphere in information processing in a clinical, therapeutic context. There is some preliminary evidence that the nondominant hemisphere is preferentially involved in information processing during hypnosis (Bowers, 1976; Hilgard & Hilgard, 1975). Edmonston (1981) showed that suggestions for relaxation are a key component in eliciting enhanced suggestibility. He has also shown that verbal suggestions for mental and physical relaxation are reliably associated with reduction in respiratory rate, skin conductance, electrodermal spontaneous activity, and other psychophysiological indications of arousal.

Relaxation instructions are one of the independent variables that increase suggestibility (Barber, 1969). Several studies (Springer, Sachs, & Morrow, 1977; Wickramasekera, 1971, 1977b) of the consequences of progressive muscular relaxation training have shown at least temporary, but small and reliable increases in hypnotizability. It would seem that increasing the precision of relaxation training with EMG feedback may increase suggestibility even more significantly. In a preliminary study (Wickramasekera, 1971) with 12, white male volunteers between the ages of 18 and 22, we found that the EMG feedback training significantly increased hypnotic susceptibility ($p = .001$) at least temporarily. Subjects were informed about the subjective sensations (tingling, floating, etc.) that typically accompany deep muscle relaxation with frontal EMG feedback and they often spontaneously verified these subjective reports. These verbal reports were not previously reported (Wickramasekera, 1971, 1973a) because they were hard to quantify. But today, I think they are an important part of the procedure, particularly if the therapist's predictions are verified in the subjective experience of the patient (Wickramasekera, 1976). They are like the side effects of drugs indicating that something important is happening. The control procedure was an auditory tape of the first six sessions of a psychiatric patient in feedback training. The feedback tone declined over time, but noncontingently.

Encouraged by these preliminary observations, we attempted replication, again using 12 white volunteer subjects and an experimental design identical to the previous study. The only differences were that in the present (Wickramasekera, 1973a) study, there were 10, 30-minute EMG feedback training sessions; the posttesting for hypnotic susceptibility was done by a research assistant who was blind to the nature (true or false) of the feedback training the subjects received. We again found that response contingent (true) feedback training increased hypnotic susceptibility significantly ($p=.001$).

In both of the studies just cited, all groups were equated on predetermined hypnotizability, and verbal instructions to the subjects were limited to taped verbal instructions that told them they were to be trained to relax, that subjective sensations could occur, and that feedback training could increase their ability to relax and experience their sensations. These studies do need independent replication with better controls,[3] but within the constraints of both our experimental (Wickramasekera, 1971, 1973a) studies and our clinical procedures with tension headache patients (Wickramasekera, 1972, 1973b), we often observe that those who succeed in learning reliably to reduce frontal EMG levels (to approximately 3uV. P-P) appear more responsive to hypnosis on posttesting on the SHSS:B (Wickramasekera, 1976) and nearly always report subjective sensations of disorientation, floating, warmth, and so forth. MacDonald (1978) found a modest increase in hypnotizability with EMG feedback training and Engstrom (1976), using an EEG alpha feedback procedure to induce relaxation, also found a significant increase in hypnotizability. Melzack and Perry (1975) found that a combination of alpha feedback and hypnotic suggestions (which probably potentiated relaxation) was most clinically efficacious. The latter studies used EEG feedback for inducing relaxation, and there may be some problems in interpreting the EEG studies (Dumas & Spitzer, 1978; Evans, 1972). In summary, the low-arousal component built into all of the previously cited six stress-reduction techniques may, in fact, increase the primary suggestibility or hypnotizability of their trainees, rendering them more responsive to the implicit or explicit suggestions in the therapy context.

Summary

Self-hypnosis and the five other psychophysiological stress-reduction techniques have some similarities. Despite varied cultural, philosophical, and historical roots, these six techniques are alike with respect to several procedural variables. It appears very likely that the active therapeutic procedures in these six stress-reduction techniques include a

---

[3]The credibility of the "false" feedback procedure I used is questionable because subjects can verify the contingency. The Radtke, Spanos, Armstrong, Dillman, and Boisvenue (1983) problems in replicating my results probably result from a failure to use my procedure, particularly to train subjects down to the criteria of frontal EMG of 3 UV. P-P or less, and the use of unskilled undergraduates as biofeedback trainers.

graduated, educational approach of self-responsibility, credibility manipulations, structuring therapeutic expectancies, increased sensory restriction, and promoting muscle relaxation. These procedural components foster patient independence and temporarily enhance hypnotizability, creating an altered state of consciousness, which may have important clincal implications. This altered state may increase receptivity to new information and verbal instructions, enable the patient to look at his stressors from multiple and fresh perspectives, stimulate self-mobilization and promote the initiation of coping efforts in a context of graduated task orientation, in which short-term goals, such as cognitive control of physiological functions, can be undertaken in a graduated fashion.

References

Adams, H. B. Therapeutic potentialities of sensory deprivation procedures. *International Mental Health Research Newsletter, VI,* 1964, *4,* 7–9.

Adams, H. B., Robertson, M. H., & Cooper, G. D. Facilitating therapeutic personality change in patients by sensory deprivation. Paper presented at the International Congress of Psychology, November, 1964.

Anastasi, A. *Psychological testing.* New York: Macmillan, 1961.

Appley, M. H., & Trumbull, R. *Psychological stress.* New York: Appleton-Century-Crofts, 1967.

Arnold, M. B. *Emotion and personality.* New York: Columbia University Press, 1969.

Azima, H., Vispo, R. H., & Cramer-Azima, F. J. Observations on analytic therapy during sensory deprivation. In P. Solomon (Ed.), *Sensory deprivation.* Cambridge: Harvard University Press, 1961.

Bakal, D. A. *Psychology and medicine.* New York: Springer, 1979.

Bandura, A. *Principles of behavior modification.* New York: Holt, Reinhart 1969.

Bandura, A. Self-efficacy: Toward a unifying theory of behavioral change. *Psychological Review,* 1977, *84,* 191–215.

Barabasz, A., Baer, L., Sheehan, D., & Barabasz, M. Three year follow up of hypnosis and REST for smoking. *International Journal of Clinical and Experimental Hypnosis,* 1986, *34,* 169–181.

Barabasz, A. F. Restricted environmental stimulation and the enhancement of hypnotizability: Pain, EEG alpha, skin conductance and temperature responses. *International Journal of Clinical and Experimental Hypnosis,* 1982, *30,* 147–166.

Barber, T. X. The effects of "hypnosis" on pain: A critical review of experimental and clinical findings. *Psychosomatic Medicine,* 1963, *25,* 303.

Barber, T. X. *Hypnosis: A scientific approach.* New York: Van Nostrand Reinhold, 1969.

Barber, T. X. *Advances in altered states of consciousness & human potentialities* (Vol. 1). New York: Psychological Dimension, 1976.

Beck, A. *A cognitive therapy and emotional disorders.* New York: International Universities Press, 1976.

Beecher, H. K. *Measurement of subjective responses: Quantitative effect of drugs.* New York: Oxford University Press, 1959.

Benson, H. *The mind/body effect*. New York: Simon & Schuster, 1979.

Blackwell, B. Minor tranquilizers, misuse or overuse? *Psychosomatics*, 1975, *16*, 28–31.

Borkovec, T. D., & Nau, S. D. Credibility of analogue therapy rationales. *Journal of Behavior Therapy and Experimental Psychiatry*, 1972, *3*, 257–260.

Bowers, K. S. *Hypnosis for the seriously curious*. New York: Norton, 1976.

Bowers, P. G. Hypnotizability, creativity, and the role of effortless experiencing. *International Journal of Clinical and Experimental Hypnosis*, 1978, *3*, 184–202.

Bowers, K., & Kelly, P. Stress, disease, psychotherapy, and hypnosis. *Journal of Abnormal Psychology*, 1979, *88*, 490–505.

Buchwald, A., & Young, R. R. Some comments on the foundation of behavior therapy. In C. M. Franks (Ed.), *Behavior therapy appraisal and status*. New York: McGraw-Hill, 1969.

Budzynski, T. Biofeedback and the twilight states of consciousness. In G. E. Schwartz & D. Shapiro (Eds.), *Consciousness and self-regulation* (Vol. 1). New York: Plenum Press, 1976.

Budzynski, T., Stoyva, J., Adler, C. S., & Mullaney, D. J. EMG biofeedback and tension headache. *Psychosomatic Medicine*, 1973, *35*, 484–496.

Cobb, J. C., & Shor, R. E. *Development of techniques to maximize hypnotic responsiveness*. Paper presented at the Meeting of the Eastern Psychological Association, Philadelphia, April 1964.

Culpan, R., & Davies, B. Psychiatric illness at a medical and surgical outpatient clinic. *Comprehensive Psychiatry*, 1960, *1*, 228–235.

Cummings, N. A. The anatomy of psychotherapy under National Health Insurance. *American Psychologist*, 1977, *32*, 711–718.

Dave, R. Effects of hypnotically induced dreams on creative problem solving. *Journal of Abnormal Psychology*, 1979, *88*, 293–302.

DePiano, F. A., & Salzberg, H. C. Clinical applications of hypnosis to three psychosomatic disorders. *Psychological Bulletin*, 1979, *86*, 1223–1235.

Dumas, R. A., & Spitzer, S. E. Influences of subject self-selection on the EEG alpha-hypnotizability correlation. *Psychophysiology*, 1978, *15*,(6) 606–608.

Edmonston, W. E. *Hypnosis and relaxation*. New York: Wiley, 1981.

Ellis, A. *Reason and emotion in psychotherapy*. New York: Lyle Stuart, 1962.

Engstrom, D. R. Hypnotic susceptibility, EEG-alpha and self regulation. In G. E. Schwartz & D. Shapiro (Eds.), *Consciousness and self-regulation*. New York: Plenum Press, 1976.

Evans, F. J. Hypnosis and sleep: Techniques for exploring cognitive activity during sleep. In E. Fromm & R. E. Shor (Eds.), *Hypnosis: Research developments and perspectives*. Chicago: Aldine, 1972.

Evans, F. J. The placebo response in pain reduction. In J. J. Bonica (Ed.), *Advances in Neurology: Vol. 4. Pain*. New York: Raven Press, 1974.

Eysenck, H. J., & Furneaux, W. D. Primary and secondary suggestibility: An experimental and statistical study. *Journal of Experimental Psychology*, *35*, 1945, 485–503.

Ferguson, P. C., & Gowan, J. *The influence of transcendental meditation on anxiety, depression, aggression, neuroticism, & self-actualization*. Paper presented at California State Psychological Association, Fresno, California, February, 1974.

Frank, J. D. *Persuasion and healing*. Baltimore: Johns Hopkins Press, 1965.

Freud, S. *Collected papers* (Vol. 1). New York: Basic Books, 1959.

Fromm, E. Quo vadis hypnosis? Predictions of future trends in hypnosis research. In E. Fromm & R. E. Shor (Eds.), *Hypnosis: Research developments and perspectives*. Chicago: Aldine, 1972.

Fromm, E., Bopxer, A. M., Brown, D. P., Hurt, S. W., Oberlander, J. Z. *The phenomena and characteristics of self-hypnosis*. Unpublished manuscript, 1981.

Goldstein, A. P. *Therapist–patient expectancies in psychotherapy*. New York: Pergamon Press, 1962.

Green, A., Green, E., & Walters, D. *Psychological training for creativity*. Paper presented at the meeting of the American Psychological Association, Washington, D.C., September, 1971.

Hebb, D. O. *A textbook of psychology*. Philadelphia: W. B. Saunders, 1966.

Herzfeld, G., & Taub, E. Suggestion as an aid to self-regulation of hand temperature. *International Journal of Neuroscience*, 1977, *8*, 23–26.

Hilgard, E. R., & Hilgard, J. R. *Hypnosis in the relief of pain*. Los Altos: William Kaufman, 1975.

Hilgard, E. R. *Hypnotic susceptibility*. New York: Harcourt, Brace & World, 1965.

Hilgard, J. R. *Personality and hypnosis: A study of imaginative involvement*. Chicago: University of Chicago Press, 1970.

Hilkevitch, A. Psychiatric disturbances in outpatients of a general medical outpatient clinic. *International Journal of Neuropsychiatry*, 1965, *1*, 371–375.

Hinkle, L. E. Ecological observations on the relation of physcial illness, mental illness and social environment. *Psychosomatic Medicine*, 1961, *23*, 289–296.

Hull, C. L. *Hypnosis and suggestibility: An experimental approach*. New York: Appleton Century, 1933.

Jacobson, E. *Modern treatments of tense patients*. Springfield, IL: Charles C Thomas, 1970.

Johnson, L. S. Self-hypnosis: Behavioral and phenomenological comparisons with heterohypnosis. *International Journal of Clinical and Experimental Hypnosis*, 1979, *27*, 240–246.

Johnson, L. Current research in self-hypnotic pneuomenology: The Chicago paradigm. *International Journal of Clinical and Experimental Hypnosis*, 1981, *29*, 247–258.

Kazdin, A. E., & Wilcoxon, L. A. Systematic desensitization and non-specific treatment effects: A methodological evaluation. *Psychological Bulletin*, 1976, *83*, 729–758.

Kazdin, A. E. Therapy outcome questions requiring control of credibility and treatment-generated expectancies. *Behavior Therapy*, 1979, *10*, 81–93.

Knowles, J. H. Responsibility for health. *Science*, 1977, *198*, 4322.

Kris, E. On preconscious mental processes. In D. Rapaport (Ed.), *Organization and pathology of thought*. New York: Columbia University Press, 1951.

Larsen, S. Strategies for reducing phobic behavior. *Dissertation Abstracts*, 1966, *26*, 6850.

Lazarus, R. S. *Psychological stress and the coping process*. New York: McGraw-Hill, 1966.

Leva, R. A. Performance of low-susceptibility Ss on Stanford Profile Scales after sensory deprivation. *Psychological Reports*, 1974, *34*, 835–838.

Levitt, E. E., Brady, J. P., Ottinger, D., & Hinesley, R. Effects of sensory restriction on hypnotizability. *Archives of General Psychiatry*, 1962, *17*, 343–345.

Lick, J., & Bootzin, R. Expectancy factors in the treatment of fear: Methodological and theoretical issues. *Psychological Bulletin*, 1975, *82*, 917–931.

Lilly, J. C. Mental effects of reduction of ordinary levels of physical stimuli on intact, healthy persons. *Psychiatric Research Report*, 1956, *5*, 1–9.

Lindsley, D. B. Psychophysiology and motivation. In M. R. Jones (Ed.), *Nebraska Symposium on Motivation*. Lincoln: University of Nebraska Press, 1957.

Ludwig, A. M. Altered states of consciousness. In C. T. Tart (Ed.), *Altered states of consciousness*. New York: Wiley, 1969.

MacDonald, H. *The effect of frontalis EMG biofeedback relaxation training on hypnotizability*. Paper presented at the Western Psychological Association annual meeting, April 1978.

Mandler, G. *Mind and emotion*. New York: Wiley, 1975.

Mason, J. A re-evaluation of the concept of "non-specificity" in stress theory. *Journal of Psychiatric Research*, 1976, *8*, 323–333.

Melzack, R., & Perry, C. Self-regulation of pain, use of alpha feedback and hypnotic training for the control of chronic pain. *Experimental Neurology*, 1975, 46, 452–469.

Orne, M. T. On the social psychology of the psychological experiment with particular reference to demand characteristics and their implications. *American Psychologist*, 1962, 17, 776–783.

Orne, M. T. Pain suppression by hypnosis and related phenomena. In J. J. Bonica (Ed.), *Advances in neurology: Vol. 4. Pain*. New York: Raven Press, 1974.

Paul, G. L. *Insight versus desensitization in psychotherapy*. Stanford: Stanford University Press, 1966.

Paul, G. L. Inhibition of physiological response to stressful imagery by relaxation training and hypnotically suggested relaxation. *Behaviour Research and Therapy*, 1969, 7, 249–256.

Pena, F. *Perceptual isolation and hypnotic susceptibility*. Unpublished doctoral dissertation, Washington State University, 1963.

Perry, C., Gelfand, R., & Marcovitch, P. The relevance of hypnotic susceptibility in the clinical context. *Journal of Abnormal Psychology*, 1979, 88, 592–603.

Radtke, L. H., Spanos, N. P., Armstrong, L. A., Dillman, N., & Boisvenue, M. E. Effects of electromyographic feedback and progressive relaxation training on hypnotic susceptibility: Disconfirming results. *International Journal of Clinical and Experimental Hypnosis*, 1983, 21, 98–105.

Raikov, V. L. The possibility of creativity in the active stage of hypnosis. *International Journal of Clinical and Experimental Hypnosis*, 1976, 3, 258–268.

Rasmussen, J. (Ed.). *Man in isolation and confinement*. Chicago: Aldine, 1973.

Roberts, A. H., Kewman, D. G., & MacDonald, H. *Voluntary control of skin temperature: Unilateral changes using hypnosis and auditory feedback*. Paper presented at Biofeedback Society meeting, Boston, March, 1972.

Rogers, M. P., Devendara, D., & Reich, P. The influence of the psyche and the brain on immunity and disease susceptibility: A critical review. *Psychosomatic Medicine*, 1979, 41, 147–164.

Ruch, J. C. Self-hypnosis: The result of heterohypnosis or vice versa? *International Journal of Clinical Experimental Hypnosis*, 1975, 23, 282–304.

Sanders, R. S., & Rehyer, J. Sensory deprivation and the enhancement of hypnotic susceptibility. *Journal of Abnormal Psychology*, 1969, 74, 375–381.

Sarbin, T. R., & Slagle, R. W. Hypnosis and psychophysiological outcomes. In E. Fromm & R. E. Shor (Eds.), *Hypnosis: Research developments and perspectives*. Chicago: Aldine, 1972.

Saward, E., & Sorenson, A. The current emphasis on preventive medicine. *Science*, 1978, 200, 889–894.

Schachtel, E. G. *Metamorphosis: On the development of affect, perception, attention, and memory*. New York: Basic Books, 1959.

Schachter, S. The interaction of cognitive and physiological determinants of emotional state. In C. D. Speilberger (Ed.), *Anxiety and behavior*. New York: Academic Press, 1966.

Schubot, E. D. *The influence of hypnotic and muscular relaxation in systematic desensitization of phobias*. Unpublished doctoral dissertation, Stanford University, 1966.

Schultz, J. H., & Luthe, W. *Autogenic training*. New York: Grune & Stratton, 1959.

Shapiro, A. Placebo effects in medicine, psychotherapy, and psychoanalysis. In A. Bergin & S. Garfield (Eds.), *Handbook of psychotherapy and behavior change*. New York: Wiley, 1971.

Smith, R. J. Study finds sleeping pills overprescribed. *Science*, 1979, 204, 287–288.

Spiegel, H. A single-treatment method to stop smoking using ancillary self-hypnosis. In I. Wickramasekera (Ed.), *Biofeedback, behavior therapy, and hypnosis.* Chicago: Nelson-Hall, 1976.

Springer, C. J., Sachs, L. B., & Morrow, J. E. Group methods of increasing hypnotic susceptibility. *International Journal of Clinical and Experimental Hypnosis,* 1977, *25,* 184–191.

Strupp, H., & Bergin, A. E. *Changing frontiers in the science of psychotherapy.* Chicago: Aldine, 1972.

Suedfeld, P. *Restricted environmental stimulation.* New York: Wiley, 1980.

Suedfeld, P. Changes in intellectual performance and in susceptibility to influence. In J. P. Zubeck (Ed.), *Sensory deprivation: Fifteen years of research.* New York: Appleton-Century-Crofts, 1969.

Surwit, R. S., Pilon, R. N., & Fenton, C. H. Behavioral treatment of Raynaud's disease. *Journal of Behavioral Medicine, 1,* 323–335.

Szasz, T. S. The myth of mental illness. *American Psychologist,* 1960, *15,* 113–118.

Tart, C. L. Introduction. In C. L. Tart (Ed.), *Altered states of consciousness.* New York: Wiley, 1969.

Valliant, G. E. Natural history of male psychological health: IV. What kinds of men do not get psychosomatic illness. *Psychosomatic Medicine,* 1978, *40,* 420–431.

Wallace, R. K., & Benson, H. The physiology of meditation. *Scientific American,* 1972, *226*(2) 84.

Weiner, H. *Psychobiology and human disease.* New York: Elsevier, 1977.

Weitzenhoffer, A. M. *General techniques of hypnotism.* New York: Grune & Stratton, 1957.

Whatmore, G. B., & Kohli, D. R. *The physiopathology and treatment of functional disorders.* New York: Grune & Stratton, 1974.

Wickramasekera, I. Effects of sensory restriction on susceptibility to hypnosis. *International Journal of Clinical and Experimental Hypnosis,* 1969, *17,* 217–224.

Wickramasekera, I. Effects of sensory restriction on susceptibility to hypnosis: A hypothesis and more preliminary data. *Journal of Abnormal Psychology,* 1970, *76,* 69–75.

Wickramasekera, I. Effects of EMG feedback training on susceptibility to hypnosis. In J. Stoyva, T. Barber, L. V. Dicara, J. Kamiya, N. E. Miller, & D. Shapiro (Eds.), *Biofeedback and self-control.* Chicago: Aldine, 1971.

Wickramasekera, I. EMG feedback and tension headache. *American Journal of Clinical Hypnosis,* 1972, *15,* 83–85.

Wickramasekera, I. Effects of EMG feedback on hypnotic susceptibility. *Journal of Abnormal Psychology,* 1973, *82,* 74–77. (a)

Wickramasekera, I. Temperature feedback for the control of migraine. *Journal of Behavior Therapy and Experimental Psychiatry,* 1973, *4,* 343–345. (b)

Wickramasekera, I. Application of verbal instructions and EMG feedback training to the management of tension headache. *Headache,* 1973, *13,* 74–76. (c)

Wickramasekera, I. Heart rate feedback and the management of cardiac neurosis. *Journal of Abnormal Psychology,* 1974, *83,* 578–580.

Wickramasekera, I. (Ed.), *Biofeedback, behavior therapy and hypnosis: Potentiating the verbal control of behavior of clinicians.* Chicago: Nelson-Hall, 1976.

Wickramasekera, I. The placebo effect and biofeedback for headache pain. *Proceedings of the San Diego Biomedical Symposium.* New York: Academic Press, 1977. (a)

Wickramasekera, I. On attempts to modify hypnotic susceptibility: Some psychophysiological procedures and promising directions. *Annals of the New York Academy of Sciences,* 1977, *296,* 143–153. (b)

Wickramasekera, I. A conditioned response model of the placebo effect: Predictions from the model. *Biofeedback and self-regulation*, 1980, *5*, 5–17.

Wickramasekera, I., Paskewitz, D., & Taube, E. *Do beliefs have biological consequences?* Paper presented at a symposium of the Biofeedback Society of America, San Diego, March, 1979.

Wolff, H. G. *Headache and other pain.* New York: Oxford University Press, 1963.

Wolpe, J. *The practice of behavior therapy.* New York: Pergamon Press, 1973.

Woolfolk, R., & Lehrer, P. *Principles and practice of stress management.* New York: Guilford Press, 1984.

Zimbardo, P., Maslach, C., & Marshall, G. Hypnosis and the psychology of cognitive and behavioral control. In E. Fromm & R. E. Shor (Eds.), *Hypnosis: Research developments and perspectives.* Chicago: Aldine, 1972.

Zubek, J. P. (Ed.), *Sensory deprivation: Fifteen years of research.* New York: Appleton-Century-Crofts, 1969.

Zukerman, M., & Cohen, N. Is suggestion the source of reported visual sensations in perceptual isolation? *Journal of Abnormal and Social Psychology*, 1964, *68*, 655–660.

APPENDIXES

A

PROBLEMS WITH HYPNOSIS AND CRUCIAL CLINICAL CONCEPTS

1. Hypnosis is generally a very safe procedure with voluntary patients, people without a psychiatric history, and with medical patients with circumscribed problems like acute pain, anxiety about specific medical procedures, and so forth. Complications (headaches, resistance, anxiety, disorientation) are likely to occur only if you are using hypnosis to alter some critical general life style issue or habit (e.g., smoking, obesity, chronic pain, posthypnotic suggestions for personality change or memory alterations) that may be important to the patient (e.g., secondary gain). Generally, patients who are acutely psychotic, paranoid, or very depressed are unlikely to be responsive to hypnosis unless you can capture and hold their attention and trust.

2. Of people who take a course in hypnosis only approximately 25% of them will still use hypnosis with any frequency 1 year later. One of the primary reasons for this is unreinforced practice. If you initially only use hypnosis with people with moderate- to high-hypnotic ability you are more likely to be using hypnosis 1 year from now. Assessing your patients hypnotic ability up front will enable you to pick patients who are more likely to profit from a hypnotic procedure and will ensure that your hypnotic behaviors are reinforced. Patients who are low in hypnotic ability are candidates for biofeedback or relaxation training. Some patients of high-hypnotic ability should initially be approached only with biofeedback or progressive muscular relaxation exercises if they are initially fearful or suspicious of the label and procedures of hypnosis.

3. Approximately 0.1% of people who take a course in hypnosis stop whatever else they were doing before (medicine, clinical psychology, OB-GYN, etc.) and limit their practice exclusively to hypnosis. Such practitioners should be viewed with caution. It is likely that the illusions of hypnosis are feeding some latent psychotic or characterological needs (power, control, intimacy) in them. Hypnosis is a reactive procedure (it alters the practitioner) and can bring out latent psychopathology in therapists. It is important for the hypnotist to ask himself who is hypnotizing who?

4. The dangers in hypnosis are in the hypnotist not in hypnosis *per se*. A sharp

knife can heal or hurt, depending on who (e.g., a surgeon or butcher) is holding the knife.

5. Skill in the induction of hypnosis is simple and easily learned. Once the trance is induced what one does with it is a function of professional knowledge, skill, and expertise. Hypnosis is like an empty syringe. What you put into the syringe is a function of matching professional knowledge and diagnosis of the patient's specific problem (etiology, psychodynamic, behavioral analysis, etc.) to specific therapeutic remedies. Hence, a broad knowledge of psychotherapy, pathophysiology, psychophysiology, psychopathology, and human behavior are very relevant to hypnotherapy.

6. Everything that occurs in counseling and psychotherapy occurs in hypnosis, only much more rapidly. Hence, the hypnotherapist should first have broad training in psychotherapy, its phenomena and in psychopathology. Because he travels faster, the hypnotherapist should know the road well and have plenty of skill in driving. Otherwise, he should take the Pinto and leave the Ferrari in the garage. Collision at high speed is more likely to be messy and painful.

7. The hypnotherapist should daily examine and clean up his motivations and soul. He should always ask himself who is hypnotizing who? You cannot both be out to lunch, somebody should be watching the store.

8. Constructs crucial to hypnosis are: the unconscious, transference, dissociation, and desynchrony.

B

BRIEF PROCEDURES TO ASSESS
HYPNOTIC ABILITY AND ATTITUDE

Hypnotic experience and behavior are a function of two components: hypnotic ability and a hypnotically receptive attitude. Hypnotic ability is the more salient of these variables and will be discussed first. Hypnotic ability is not significantly correlated with any known personality variable. It is now clear that hypnotic ability is a subject variable that has important clinical implications for both therapy outcome and vulnerability to the development of stress-related mental and physical disorders. Hence, it is both clinically and theoretically useful to secure a valid and reliable measure of this subject variable even if hypnosis *per se* is never used in therapy. Generally about 60% of superior hypnotic subjects and only 3% of low-hypnotic ability subjects can significantly alter pain perception. Ideally such a measure should also be brief, nonreactive, simple to administer and unobtrusive to ensure its maximal utility in clinical practice. A nonreactive hypnotic measure will be uncontaminated by patient's attitudes and beliefs about hypnosis.

In fact the simplest, briefest and least reactive and unobtrusive (covert) procedure, the "Eye-Roll sign," has the lowest validity. At the other end of the spectrum is the SHALIT (Hilgard, Crawford, & Wert, 1979) which has satisfactory validity, and reliability, is brief (6 min) and simple to administer but which is transparently a test of hypnotic ability. Hence it is both a reactive and obvious test of hypnotic ability.

The eye-roll (ER) sign is hypothesized to be a biological marker of the capacity to experience hypnosis. The ER is determined from the amount of sclera (white part of eye) visible between the lower border of the iris and the lower eyelid when the patient looks upward as high as possible and slowly closes his eyelids. Spiegel (1972) himself reported this sign to be a false positive indicator of hypnotic capacity 25% of the time and that this false positive rate may be due to some type of "attentional impairment" (e.g., situational, psychopathological, neurologic). Hilgard (1982) and others have empirically challenged the validity of this clinically useful sign. But there are several empirical studies (Frischholz, Fisher, Spiegel, Tryon, Vellois, & Maruffi, 1980) supporting the continued cautious use of it in clinical practice. For example, one study (Frischholz *et al.*, 1980) found a significant correlation of 0.44 between the ER sign and the Stanford

Scale Form C and a separate analysis found a significant correlation of 0.49 between the ER sign and the Stanford Form C. I have found the ER sign a clinically useful screening device on which we continue to collect data (see Figure 30).

The ability to accurately estimate a patient's hypnotic ability covertly and nonreactively has great value in clinical practice. First, because it enables the clinician who knows the scientific literature of hypnosis to make many accurate predictions and postdictions about a specific patient in the initial sessions. The therapist's knowledge of the base rates of certain experiences and potential behaviors (you can wake up without an alarm at a preselected time, you are likely to cry at movies, you can fall asleep easily in a variety of places, you spend time in fantasy, you had transitional objects in childhood) in people of high- and low-hypnotic ability may grasp the patient's attention and interest, enhancing the therapist's social-influence value in the critical first few sessions of therapy. A therapist's enhanced attention value may potentiate his ability to influence the patient's past and present perceptions. Clinical lore and empirical research have confirmed the critical importance of the first few therapy sessions for positive therapy outcome. The subtle therapist who can make uncannily accurate predictive and postdictive statements to a patient early in therapy enhances the therapist's stimulus value, even if he or she never uses hypnosis in therapy. The patient feels quickly understood. The patient is likely to see the therapist as having specialized knowledge and being trustworthy. A patient is more likely to follow the instructions of such a therapist. A sense of hope, trust, and mystery is sometimes a prerequisite to mobilize a demoralized patient. This sense of strength and mystery can be used to mobilize a patient to take the initial steps to become an active participant in his or her own rehabilitation.

Second, it is useful to know to what extent your patient typically uses the hypnotic mode of information processing in everyday life. It is important to elicit this information without exposing the patient to the prospect of failure on a hypnosis test. This information is useful even if you never label the interventions you use as "hypnotic." For the patient who easily and often uses the hypnotic mode of information processing, the prescription and administration of, for example, an active medication can be a type of neutral "waking" hypnotic induction. The ritual of prescription writing and delivery can be used to secure eye contact with the patient and to give direct clear and simple verbal suggestions to potentiate the effects of even small quantities of, for example, sleep, pain, or antianxiety medication. In the case of the patient who accesses the hypnotic mode easily (high-hypnotic ability patients) special care should be taken in interview and communication to avoid inadvertently delivering negative suggestions or to cause iatrogenic illness. If negatively engaged, the patient of high hypnotic ability can be a formidable antagonist; one who is creatively resistant, unpleasant, and very difficult to deal with; one who can frustrate the best efforts and clinical efficacy of chemical and surgical procedures of scientifically demonstrated potency. The ability to match clinical procedures (e.g., autogenic training, meditation, progressive muscular relaxation, twilight learning, biofeedback, sensory restriction) to receiver characteristics (patient vari-

Name: _____Sex: M   F

Age: _____Date: _____Hand: L   R   Amb

SPIEGEL EYE-ROLL TEST FOR HYPNOTIZABILITY

Eye-roll test (squint)   Eye-roll test for hypnotizability

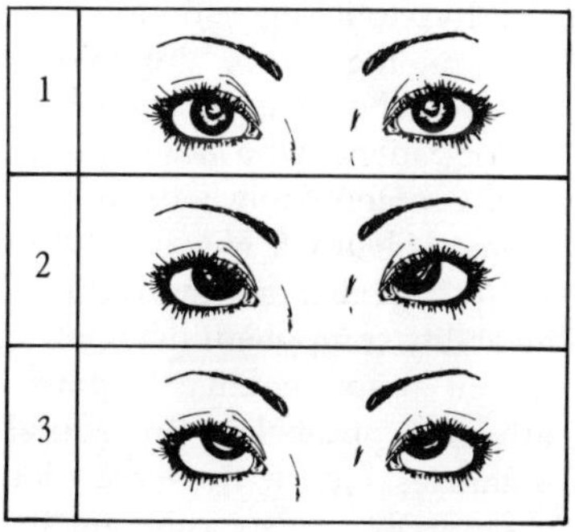

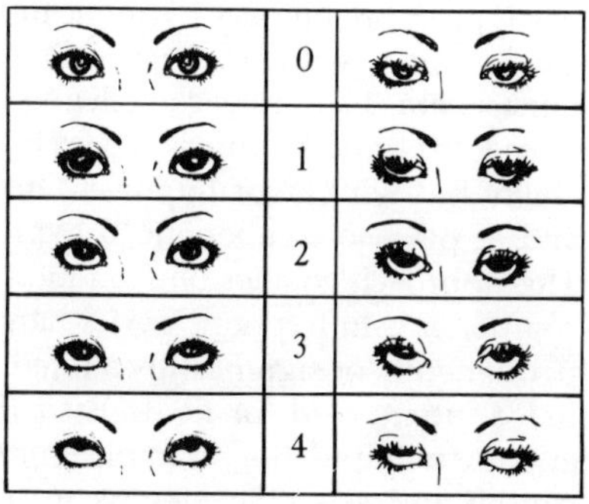

Total score = Up-gaze + roll + squint

_____ = _____ + _____ + ____

1. Hold your head looking straight forward.
2. While holding your head in that position, look upward toward your eyebrows—now, toward the top of your head (up-gaze).
3. While continuing to look upward, at the same time close your eyelids slowly (roll).
4. Now open your eyes and let your eyes come back into focus.

Figure 30. The Spiegel Eye-Roll Test for Hypnotizability.

ables) may have practical value (Zillmer & Wickramasekera, 1987). It is more heuristic to match patients to procedures rooted in empirical research on established mechanisms and process variables, rather than on labels and theories. For example, a patient who has good hypnotic ability, but is technologically and quantitatively minded and skeptical of hypnosis *per se* (negative hypnotic attitude), should be a good candidate for "delayed biofeedback." Delayed biofeedback involves verbally instructing the patient to relax and withholding for example immediate EMG feedback. But providing the feedback after 2–3 minutes of delay, either visually (on a strip chart recorder) or digitally, as an integrated average of a time period. It is replicated finding that immediate auditory EMG feedback initially interferes with relaxation learning of good hypnotic subjects (Qualls & Sheehan, 1981). I have found that delayed quantitative (e.g., EMG strip chart data) feedback provides high credibility confirmation of the good hypnotic subject's natural ability to manipulate his physiology. In fact, it does so in a manner that has high credibility for the hypnotically skeptical person, thus motivating him to further practice and refine his relaxation skill. Labeling the procedure "delayed biofeedback" enables the therapist to still access instructionally the patient's hypnotic ability, but to avoid the likely mobilization of the patient's skepticism and resistance if the *label* hypnosis had been used. The patient with low hypnotic ability has been shown to learn to drop his frontal EMG signal (relaxation) most rapidly with immediate EMG biofeedback (Qualls & Sheehan, 1981). If a patient with low-measured-hypnotic ability has a strongly positive attitude toward hypnosis, the biofeedback procedure may be presented as a type of preliminary hypnotic induction. In fact, hypnotic suggestions can be given along with the immediate biofeedback training procedure (Wickramasekera, 1976) thus capitalizing on the separate placebo components of both biofeedback and hypnosis. There is evidence that for patients who lack hypnotic ability but who favor hypnosis, there may still be a potentiating motivational and/or placebo component to hypnotic suggestions (Hilgard & Hilgard, 1975). This approach enables one to rationally utilize both the ability and motivational components in hypnotic performance. While the ability component may not be permanently or significantly altered, the motivational component may be potentiated, attenuated, or neutralized through creative use of labeling procedures and the manipulation of implicit or explicit expectancies. Hence, there are good clinical and scientific reasons to nonreactively or unobtrusively estimate the hypnotic ability of a patient.

Third, if a patient is found to have low-hypnotic ability but has a positive attitude toward hypnosis, there is some evidence that certain psychophysiological procedures may at least temporarily increase hypnotic ability. In fact, these pretreatment procedures may be indicated for the majority of patients, because only about 10% of the population has high-hypnotic ability. These procedures include sensory restriction, alpha and EMG feedback training, and theta feedback training. All these psychophysiological procedures, which are the pretreatment procedures of choice for all patients with low-hypnotic ability, probably work through temporarily changing the patient's level of physiological arousal and inducing a relative inhibition of critical analytic brain functions.

Practically, then, one should start by making two assessments. First, determine with a simple visual analogue rating scale how positively, neutrally or negatively the patient feels about hypnosis, and how much hypnotic ability (high, moderate, or low) the patient thinks he or she has. Positive attitudes toward hypnosis and self-predictions of hypnotic ability have been found to modestly predict hypnotic performance. If the patient has a negative attitude toward hypnosis the specific sources of the negativity should be investigated. For example, is it based on misinformation (fear of unconsciousness, "afraid I will blurt out personal or private information," only the weak-minded can be hypnotized, absolute hypnotist control of subject in the hypnotic state) or a negative personal experience with hypnosis. These negative attitudes can often be at least neutralized by counterinformation from high credibility sources. Second, it is necessary to get a valid and reliable unobtrusive measure of hypnotic ability. This measure could be used to enhance the therapist's stimulus value through therapist statements that seem uncannily accurate in a predictive and/or postdictive sense, even if hypnotic procedures are never used with the patient. In the event that the patient has low- or high-hypnotic ability clinical interventions can be planned more economically and rationally than if the information on hypnotic ability was unavailable. For example, pretreatment procedures are redundant with high-hypnotic ability subjects.

Currently there are no well-established, valid and reliable, brief, and covert measures of hypnotic ability. But there are several promising signs and brief verbal procedures that can be used in a clinical research context to covertly and nonreactively estimate a patient's hypnotic ability. When several of these signs and procedures are positive, I have greater confidence in the prediction of individual hypnotic ability.

References

Bakan, P. Hypnotizability, laterality of eye movement and functional brain asymmetry. *Perceptual and Motor Skills*, 1969, *28*, 927–932.

Day, M. E. An eye-movement phenomenon relating to attention, thought, and anxiety. *Perceptual and Motor Skills*, 1964, *19*, 443–446.

Ehrlichman, H., & Weinberger, A. Lateral eye movements and hemispheric asymmetry: A critical review. *Psychological Bulletin*, 1978, *85*, 1080–1101.

Engstrom, D. R. Hypnotic susceptibility, EEG-alpha and self-regulation. In G. E. Schwartz & D. Shapiro (Eds.), *Consciousness and self-regulation*. New York: Plenum Press, 1976.

Frischholz, E. J., Fisher, S., Spiegel, H., Tryon, W. W., Vellios, A. T., & Maruffi, B. L. The relationship between the hypnotic induction profile and the Stanford Hypnotic Susceptibility Scale, Form C: A replication. *American Journal of Clinical Hypnosis*, 1980, *22*, 185–196.

Gur, R. C., and Gur, R. E. Handedness, sex, and eyedness as moderating variables in the relation between hypnotic susceptibility and functional brain asymmetry. *Journal of Abnormal Psychology*, 1974, *83*, 635–643.

Hilgard, E. R. Illusion: The eye-roll sign is related to hypnotizability. *Archives of General Psychiatry*, 1982, *39*, 963–966.

Hilgard, E. R., & Hilgard, J. R. *Hypnosis in the relief of pain*, (Vol. 1). Los Altos, CA: Kaufmann, 1975.

Hilgard, E. R., Crawford, H. J., & Wert, A. The Stanford Hypnotic Arm Levitation Induction and Test (SHALIT): A six minute hypnotic induction and measurement scale. *International Journal of Clinical and Experimental Hypnosis*, 1979, *27*, 111–124.

Morgan, A. H., McDonald, P. J., & MacDonald, H. Differences in bilateral alpha activity as a function of experimental task with a note on lateral eye movements and hypnotizability. *Neuropsychologia*, 1971, *9*, 459–469.

Perry, C., & Laurence, J. R. Hypnotic depth and hypnotic susceptibility: A replicated finding. *International Journal of Clinical and Experimental Hypnosis*, *28*, 272–280.

Perry, C., & Laurence, J. R. Montreal norms for the Harvard Group Scale of Hypnotic Susceptibility, Form A. *International Journal of Clinical and Experimental Hypnosis*, 1982, *30*, 167–176.

Qualls, P. J., & Sheehan, P. W. Electromyograph biofeedback as a relaxation technique: A critical appraisal and reassessment. *Psychological Bulletin*, 1981, *90*(1), 21–42.

Spiegel, H. An eye-roll test for hypnotizability. *American Journal of Clinical Hypnosis*, 1972, *15*(1), 25–28.

Teitelbaum, H. A. Spontaneous rhythmic ocular movements: Their possible relationship to mental activity. *Newcology*, 1954, *4*, 350–354.

Tellegen, A. & Atkinson, G. Openness to absorbing and self-altering experiences ("absorption"), a trait related to hypnotic susceptibility. *Journal of Abnormal Psychology*, 1974, *83*, 268–277.

Wickramasekera, I. Effects of EMG feedback training on susceptibility to hypnosis: preliminary observations. *Proceedings of the 70th Annual Convention of the American Psychological Association*, 1971, *6*, 787–795, (summary).

Wickramasekera, I. The effects of EMG feedback on hypnotic susceptibility: More preliminary data. *Journal of Abnormal Psychology*, 1973, *82*, 74–77.

Wickramasekera, I. (Ed.) *Biofeedback, behavior therapy, and hypnosis.* Chicago: Nelson-Hall, 1976.

Wickramasekera, I. Development of a self-report measure of hypnotic ability: Preliminary findings. Paper presented at the 16th Annual Meeting of the Biofeedback Society of America, New Orleans, 1985.

Wilson, S. C. & Barber, T. X. The fantasy-prone personality: Implications for understanding imagery, hypnosis, and parapsychological phenomena. In A. A. Sheikh (Ed.), *Imagery: Current therapy research and application.* New York: Wiley, 1982.

Zillmer, E. A. & Wickramasekera, I. Biofeedback and hypnotizability: Initial treatment considerations. *Clinical Biofeedback and Health*, 1987, *10*(1), 26–33.

C

UNOBTRUSIVE PROCEDURES

The first two unobtrusive procedures presented to estimate hypnotic ability will be psychophysiological ones. Such procedures appear objective, quantitative, and are potentially high credibility sources of information for patients.

Low Frontal EMG with Eyes Closed

Since the early 1970s, (Wickramasekera, 1971, 1973, 1976) we have observed a subset of patients who show a marked discrepancy in their frontal EMG with eyes open and eyes closed (not asleep). In the eyes closed condition, when asked to relax, there is a significant and rapid drop in the frontal EMG in the absence of any present or prior verbal relaxation training or feedback training. Most of these people who can rapidly drop frontal EMG without prior training turn out to have moderate- to high-hypnotic ability. We have found that immediate EMG feedback for these subjects only interferes with their natural ability to further drop the frontal EMG signal. But that delayed feedback (after 2 or 3 minutes trial) that objectively confirmed their subjective experience of relaxation, is strongly motivating and is adequate to refine their development of a reliable physiological relaxation skill. The observation of a correlation between the ability to rapidly drop the frontal EMG signal and subsequently measured good hypnotic ability lead me to predict and test the hypothesis (Wickramasekera, 1971, 1973) that people who were trained to drop their frontal EMG would at least *temporarily* increase in hypnotic ability. A recent study which failed to replicate my observations did not control for the skill of the biofeedback trainer.

In the clinical situation we often observed patients who were initially quite resistant to psychosocial influence procedures (e.g., psychotherapy, behavior therapy) become increasingly receptive as their ability to lower their frontal EMG increased, almost as if they were removing body armor. We assumed that reducing muscle tension in at least the upper part of the body seemed to reduce defensiveness and increase the patients openness to fresh ways of perceiving problems in living. Wilson and Barber (1982) have recently reported that all of a subset of superior hypnotic subjects who were also in clinical or experimental biofeedback were found to report a superior ability to control several biological functions. In summary, then, it appears that at least the ability to rapidly and reliably drop frontal EMG may be related in some subjects to superior hypnotic ability.

EEG Alpha Density and Hypnotic Ability

It appears that the ease with which alpha density can be increased by a subject predicts how easily the subject will enter hypnosis (Engstrom, 1976). These studies have mostly measured alpha recorded from a single occipital site. Paskewitz has confirmed these findings of a moderate relationship between EEG alpha density and hypnotic ability. He suggests that the relationship will hold best for "alpha dynamics" rather than "alpha level *per se.*" This means that volitional changes in alpha density under varied conditions of situational stimulation will be the best predictor of cognitive hypnotic ability as measured by SHSS Forms C. Practically, the proportion of the time that the EEG alpha rhythm (8–12 cPS) appears will roughly predict cognitive hypnotic ability. Subjects who are high on "imagery" items are particularly likely to show good alpha base rates. Subjects who show a higher proportion of alpha both in and out of hypnosis will be found to be better hypnotic subjects. In conclusion, it is worth noting that a recent review by Evans questions the validity of a straightforward and simple relationship between hypnosis and alpha density.

The Conjugate Lateral Eye Movement Test

In a face-to-face situation, individuals typically move their eyes either to the left or right before answering a question requiring reflective thought and most individuals have a preferred direction of eye movement in the above situation. The initial observations of individual consistency in conjugate lateral eye movement (CLEM) was made by Teitelbaum (1954) and Day (1964). It has since been extensively tested and is now well established (Ehrlichman and Weinberger, 1978). It appears that the majority of the population (70%) have a consistent preference for either left or right eye movement during reflective thought, but that about 30% do not have a consistent preference. First, the interrater reliability of CLEM responses using both live and recorded (videotape) observation is quite high ($r = 0.96$). Second, split-half reliability of responses to items administered in the *same session* is also high ($r = 0.83$). *Between sessions* it ranges between $r = 0.65$ to 0.78. *Across situations* (face-to-face versus videotape monitoring) the CLEM response is also stable ($r = 0.77$). The above empirical findings are secure, independent of any inferences about (a) hemispheric activation or (b) the psychological correlates of CLEM. It is also important to note that there is as yet no independent EEG evidence that the stimulus questions used in CLEM studies differentially activate the left and right hemispheres. (See Figure 31.)

The discovery of reliable psychological correlates of left and right CLEMs makes it a clinically useful psychological test independent of any assumption about hemispheric activation. The association between left or right CLEM and certain psychological features is somewhat less secure than the CLEM phe-

THE CONJUGATE LATERAL EYE MOVEMENT TEST

	R	L	S	↑	↓
1					
2					
3					
4					
5					
6					
7					

CLEM: Hypothesis: Direction of eye movement is a consequence of asymmetrical activation of contralateral hemisphere.

SHSS = 0   SHSS = 12

1. VE: When you picture your father's face, what emotion (feelings) strikes you first? (visual, emotional)
2. VNE: On the face of a quarter does G. Washington's face look to the right or left? (visual, nonemotional)
3. VE: For you, is anger or hate a stronger emotion? (verbal, emotional)
4. VNE: What is the primary difference between the words recognize and remember? (verbal, nonemotional)
5. How many edges (sides) on a cube? (spatial)
6. If a person is facing the rising sun, on which side of the person is south (where is south in respect to the person)? (spatial)
7. Al is smarter than Sam. Al is duller than Rick. Who is the smartest? Rick (verbal)

Figure 31. The Conjugate Lateral Eye Movement Test (CLEM): A working format.

nomena itself. Several investigations have found that a preponderance (over 70%) of left CLEMs are associated with superior hypnotic ability (Bakan, 1969; Gur & Gur, 1974; Morgan, McDonald, & MacDonald, 1971). This relationship between hypnotic ability and left CLEMs is most secure only for right-handed males. Indirectly related findings pertinent to left CLEMs are: (a) left CLEMs are more involved with feelings and "inner" experience; (b) left CLEMs are more strongly related to "inner attentiveness"; (c) they are associated with more psychosomatic symptoms and more frequent use of defenses like repression, reaction formation, and denial; (d) left CLEMs are more responsive to persuasion; (e) children who are left movers were likely to use more adjectives than nouns; (f) two studies have found that emotionally laden questions elicit more left CLEMs; and (g) one study found that right-handed males with left CLEMs were superior both before and after training on a visceral-self perception task (heart beat discrimination) to R-CLEMs. These observations are clear and reliable. The apparent consistency of this pattern of psychological findings lends credibility to the view that left CLEMs may have some cross-situational behavioral and psychological consistencies.

It is important to note that currently these relationships are well supported only for right handed males. It has been found that administering the procedure with the tester in front of the subject (face to face) increases the directional consistency of CLEM responding. The tester should sit no closer than approx-

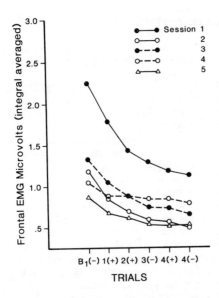

Figure 32. Learning curves for subject scoring highest on absorption scale. (90%) Note that highly hypnotizable people (subjects with high scores on absorption scale) have low frontal EMG and seem to learn in a more orderly manner than subjects low in hypnotizability. Minus (−) refers to trials without EMG auditory feedback and plus (+) refers to trials with EMG auditory feedback. From Wickramasekera (1978) unpublished data.

imately 1.22 m or what has been called "social consultative distance," since eye contact is greater at 1.8 m than 0.6 m. It appears that asymmetry in the subject's visual field can exert some influence on CLEM responses and should be avoided.

Scoring of responses. If I use the numbers on the face of a clock to represent direction of eye movements, we have left CLEMs (1,2,3,4,5) and right CLEMs

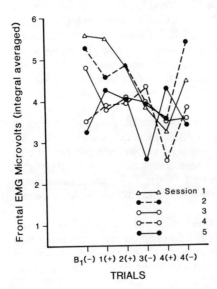

Figure 33. Learning curves for subject scoring lowest on absorption scale. (10%)

(11,10,9,8,7). Stares (looking straight ahead) and especially vertical eye movements (up and down) appear to be mainly stimulated by spatial questions, and may, therefore, be regarded as left eye movements in 95% of right-handed males. I have found this procedure of some value when it confirms independent findings from other procedures estimating hypnotic ability. These test questions are rephrased from previous CLEM investigators.

Experience Inventories

Shor pioneered in the study of experience inventories. These self-report inventories are less obtrusive than standard hypnotic tests like the Stanford. It has been found that extensive use of (a) fantasy (involvement in imagination or day dreams) and (b) the ability to make one's mind blank as in posthypnotic amnesia are major orthogonal components in hypnotic ability. The ability to reversibly alter memory functions (selective amnesia, source amnesia, etc.) may also be related to the ability to voluntarily program states of consciousness (e.g., to take naps, to wake up at a preselected time before the alarm goes off, to do lucid dreaming, to dream on preselected topics). Hence, inquiring about the extent of fantasy use, memory functions and alterations in states of consciousness in the patient's everyday life may predict hypnotic talent.

Other smaller, but critical, components in hypnotic talent appear to be empathy, the effortless occurrence of images or creative ideas, the capacity for attention and absorption, ability to alter physiological functions (EMG, EEG, heart rate, blood pressure, temperature, etc.), parapsychological verbal reports, hypersensitivity to sensory stimuli, and so forth. I have made my own and experimented with several revisions of previous self-report experience inventories that verbally sample several domains relevant to hypnotic talent.

The Wickram Experience Inventory (Wickramasekera, 1985) is the most recent revision of several previous self-report scales. It samples several domains that appear to be relevant to hypnotic talent. The Wickram Experience Inventory (WEI) is printed in Appendix D.

The Absorption Scale (Tellegen & Atkinson, 1974), which samples a domain called *absorption*, correlates with measured hypnotic ability about 0.43. Subjects scoring high or low on this scale are very likely to be good or poor hypnotic subjects, respectively. Figures 32 and 33 illustrate the process of EMG biofeedback low-arousal learning. Note that the high-absorption (high-hypnotic ability) subject has lower frontal EMG at a baseline level and appears to learn in a more orderly fashion than the subject low on absorption (low on hypnotic ability). The plus and minus signs refer to trials with (+) and without (−) EMG feedback.

Curiously, in spite of certain psychometric problems with the current WEI (examples: small and uneven number of items, etc.), it appears from three preliminary empirical studies and clinical experience that the base rate of risk for parapsychological-verbal reports is the best predictor of superior hypnotic ability (Wickramasekera, 1985, 1986).

References

Wickramasekera, I. Development of a self-report measure of hypnotic ability: Preliminary findings. Paper presented at a meeting of the Biofeedback Society of America, New Orleans, March, 1985.

Wickramasekera, I. Risk factors for parapsychological verbal report, hypnotizability, and thematic complaints. Paper presented at a meeting of the Parapsychology Foundation, Washington, D.C., November, 1986.

D

WICKRAM EXPERIENCE INVENTORY[1]

Please read the following before completing the attached questionnaire.

Some people who are productive and well adjusted may have exceptional experiences and abilities. Because these are unusual, they may have learned to conceal these experiences and abilities from others. Scientific investigation of these abilities is important because of their potential applicability to a wide variety of problems and solutions. Therefore, we would appreciate your honest and candid responses to the questions below. This information will be held in the strictest confidence.

---

[1]From Wickramasekera, 1985. Paper presented at a meeting of the Biofeedback Society of America, New Orleans, LA, March. Reprinted by permission. Several items were revised or borrowed from previous experience inventory scales and prior research. (Examples: Shor et al., 1962; As, 1963; Tellegem & Atkinson, 1974; Wilson & Barber, 1982; Evans, 1977; etc.)

Name _____Date _____

Wickram Experience Inventory

1. For most of my life, even when I have been away from home, I have been able to fall asleep in 2 or 3 minutes.   True   False

2. I am usually able to take naps in a variety of situations (e.g., bus, plane, train, car, classroom) if I want to.   True   False

3. I have been able to change a dream while it was happening.   True   False

4. I can get so wrapped up in natural beauty like a sunset, mountain, or wild flower that I temporarily forget where I am or what I am doing.   True   False

5. As a child or adolescent I was able to use fantasy to block out pain, criticism, or punishment.   True   False

6. I could entertain myself for long periods of time with fantasy without feeling lonely as a child.   True   False

7. I can imagine things vividly if I choose to.   True   False

8. As a child I had an "imaginary playmate" that carried on a life of its own through me.   True   False

9. Sometimes I can smell, taste, or feel something that is not there just by choosing to.   True   False

10. I have become so involved in the characters of plays, books, movies, or television shows that I actually respond to the events in their stories as they do.   True   False

11. Sometimes my fantasies are so vivid that I actually feel like they are happening.   True   False

12. My earliest memory is that of life events, which occurred before I was three (3) years old.   True   False

13. I sometimes have dreams or fantasies which actually occur at a later time.   True   False

14. I frequently have had what could be called "psychic experiences," such as sensing when an important phone call or letter will arrive or knowing things about people that I have not previously learned.   True   False

15. I have very vivid sensory experiences.   True   False

16. (For women) Once, I thought I was pregnant and had some of the physical signs of pregnancy, but turned out not to be pregnant.   True   False

17. I seem to pay more attention to remembering how things taste, feel, and smell than most people do.   True   False

18. When I am with strangers, I sometimes pretend to be someone else. True False

19. Just before falling asleep or waking up, I experience very vivid visual images. True False

20. Life would not be worth living if I could not take time out for fantasy. True False

21. Often I am so absorbed in a task that I completely lose track of time and become forgetful of other responsibilities or necessities, such as eating and sleeping. True False

22. I tune into other people's feelings, sometimes to the extent of physically experiencing their pain, joy, sadness, and excitement. True False

23. People are often surprised at how accurately I can sense their deepest feelings. True False

24. I believe that it is possible for the dead to make their presence known to the living. True False

E

Wickram's Modification of the Spiegel Hypnotic Induction Procedures

Have the patient sit up comfortably in the chair, feet on the floor, hands on their lap.

Script

Do you want to become hypnotized (relaxed)? Yes or no. If yes: Keep your thoughts on my words, try to picture in your mind the things that I say and permit them the freedom to affect you.

Now, I'm going to show you a relaxation (self-hypnosis) technique. On the count of "1" I want you to do one thing, on the count of "2" I want you to do two things, and on the count of "3" I want you to do three things.

Ready now, "1," look up into your eyebrows, all the way up into your head. "2," while *keeping* the eyes up there, close the lids slowly and take in a deep breath, "3," relax your eyes, breathe out, and concentrate on a sensation of sinking, sinking all the way down into the chair.

It feels so good just to sit back there and to listen to my voice talking to you as you relax all over, just to let your body go limp and loose. Limp and loose like a rag doll. Relax your eyes, relax your forehead, your jaws. Picture your forehead and scalp becoming smoother and smoother as the relaxation deepens. You can start to let go of all cares and worries at this time, only my voice and what I am saying to you seems important at this time. Everything else can go far away. Keep your thoughts on my words, picture in your mind the things I say and permit them the freedom to affect you. That's right, let your jaw hang loose and your teeth separate. Let the relaxation spread down, down your throat, down your neck. Relax your left shoulder, now your right shoulder. That's right, let the relaxation spill into your chest, just let your body go limp and loose. There is nothing to accomplish, there is no one to please. Just an opportunity to let go of all your cares, of all your worries, to permit them the freedom to go far, far away, while you keep your thoughts on my words, only my words and what I am saying to you is important at this time, everything else is going further and further away. Fading away in the distance.

Now with each breath you breathe out you can relax even more as you sink deeper and deeper into this pleasant relaxed state in which nothing can bother you. Listening only to my voice, breathing out freely and rhythmically seems to allow you to sort of dissolve or melt into the chair. The chair is strong, it can hold your body safely as you sink deeper and deeper into this pleasant, relaxed state.

Relax your shoulders, your upper back, your lower back, your buttocks, tummy and hips as you begin to let go even more like lights being turned off in a building one by one. Different parts of your body may start to let go even more as you sink deeper and deeper into this pleasant state.

Now relax your feet, your toes, your legs and knees as a sensation of heaviness or numbness can come into parts of your body, as you settle deeper into this pleasant state. At times you may even notice sensations of lightness or tingling coming into parts of your body as you relax even more deeply. As you relax like that you can imagine a nice warm blanket being drawn up your body from your toes and feet over your legs and knees and thighs, across your tummy and up to your chest. There is nothing to accomplish, nothing to prove, just the freedom to relax, to let go and to be yourself while you sink deeper and deeper into this pleasant state in which your nerves will grow stronger and steadier because of this deep relaxation. So that you will notice in the coming days, weeks and months that things that used to rattle you, or got you shook up, cannot touch you quite as easily anymore. You seem to bounce back more easily, more quickly than before.

In a few moments I will count back from 5 to 1. At the count of one, you will open your eyes feeling relaxed, refreshed, and fine all through your mind and body. 5, 4, 3, 2, 1. Open your eyes.

F

INFORMAL CLINICAL TESTING FOR HYPNOTIC ABILITY WITH TEST SUGGESTIONS

To limit the patient's experience of "failure" with the therapist and to protect the therapist from "placebo sag" (drop in social reinforcer effectiveness) the following test suggestions can be tried (a) with a formal hypnotic induction or (b) after simply asking the patient to close his or her eyes and to attend carefully to your words. Items are arranged in order (least to most) of empirically determined difficulty (Perry & Laurence, 1982). Each item passed is subjectively impressive and can in the short run enhance the patient's willingness to attend to and fantasize about the potency of the procedure. In the long run, it makes the patient aware that he or she is pregnant with possibilities for cognitive self-control of unsuspected behavioral and biological functions.

Easy Test Suggestions

1. Hand lowering
2. Hands coming together
3. Finger lock
4. Arm rigidity

Please close your eyes, relax, and listen very carefully to what I am going to say to you now. Please picture in your mind what I am saying and permit yourself the freedom to let happen whatever you find is happening, even if it is not what you expect. Just concentrate and let it happen.

1. Hand lowering
Hold your left hand and arm straight out in front of you, palm facing the floor. Left hand straight out, palm facing downward. I want you now to concentrate on this hand and arm. I want you to notice the sensations and feelings in the hand and arm and what is happening to it. I want you to pay close attention to this hand and arm because something very interesting is about to happen to that hand and arm. It is starting to get heavy, heavier and heavier like lead. As if

a weight were pulling the hand and arm down, down. As I count from 1 to 10 it begins to get heavy and goes down more and more like lead. 1 down, 2, pulling down more and more, 3, down, 4, down, 5, heavier and heavier, 6, 7, down more and more down, 8, down, 9, down, 10, down. Fine, your hand and arm are perfectly normal now. Keep your eyes closed and allow yourself the freedom to relax deeply.

2. Hands coming together

Now hold both your hands and arms straight out in front of you, palms facing each other, hands about 1 foot apart. Now I want you to think or imagine a force pulling your hands together. As you think of this force pulling your hands together, you will begin to notice a force pulling them together, drawing them together, as if a force were acting on them, drawing them closer and closer together and as you recognize this force it seems to grow even stronger pulling and pushing them together. I will now begin to count from 1 to 10 and with each count they will be drawn closer and closer together until they will touch. I wonder if they will touch by the time I reach 10. 1, moving, 2, closer, 3, 4, closer now and getting closer all the time, 5, 6, 7, very close now and getting closer, 8, 9, 10. Fine, your hands and arms are perfectly normal now, keep your eyes closed and permit yourself the freedom to relax even deeper now.

3. Finger lock

I want you to press your palms together, interlocking your fingers. Fingers tightly interlocked together, tightly interlocked together, so tightly stuck together, locked together that you wonder very much if you could take your hands apart. Your hands are stuck together, locked together, tightly interlocked. In a few moments I will ask you to try to take your hands apart. When I ask you to try you will find it difficult because they are stuck, interlocked together. You might try later when I ask you to, but I think it will be too much of an effort even to try. Your hands are locked, stuck together, please try to take them apart. I think you will find it very difficult. You can take your hands apart easily now, they are not locked, take them apart, relax, and let yourself sink even deeper into the comfort and well-being of this pleasant state.

4. Arm rigidity

I want you to hold your left hand and arm straight out in front of you. Left arm reaching straight out in front of you. I want you now to make a tight fist with this hand. Left arm straight out in front of you with a very tight fist. Make your fist tighter, and now you notice something very interesting, a feeling of stiffness, rigidity, coming into the arm, hand and fist. A creeping feeling of stiffness is coming into your arm and hand. Now a feeling of stiffness is coming into your arm and forearm, they are becoming stiff and rigid like a bar of iron, and you know how difficult it is to bend a bar of iron like your arm and hand. In a few moments I will ask you to try to bend your arm, and I think you will find it very difficult. In fact, it may even get stiffer as if something is pulling the arm even stiffer. Now as I stroke it and count from 1 to 10 it grows stiffer and becomes like a bar of iron. 1, 2, 3, 4, very stiff, so rigid like a bar of iron, 6, 7, 8, 9, 10. Try to bend it and see how difficult it is as it grows stiff when you try to bend it. Just try. Now, relax your arm and hand and as they relax let your whole body relax even more. Permit yourself the freedom to settle even more comfortably into this pleasant, relaxed state in which there is nothing to accomplish, no one to please, just the freedom to relax, let go and be yourself. It can feel so good just to lay back and listen to my voice talking to you. You have no cares, no worries, only my voice and what I am saying seems important at this time, everything else seems to be fading away, far away.

Reference

Perry, C. & Laurence, J. R. 1980. Hypnotic depth and hypnotic susceptibility: A replicated finding. *International Journal of Clinical and Experimental Hypnosis, 28,* 272–280.

G

SUBJECTIVE RESPONSE INQUIRY

Inquire About Subjective Responses During Biofeedback or Hypnosis[a]
(Administer after each low-arousal episode and draw patient's attention to reliable subjective feedback sensations)

1. Name _____ Date _____
2. How would you rate the session in general?
   Poor 0 1 2 3 4 5 6 7 8 9 10 Excellent
3. Were you able to relax? Yes No If not, what were the obstacles?

_____

4. Did you experience any of the following sensations in any parts of your body during the relaxation?

	Not at all	Slightly	Moderately	Definitely
a. heaviness	(0)	(1)	(2)	(3)
b. numbness	(0)	(1)	(2)	(3)
c. tingling	(0)	(1)	(2)	(3)
d. floating	(0)	(1)	(2)	(3)
e. pulsing	(0)	(1)	(2)	(3)
f. body or body parts expanding, contracting, or bobbing	(0)	(1)	(2)	(3)
g. spatial displacement of parts of body (e.g., hands not there, or above or below where they are)	(0)	(1)	(2)	(3)

5. Emotional feelings that occurred. Did you experience any of the following?
   1. fear   2. comfort   3. sadness   4. calm   5. anxiety
   6. joy   7. pleasure   8. other _____

281

6. Did you have any brief, unexpected or surprising thoughts, sensory impressions (colors, etc.) pictures, or images? (theta state)
   1. visual   2. auditory   3. spatial   4. smell   5. taste
   6. tactile   7. other _____
7. Did you become drowsy?   Yes   No
8. Was there anything that you liked or disliked about this session?

---

[a]Adapted from Green and Green, 1977.

H

WICKRAMASEKERA'S DIAGNOSTIC INTERVIEW FOR HEADACHE[1]

1. *Etiologic, Associated or Precipitating Factors* (Check and inquire)
   A. Sustained muscle contraction of head, face and neck (tension headache).
   B. Dilation of cranial arteries with sterile local inflammatory reaction (migraine headache patients appear to have very labile vascular systems).
   C. Organic dseases and trauma of skull, brain, meninges, arteries, veins, eyes, nose, ears, and paranasal sinuses.
   D. Hypertension.
   E. Psychological factors (chronic depression, anxiety, perfectionism, rigidity, inhibited rage).
   F. Allergies (seasonal, substances or food), fatigue, loss of sleep, menstruation, bright lights, high humidity, high altitude, hunger (hypoglycemic reaction, foods and drugs that contain tyramine and certain other substances (for example, histamine, alcohol, oral contraceptives, hormonal therapy) inhaling nitrates and carbon monoxide.

2. *Headache History* (Inquire and note)
   A. How many types of headaches does the patient complain of? For example, tension, migraine, cluster, sinus headaches, etc.
   B. Onset prior headache history, yes or no (age at onset _____, time of day or waking from sleep _____, gradual or sudden, weekends, vacations).
   C. Course of headache (has become worse, improved, stayed the same, length of periods of remissions (days, weeks, months, years).
   D. Location at onset (unilateral, bilateral, generalized, focal, alternate sides).
   E. Frequency, 1. Episodes per day (1,2,3) 2. Per week (1,2,3,4,5,6) 3. Per month (1,2,3,4) 4. Continuous (change only in intensity) 5. Clusters (duration 8–12 weeks) and remission (duration).
   F. Seasonal (spring, summer, fall, winter).
   G. Duration. Does the headache last for a few minutes, few hours (1–24), few days (2,3,4,5)?
   H. Type of pain. Is the pain dull, tight, steady, pulsating, throbbing, or deep and boring, excruciating (considers suicide)?

[1]From Wickramasekera, 1976. Reprinted by permission.

I. Prodromata (warning signs) visual defects (blind spots, flashing lights, fortification spectra, hallucinations, ataxia, or vertigo present).

J. Associated symptoms (photophobia, nausea, vomiting, lacrimation, cranial tenderness, hypersensitivity to sound, nasal congestion, and anorexia, unilateral flushing of painful side of face).

K. Sleep and sexual habits (Delays in falling asleep, frequent awakening, early awakening, primary or secondary orgasmic dysfunction, premature ejaculation or erectile dysfunction, or other sexual problems present?)

L. Family history (Is there a positive family history of headaches with similar symptoms?) brother, sister, father, mother.

M. Previous physical and neurological examinations. What previous physical and neurological examinations have been done? What previous laboratory tests have been completed (skull X rays, brain scan, EEC, spinal puncture, etc.)?

N. Medications and response to them. What medications is the patient taking, antidepressants (Elavil, Tofranil), Ergotamine tartrate, reserpine, hormone therapy (menopause, birth control), any analgesic abuse?

O. Frontal EMG Level: eyes open;   eyes closed;   stress;   eyes open;   eyes closed.

P. Hand temp: Left;   Right.

Q. Diagnosis.

I

HYPNOTIC PROCEDURE TO REDUCE HEADACHE PAIN

Hypnotic Procedure to Reduce Headache Pain

The following procedure is most likely to be effective with a severe chronic vascular or muscular headache only if applied in the early stages of headache onset. Ask the patient the following questions or provide the following instructions.

1. Do you want to reduce or eliminate this headache pain that you now have? Yes or No.
2. If "no" abort following procedure, proceed with psychotherapeutic exploration of meaning and reasons for "no."
3. If "yes" proceed as follows. Give the pain an intensity rating between 0–1 (slight) and 10 (very painful). Use 1,2,3, technique to relax patient.
4. At termination of 1,2,3 technique say, "Imagine the space between your eyes. When you can do this raise your right finger."
5. (When right finger goes up) Imagine this space getting wider and wider as I count from 1 to 5 and as you relax deeper.
6. Imagine the space between your ears. When you can do this raise your right finger.
7. (When right finger goes up) imagine this space getting wider and wider as I count from 1 to 5 and as you relax deeper and deeper.
8. Now tell where in your head is the pain located (e.g., forehead, between eyes, back of head, etc.)?
9. Now what is the size and shape of your pain (e.g., large, small, etc.)?
10. Now what is the color of the pain (red, blue, pink, purple, etc.)?
11. Now imagine the pain shrinking in size and fading in color around the edges as I count slowly from 1 to 10 and as you relax even more deeply.
12. As I count backward from 5 to 1 you will open your eyes and come out of hypnosis feeling relaxed and refreshed. 5, 4, 3, 2, 1.
13. On the 10 point scale of pain intensity, please give me a rating of your current pain level.

J

IN VITRO DESENSITIZATION (SD) PROCEDURE

1. Patient is first trained in deep relaxation with 1,2,3 procedure or progressive muscle relaxation technique.
2. Patient is asked to briefly (2 or 4 lines) list on reporter note cards all prior, present, or anticipated situations relating to a specific unpleasant or phobic situation. These should be situations of mild, moderate and intense anxiety and at least 2 or 3 of each intensity level. (This procedure is anxiety provoking and may require support).
3. These note cards (e.g., $n = 15$) are to be brought to the therapy session arranged in order of phobic intensity from 1 least to 15 most. (This procedure is anxiety provoking.)
4. The patient is asked to go into the relaxed state with the 1,2,3 technique and when deeply relaxed and ready to start the SD procedure, he is asked to signal relaxation with right forefinger.
5. The subject is then told "Now, I want you to try to picture the following scene as vividly and clearly as you can while relaxing deeply. If you should feel even the slightest tension or uneasiness when picturing the scene, signal me by raising your left forefinger. If left forefinger is not raised for at least 15 seconds twice consecutively, proceed to next anxiety hierarchy.
6. If the left finger goes up at any time before 15 seconds say, "Switch it off completely and go down deeper into relaxation. When you are deeply relaxed again and all the previous anxiety has passed, let me know by raising your right forefinger. The previous hierarchy item is repeated until it does not evoke left finger response for two 15-second trials consecutively.
7. After two extinction trials ($-15''$, $-15''$) proceed to next item on anxiety hierarchy.
8. Concurrent frontal EMG monitoring during SD can at times provide impressive physiological tracking of the desensitization process (Wickramasekera, 1976, p. 93).

K

BACKGROUND QUESTIONNAIRE

The purpose of this questionnaire is to obtain rapidly a comprehensive picture of your background. In scientific and medical work records are necessary, since they permit a rapid and more complete review of your situation.

DATE: _____

1. *GENERAL*

Name: _____

Address: _____

Telephone numbers: Home: _____ Work: _____

Age: _____ Education: _____ Sex: _____

Occupation: _____ Name of employer: _____

With whom are you now living? First name and age (children & adults) _____

_____

Do you live in a house, hotel room, apartment, etc.? _____

Marital status: single, married, remarried, separated, divorced, widowed. (Circle answer)
How strongly do you want treatment for your problem? Very much, much, moderately.
Could be without it, if necessary. (Circle one answer.)
Name of insurance company and policy number: (optional information) _____

_____

2. *CLINICAL*
State in your own words the nature of your chief problem. (Be specific). _____

_____

289

State related problems. _____

_____

Approximately how many years or months ago did your problem start? _____

Has it gotten worse, better, or stayed the same since it started? _____

_____

Names and dates of the professional people you have consulted about this
problem: _____

_____

_____

Name of the person who referred you to this office _____

What is the longest period of remission that you have experienced (i.e.. period
of time when you have been free of your symptoms)? _____

What do you think is the *real* cause of your problem? _____

_____

_____

L

BEHAVIORAL MEDICINE CLINIC AND STRESS DISORDERS RESEARCH LABORATORY
Statement of Procedures

1. During your treatment you may need to continue under medical management of any organic disease. We may have to consult verbally or in writing with your referring physician or other health service providers involved in your treatment. By signing this form you are giving us permission to do so. Other than this your records will be kept confidential within the limits prescribed by law.

2. This Clinic is part of the Medical School and is involved in the education and training of physicians and psychologists. Therefore, trainees may be in the room or participating in your treatment. You have the right to withdraw your permission for this at any time.

3. This Clinic is also a research facility. We may request your permission to electronically record portions of your treatment or to use material from your case in research publications. In all these instances all identifying information (name, address, etc.) will be removed. Its intended use will be explained to you. You have the right to deny permission for this.

4. After the active part of your treatment is completed, you will be placed on follow-up status for a 5-year period. Your appointments will become less frequent (once a month, then once in three months, and finally, once in six months). This allows us to help you prevent your problem from recurring, and protects the time and effort you have invested in your treatment.

5. No experimental procedures will be used without your complete knowledge and consent.

6. If there are any sections of the above you do not consent to please delete each and attach your signature. We will need to discuss these with you.

I have carefully read and understand the above and I hereby freely give consent to the above provisions and agree to cooperate fully with the assessment and treatment of my problem.

Signature _____ Date _____
(Patient, Parent, or Guardian)

Witness _____ Date _____

M

BEHAVIORAL MEDICINE CLINIC AND STRESS DISORDERS RESEARCH LABORATORY
Assessment for Admission

As part of your assessment for admission into the Behavioral Medicine Program, you will be completing the series of evaluations described below.

1. *Self-report questionnaires.* This packet contains 11 simple questionnaires that you will complete here at the clinic. The average amount of time required to take them is 1 to 1½ hours. The results of these tests will help us determine if our treatment will be beneficial to you, and all results will be described to you at your feedback appointment.

   Self-report questionnaire appointment: _____

2. *Harvard Hypnotic Susceptibility Scale.* This standard procedure is used at several major medical centers to determine an individual's level of hypnotic ability. During the procedure, you will be asked to perform some simple tasks; no personal questions will be asked and you will not be asked to answer any questions verbally. Following the procedure, you will answer questions in a response booklet about the things you experienced during the test. Please read and complete the information in the hypnosis handout and bring it with you to this evaluation. The procedure lasts 1½ hours. If you are delayed in keeping your appointment, it may have to be rescheduled.

   Harvard hypnotic scale appointment: _____

3. *Psychophysiological Profile.* This procedure involves placing sensors on your skin to record certain physiological processes (blood pressure, muscle tension, heart rate, skin temperature and conductance) under different conditions. The sensors are placed on the skin surface and the skin is not broken. The procedure is completely painless and usually does not require removal of any clothing.

   Our blood pressure monitor can take readings through a shirt or blouse of normal weight materials. Please DO NOT wear heavier materials such as cable knit sweaters or sweatshirts. Certain sensors may be placed on your forehead and held by a band placed around your head. Your forehead will be wiped with an alcohol swab. If you wear make-up on your forehead, this will remove it. The band might also disturb certain hairstyles. You may wish to bring anything you need to repair your makeup and hairstyle afterward.

This procedure often takes the entire scheduled hour and cannot be interrupted once it begins. If you are delayed in keeping your appointment, it may have to be rescheduled for another day.

Psychophysiological profile appointment:

4. *Feedback.* At this appointment all evaluation results will be discussed with you and any future treatment will be outlined.

Feedback appointment: _____

5. *Follow-up.*
   A. Upon completion of active treatment you will be required to repeat the above evaluations (Self-report Questionnaires, Harvard Hypnotic Susceptibility Scale, Psychophysiological Profile) to enable us to measure the progress you have made during the period of treatment.
   B. After your period of intensive treatment is over, we will need to see you once a month for a period of one year and then once in three to six months for four years. The purpose of these follow-ups is to ensure that occasional relapses, which are very common with stress disorders, do not become transformed once again into chronic problems which are much more difficult to reverse. This follow-up also ensures that we are able to monitor any further progress you make after the termination of your treatment and in a sense is a preventative way you can protect your initial investment. Our research has shown that if you are able to be relatively symptom free for a period of at least five years it is very unlikely that you will ever again develop chronic problems in these areas.

N

PSYCHOPHYSIOLOGICAL PROFILE[1]
(Wickramasekera—1976)

Name   Sex: M/F   Age   Hand: R/L/AMB   Date
CLEM L   R   S   E.R. 0, 1, 2, 3, 4

	1	2	3	4	5
BP Left upper arm	D S	D S	D S	D S	D S
	eyes open	eyes closed	stress (30 sec)	eyes open	eyes closed
Pulse (bpm) Right hand Finger 1	Hi Low x̄ SD	Hi Low x̄ SD	Hi Low x̄ SD	Hi Low x̄ SD	Hi Low x̄ SD
Temp (°F) Right hand Finger 2 Med. phalanx	Hi Low x̄ SD	Hi Low x̄ SD	Hi Low x̄ SD	Hi Low x̄ SD	Hi Low x̄ SD
SCR Right hand Fingers 3 & 4 Med. phalanx	Hi Low x̄ SD	Hi Low x̄ SD	Hi Low x̄ SD	Hi Low x̄ SD	Hi Low x̄ SD
EMG (uv) Frontalis −3	Hi Low x̄ SD	Hi Low x̄ SD	Hi Low x̄ SD	Hi Low x̄ SD	Hi Low x̄ SD
Respiration: RPM Amplitude Pattern Holding					

[1]From Wickramasekera, 1976. Reprinted by permission.

SELECTED BIBLIOGRAPHY

Achterberg, J., & Lawlis, G. F. *Imagery of cancer*. Champaign, IL: Institute for personality and ability testing, 1978.

Aronoff, G. M. [Editorial]. *Clinical Journal of Pain*, 1985, *1*, 1–3.

Bakal, D. A. *Psychology and medicine*. New York: Springer, 1979.

Bandura, A. *Principles of behavior modification*. New York: Holt, Rinehart & Winston, 1969.

Benson, H. *The mind/body effect*. New York: Simon & Schuster, 1979.

Blackwell, B. Minor tranquilizers, misuse or overuse? *Psychosomatics*, 1975, *16*, 28–31.

Blumberg, E. M., West, P. M., & Ellis, F. W. MMPI findings in human cancer. In W. G. Dahlstrum & G. S. Welsh (Eds.), *Basic readings on the MMPI in psychology and medicine*. Minneapolis, MN: University of Minnesota Press, 1956.

Bonica, J. J., & Fordyce, W. E. Operant conditioning for chronic pain. In J. J. Bonica, P. Procacci, & C. A. Pagni (Eds.), *Recent advances on pain*. Springfield, IL: Charles C Thomas, 1974.

Borkovec, T. D., & Nau, S. D. Credibility of analogue therapy rationales. *Journal of Behavior Therapy and Experimental Psychiatry*, 1972, *3*, 257–260.

Bowers, K. S. *Hypnosis for the seriously curious*. New York: Norton, 1976.

Budzynski, T. Biofeedback and the twilight states of consciousness. In G. E. Schwartz & D. Shapiro (Eds.), *Consciousness and self-regulation* (Vol. 1). New York: Plenum Press, 1976.

Canter, A., Imboden, J. B., & Cluff, L. E. The frequency of physical illness as a function of prior psychological vulnerability and contemporary stress. *Psychosomatic Medicine*, 1966, *28*, 344–350.

Cobb, B. Emotional problems of adult cancer patients. *Journal of the American Geriatrics Society*, 1959, *1*, 274–285.

Culpan, R., & Davies, B. Psychiatric illness at a medical and surgical outpatient clinic. *Comprehensive Psychiatry*, 1960, *1*, 228–235.

Cummings, N. A. The anatomy of psychotherapy under National Health Insurance. *American Psychologist*, 1977, *32*, 711–718.

Evans, F. J., Orne, E. C., & Markowsky, P. A. *Punctuality and hypnotizability*. Paper read at Eastern Psychological Association, Boston, MA, April, 1977.

Ferguson, P. C., & Gowan, J. *The influence of transcendental meditation on anxiety, depression, aggression, neuroticism, & self-actualization*. Paper presented at California State Psychological Association, Fresno, CA, 1974.

Fineberg, H. V. Paper presented at the Sun Valley National Forum, Sun Valley, ID, August 1–5, 1977.

Gerwitz, J. L., & Baer, D. M. The effect of brief social deprivation on behaviors for a social reinforcer. *Journal of Abnormal and Social Psychology,* 1958, *56,* 49–56.

Green, A., Green, E., & Walters, D. *Psychological training for creativity.* Paper presented at the meeting of the American Psychological Association, Washington, DC, September, 1971.

Hamberg, D. A. Health and behavior [Editorial]. *Science,* 1982, *217,* 399.

Hilkevitch, A. Psychiatric disturbances in outpatients of a general medical outpatient clinic. *International Journal of Neuropsychiatry,* 1965, *1,* 371–375.

Holmes, T. H. *Schedule of recent events.* Seattle, WA: University of Washington Press, 1981.

Horder, T. J. In M. S. Straus (Ed.), *Familiar medical quotations.* Boston, MA: Little, Brown, & Company, 1968.

Imboden, J. B., Canter, A., & Cluff, L. E. Brucellosis. *Archives of Internal Medicine,* 1959, *103,* 406–414.

Kazdin, A. E. Therapy outcome questions requiring control of credibility and treatment-generated expectancies. *Behavior Therapy,* 1979, *10,* 81–93.

Kazdin, A. E., & Wilcoxon, L. A. Systematic desensitization and nonspecific treatment effects: A methodological evaluation. *Psychological Bulletin,* 1976, *83,* 5, 729–758.

Kissen, D. M. Psychosocial factors, personality, and lung cancer in men aged 55–64. *British Journal of Medical Psychology,* 1967, *40,* 29.

Kissen, D. M., & Eysenck, H. J. Personality in male lung cancer patients. *Journal of Psychosomatic Research,* 1962, *6,* 123.

Krippner, S. Experimentally induced telepathic effects in hypnosis and nonhypnosis groups. *Journal of the American Society for Psychical Research,* 1968, *62,* 387–398.

Larsen, S. Strategies for reducing phobic behavior. *Dissertation Abstracts,* 1966, *26,* 6850.

LeShan, L. An emotional life history pattern associated with neoplastic disease. *Annals of the New York Academy of Sciences,* 1966, *124,* 160.

Lick, J., & Bootzin, R. Expectancy factors in the treatment of fear: Methodological and theoretical issues. *Psychological Bulletin,* 1975, *82*(6), 917–931.

Ng, L. K. Y., & Bonica, J. J. *Pain, discomfort and humanitarian care.* New York: Elsevier, 1980.

Pless, I. B., & Roghmann, K. J. Chronic illness and its consequences: Observations based on three epidemiologic surveys. *Journal of Pediatrics,* 1971, *79,* 351–359.

Rahe, R. H. Longitudinal study of life change and illness onset. *Journal of Psychosomatic Research,* 1967, *10,* 355.

Rahe, R. H., & Arthur, R. J. Life-change patterns surrounding illness experience. *Journal of Psychosomatic Research,* 1968, *11,* 341–345.

Rogers, M. P., Devendara, D., & Reich, P. The influence of the psyche and the brain on immunity and disease susceptibility: A critical review. *Psychosomatic Medicine,* 1979, *41*(2), 147–164.

Schachter, S. The interaction of cognitive and physiological determinants of emotional state. In C. D. Speilberger (Ed.), *Anxiety and behavior.* New York: Academic Press, 1966.

Schubot, E. D. *The influence of hypnotic and muscular relaxation in systematic desensitization of phobias.* Unpublished doctoral dissertation, Stanford University, 1966.

Shor, R. E., & Orne, E. C. *Manual: Harvard Group Scale of Hypnotic Susceptibility, Form A.* Palo Alto, CA: Consulting Psychologists Press, Inc., 1962.

Smith, R. J. Study finds sleeping pills over-prescribed. *Science,* 1979, *204,* 287–288.

Struening, E., & Guttentag, M. (Eds.). *Handbook of evaluation research.* Beverly Hills, CA: Sage, 1975.

Strupp, H., & Bergin, A. E. *Changing frontiers in the science of psychotherapy.* Chicago: Aldine, 1972.

Surwit, R. S., Pilon, R. N., & Fenton, C. H. Behavioral treatment of Raynaud's disease. *Journal of Behavioral Medicine*, 1978, *1*(3), 323–335.

Weitzenhoffer, A. M., & Hilgard, E. R. *Stanford Hypnotic Susceptibility Scale Form C.* Palo Alto, CA: Consulting Psychologists Press, Inc., 1962.

Wickramasekera, I. Reinforcement and/or transference in hypnosis and psychotherapy: A hypothesis. *American Journal of Clinical Hypnosis*, 1970, *12*(3), 137–140.

Wickramasekera, I. Application of verbal instructions and EMG feedback training to the management of tension headache. *Headache*, 1973, *13*, 74–76.

Wickramasekera, I. Heart rate feedback and the management of cardiac neurosis. *Journal of Abnormal Psychology*, 1974, *83*, 578–580.

INDEX